A Visual Encyclopedia of
UNCONVENTIONAL
MEDICINE

A Visual Encyclopedia of
UNCONVENTIONAL
MEDICINE

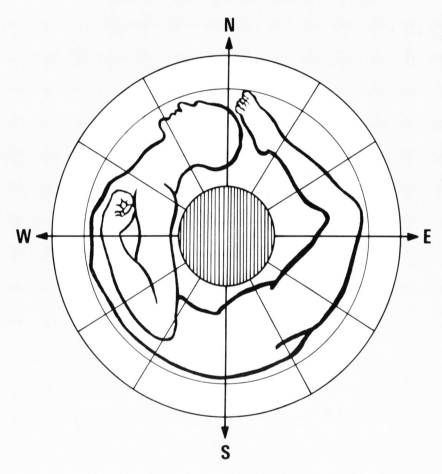

Edited by Ann Hill

CROWN PUBLISHERS INC., NEW YORK

Acknowledgements

The Publishers would like to thank C. Maxwell Cade for kindly allowing them to photograph and reproduce charts used in his Biofeedback courses. Sidney Rose-Neil generously lent a number of photographs of therapies in practice at Tyringham Naturopathic Clinic. A. Nelson & Co, the homoeopathic pharmacists, were most hospitable in allowing photographs to be specially taken at their laboratory. Mary Hayley collected much useful information in California.

Photographs, illustrations and diagrams were provided by the following : Arica Institute 198, 199 ; Audio Ltd 191, 195 ; Associated Press 52, 53 ; Bayly, Doreen 61, 62, 63 ; Bhatt, Amidhar 17 ; Bluestone Clinic 99 ; Breen, Alan C. 74, 75, 76 ; Camera Press 196, 197 ; Community Health Foundation 64, 66, 67 ; Copen, Dr Bruce 172 ; Crawford, J. 25 (bottom) ; Dawes, Christopher, 126, 130, 131, 137, 138, 148, 225, 226, 227, 228, 229, 232, 233, 234 ; Delawarr Laboratories 167 ; Dyer, Michael 24, 25, 26, 57, 58, 59, 68, 70, 71, 72, 175 ; Evans, Mary, Picture Library 22, 109 (below) ; Finnish Tourist Board 88, 89 ; Forbes, Lieutenant-Colonel 104 (below) ; Francis, Karl 46, 47 ; Gemeentemuseum, The Hague 31 ; Gollancz, Victor Ltd 220 ; Goulden, Henry 29 ; Hutchinson, Ronald 221, 224 ; Larsen, John 39 ; Malim, Lydia 34, 35, 37, 38, 84, 86, 87, 96, 97, 132, 133, 144, 179 ; Mansell Collection 106 (bottom), 188 ; McCausland, Marcus 181 ; Mims Magazine 73 ; Nest, Franz 205 ; Nightingale, M. J. 100 ; Nixon, Sandy 209, 210 ; Northern Institute of Massage 82, 83 ; Radio Times Hulton Picture Library 93, 94, 105, 107 (top), 108 (top), 109 (top), 110 (centre), 176, 177, 186, 187 ; Rae, Malcolm 28 ; Robinson, Michael 13, 14, 23, 36, 101, 102 ; Rutherford, Meg 16, 120, 121, 122 ; Schoepflin, Albert 201 ; Sculfor, Leslie 218 ; Snellgrove, Brian 48, 49, 50, 51 ; Tansley, David 163, 164, 165, 166, 168, 169, 170, 171 ; Tracey, John 78, 79 ; Topham, John Picture Library 174 ; Tyringham Naturopathic Clinic 42, 56, 90, 91, 98, 108 (bottom), 110 (top right), (below left) ; De Vorss & Co 44 ; Wadley, Nicholas 211, 213, 214, 216, 217 ; Walker, Professor 104 (above) ; Yoga Today 222, 223.

Published in the USA in 1979 by Crown Publishers, Inc., New York

First published in Great Britain by Triune Books Ltd, 1978

Created, designed and produced by Trewin Copplestone Publishing Ltd, London

Printed in Italy by New Interlitho Spa, Milan

Library of Congress Cataloging in Publication Data :
MAIN ENTRY UNDER TITLE :
A VISUAL ENCYCLOPEDIA OF UNCONVENTIONAL MEDICINE.
     1.   THERAPEUTIC SYSTEMS.   I HILL, ANN.
R733.V57   615'.53   78–14009
ISBN 0–517–53613–7
ISBN 0–517–536145 PBK.

Contributors

Joel Badaines Ph D
Member of the British Psychological Association
Executive Member of the Drama Therapy Association

Doreen E. Bayly
Certified Reflexologist (USA)
Lecturer on Compression Massage

Charles E. Belyea
Teacher of T'ai Chi Ch'uan

Sybil Beresford-Peirse LRAM LGSM (MT)
Director of Music Therapy and Training
Nordoff Music Therapy Centre

Geoffrey Blundell
Researcher into Biofeedback instrumentation

Peter Blythe
Consultant Hypnotist and Psychotherapist

David Boadella BA, M Ed
Consultant Therapist, Centre for Bioenergy, London
Editor, *Self and Society*

Alan C. Breen DC
Lecturer in Therapeutics, Anglo-European College of
Chiropractic

H. Bryn Jones ND, MCS
Co-founder of Somatography Training

Brian H. Butler BA, LCSP (Phys), MFPhys
Consultant Therapist in Naturopathy, Lecturer in Applied
Kinesiology

John H. Crook Ph D, D Sc
Department of Psychology, University of Bristol

James A. Dyson MRCS, LRCP
Member, Anthroposophical Medical Association (UK)
Member, Medical Section, University for Spiritual Science,
Goetheanum, Dornach

Ursula Fausset
Gestaltist

Tom Feldberg
Director, Quaesitor Outside Projects, London

F. Fletcher Hyde B Sc, FNIMH
Director of Research, National Institute of Medical
Herbalists
Chairman, British Herbal Pharmacopoeia

Karl A. Francis MFPhys(Lond) LCSP (Assoc)
Principal, The Acacia House Centre for Education,
Philosophy and Healing

Theo Gimbel DCE
Director of Research, Hygeia Studios (Colour-Light-Art
Research Ltd) Avening, Gloucestershire

George Hall Ph D, Ll D
Director of Education, The Human Cybernetics
Organization, London

John Heron BA
Hon. Project Director, Human Potential Research Project
Assistant Director (Medical Education) British Postgraduate
Medical Federation

Carlotta Hollmann BA
Member, General Anthroposophical Section, University
for Spiritual Science, Goetheanum, Dornach

Roger Horrocks, Ph D
Lecturer in Psychology, Encounter Group Leader

Felicity Ling MA, B Ed
Lecturer in Dance and Dance Therapy

John R. Mansfield MRCS, LRCP, DRCOG
Specialist in Clinical Ecology

Marika McCausland
Secretary, Health for the New Age

Michael McDonald B Sc, C Eng, MIEE
Director, Biocal Ltd

Alan Moyle ND, MBNOA
Registered Naturopath and Osteopath

Roger Newman Turner ND, DO, MBNOA, M Ac A
Registered Naturopath, Osteopath and Acupuncturist

M. J. Nightingale DO, ND, Lic A, MBEOA, MGN, M Ac A,
LCSP (Phys)
Registered Naturopath, Osteopath and Acupuncturist

Stephen Pirie ND, DO, MBNOA, MSO
Registered Osteopath and Naturopath

Michael Reddy Ph D
President, European Association for Transactional
Analysis

Peter Robinson BA
Arica student

Michael Ronan
Secretary, the Bates Association of Eyesight Training

Sidney Rose-Neil
Chairman, British Acupuncture Association
Director, Tyringham Naturopathic Clinic

Manning D. Ross

A. J. Ruffhead
Technical Director, New Era Laboratories

Peter B. Smith Ph D
Lecturer in Social Psychology, University of Sussex

Brian J. Snellgrove BA
Researcher and Lecturer on Kirlian Photography,
Counselling and Healing

Valerie Soukup
Curative Eurythmy Diploma, Goetheanum, Dornach,
Switzerland

Christopher Stevens
Researcher of the Alexander Technique

William Swartley Ph D
Founder, International Primal Association

David V. Tansley DC
Chiropractor and researcher into radionics and
energy fields

John B. Tracey MB, BChir
Originator and Practitioner of Impact Therapy

Robert Tisserand
Proprietor, Aromatic Oil Company, Oxford

Nora Weeks (the late)
Dr Edward Bach Centre

Aubrey T. Westlake BA, MB, B Chir, MRCS, LRCP
Fellow of the Institute of Psionic Medicine

Geoffrey Whitfield
Training Coordinator, British Association for
Bioenergetic Analysis

H. W. Williams DO, DC, ND
Registered Osteopath, Chiropractor, Naturopath

K. Woodward FLCSP (Phys), FAB Th, M Soc P
Principal, Northern Institute of Massage

Vivian Worthington
Secretary-General, The British Wheel of Yoga

Contents

Contents

Reading List

GENERAL

Annett, Stephen (ed) *The Many Ways of Being* Sphere
Books, 1976
Blythe, Peter *Drugless Medicine* Arthur Barker, 1974
Burr, H. S. *Blueprint for Immortality* Neville Spearman,
1972
Carlson, R. J. *The End of Medicine* John Wiley & Sons, 1975
Ferguson, Marylin *The Brain Revolution* Davis-Poynter,
1974
Forbes, H. A. W. *Try Being Healthy* Langdon Books, 1976
Gowan, John Curtis *Trance, Art and Creativity* Available
from the author at 9030 Darby Avenue, Northridge,
California 91324
Hulke, M. (ed) *The Encyclopedia of Alternative Medicine
and Self Help* Hutchinson, 1978
Illich, I. *Medical Nemesis: The Expropriation of Health*
Calder & Boyars, 1975
Inglis, Brian *Fringe Medicine* Faber, 1964
Liss, Jerome *Free to Feel: Finding Your Way Through the
New Therapies* Wildwood House, 1974
Maslow, Abraham H. *The Farther Reaches of Human
Nature* Penguin, 1976
Powell, Eric F. W. *The Natural Home Physician* Health
Science Press, 2nd edition, 1978
Tart, Charles T. (ed) *Altered States of Consciousness*
Doubleday Anchor, 1972
Weil, A. W. *The Natural Mind* Cape, 1973

THE ALEXANDER TECHNIQUE

Barlow, Wilfred *The Alexander Principle* Gollancz, 1973
Maisel, E. (ed) *The Alexander Technique* Thames &
Hudson, 1974. Published in the US by Delta under the
title *The Resurrection of the Body*
Pierce Jones, Frank *Body Awareness in Action* Schocken
Books, 1976

ANTHROPOSOPHICAL MEDICINE

Bott, Victor *Anthroposophical Medicine: an Extension of
the Art of Healing* Rudolf Steiner Press, London, 1978
Davy, John (ed) *Work Arising from the Life of Rudolf
Steiner* Rudolf Steiner Press, London, 1975
Hemleben, Johannes *Rudolf Steiner: a documentary
biography* Goulden, East Grinstead, 1975
Steiner, Rudolf *The Anthroposophical Approach to
Medicine* London, 1928

AROMATHERAPY

Maury, Marguerite *The Secret of Life and Youth*
Macdonald, 1964
Tisserand, R. B. *The Art of Aromatherapy* C. W. Daniel,
1977
Valnet, Jean *Aromatherapy* C. W. Daniel, 1978

AUTOGENIC TRAINING

Luthe, W. *Autogenic Training: method, research and
application in medicine in Altered States of
Consciousness* Ed Charles T. Tart. Doubleday
Anchor, 1969
Rosa, Dr Karl Robert *Autogenic Training* Saturday Review
Press/E. P. Dutton, 1976
Schulz, J. H. and Luthe, W. *Autogenic Training: a
psychophysiologic approach in psychotherapy*
Grune & Stratton, New York, 1959

THE AURA

Kilner, Dr W. J. *The Human Atmosphere* George
Routledge, 1920
Leadbeater, C. W. *The Chakras* Theosophical Publishing
House, 1927, reprinted Quest Books, 1974
Leadbeater, C. W. *Man Visible and Invisible* Theosophical
Publishing House, 1920, reprinted Quest Books, 1974
Ousley, L. G. J. *The Science of the Aura* L. N. Fowler,
London, 1949, revised ed 1960

AUTO-SUGGESTION

Baudouin, Charles *Suggestion and Auto-suggestion* Allen
& Unwin, 1921

AYURVEDIC MEDICINE

Bhattacharya, Dr B. *The Science of Tridosha* Gotham
Books, New York
Thakkur, Chandrashekhar G. *Introduction to Ayurveda*
ASI Books, New York, 1976

BACH FLOWER REMEDIES

Bach, Edward *The Twelve Healers* C. W. Daniel, 1933,
15th impression, 1977
Weeks, Nora *The Medical Discoveries of Edward Bach,
Physician* C. W. Daniel, 1973
Wheeler, F. J. *The Bach Remedies Repertory* C. W. Daniel,
1952, reprinted 1977

BATES METHOD OF EYESIGHT TRAINING

Benjamin, H. *Better Sight Without Glasses* Thorsons, 1921,
4th edition, 1977
Bates, W. H. *Perfect Sight Without Glasses* New York, 1920
Huxley, Aldous *The Art of Seeing* Chatto & Windus, 1943

BIODYNAMIC PSYCHOLOGY

St John, Ian (ed) *Biodynamic Psychology: Collected
Papers* Centre for Bioenergy, Acton, London, 1978

BIOENERGETICS

Lowen, Alexander *Bio-energetics* Coventure, London,
1976
Lowen, Alexander *The Betrayal of the Body* Collier
Macmillan, 1967
Lowen, Alexander *The Language of the Body* Collier
Macmillan, 1971

BIOFEEDBACK

Barber, Theodore X. et al *Biofeedback and self-control:
An Aldine Reader* Aldine-Atherton, 1970
Blundell, Geoffrey *EEG Measurement* Audio Ltd, London,
1977
Blundell, Geoffrey *The Omega I ESR Meter* Audio Ltd,
London, 1977
Brown, Barbara *Stress and the Art of Biofeedback* Bantam
Books, 1978
Cade, C. Maxwell and Coxhead, Nona *The Awakened
Mind* Heinemann, London and Delacourt, New York,
1979

BIORHYTHMS

Gittelson, Bernard *Bioryhthm: a personal science* New
York: Arco, London: Futura, 1975
Thommen, George, S. *Is This Your Day?* Crown, New
York, 1973

CHIROPRACTIC

Bach, Marcus *The Chiropractic Story* DeVorss & Co, Los
Angeles, 1968
Hippocrates Volume III 1968 edition, Loeb Classical
Library, Heinemann
Schafer, R. C. *Chiropractic Health Care* Foundation for
Chiropractic Education and Research, 3209 Ingersoll
Avenue, Des Moines, Iowa 3rd edition, 1977

CO-COUNSELLING

Evison, R. and Horobin, R. *How to Change Yourself and
Your World* 5 Victoria Road, Sheffield, England, 1977
Heron, J. *Reciprocal Counselling* Human Potential
Research Project, University of Surrey, 1974
Heron, J. *Catharsis in Human Development* British
Postgraduate Medical Federation, 1977
Heron, J. *Co-counselling Teachers' Manual* British
Postgraduate Medical Federation, 1978
Jackins, Harvey *The Human Side of Human Beings*
Rational Island Publishers, Seattle, 1965
Jackins, Harvey *The Human Situation* Rational Island
Publishers, Seattle, 1973
Jackins, Harvey *Fundamentals of Co-counselling Manual*
Rational Island Publishers, Seattle, 1970

COLOUR THERAPY

Gimbel, Theo *Healing Through Colour* C. W. Daniel, 1978

CURATIVE EURYTHMY

Glas, Dr Maria *Experience in Remedial Eurythmy*
Published privately, 1971
Kirchner-Bockholt, Dr M. *Fundamental Principles of
Curative Eurythmy* Rudolf Steiner Press, 1978
Steiner, Rudolf and Wegman, Ita *The Fundamentals of
Therapy* 1967

CYMATICS

Bhattacharyya, B. *The Science of Cosmic Ray Therapy or
Teletherapy* K. L. Mukhopadhyay, Calcutta, 1972,
revised edition 1977
Capra, F. *The Tao of Physics* Fontana, 1976
Ghyka, M. *The Geometry of Art and Life* Sheed & Ward,
1945
Hambridge, J. *Dynamic Symmetry in Composition* Yale
University Press, 1948
Jenny, H. *Cymatics* Basileus Press, Basle, 1966
Kayser, H. *Harmonia Plantarium* B. Schwabe & Co, Basle,
1943
Ostrander, S. and Schroeder, L. *PSI: Psychic Discoveries
Behind the Iron Curtain* Sphere Books, 1970,
reprinted 1977
Thompson, D'A *On Growth and Form* Cambridge, 1942
Watson, L. *Supernature* Hodder & Stoughton, 1973

DANCE THERAPY

Bernstein, P. *Theory and Methods in Dance Movement
Therapy* Kendall/Hunt, Iowa, 1972
Laban, R. *Modern Educational Dance* Macdonald & Evans,
1948
Schoop, T. *Won't You Join the Dance?* National Press,
USA, 1974

ENCOUNTER

Blank, L. et al (eds) *Confrontation: Encounter in Self and
Interpersonal Awareness* Collier-Macmillan, 1971
Rogers, Carl R. *On Encounter Groups* Penguin, 1973
Schutz, William C. *Elements of Encounter* Joy Press, 1973

ENLIGHTENMENT INTENSIVE

Kapleau, Philip *The Three Pillars of Zen*
Love, Jeff *The Quantum Gods* Compton Russell Element,
1976

GESTALT

Fagan, Joen and Shepherd, Irma Lee *Life Techniques in
Gestalt Therapy* Science and Behaviour Books, 1970
Perls, Frederick S. *Gestalt Therapy Verbatim* Real People
Press, 1969
Perls, Frederick S. *The Gestalt Approach and Eye
Witness to Therapy* Science and Behaviour Books,
1973
Stevens, John O. (ed) *Gestalt Is* Real People Press, 1975

HEALING

Ash, M. *Handbook of Natural Healing* Cans Press, 1977
Edwards, H. *Spirit Healing* Healing Publishing Co, 1960
Gallert, M. L. *New Light on Therapeutic Energies* James
Clarke, 1966
King, George *You Too Can Heal* Aetherius Society, 1976
Le Shan, L. *The Medium, the Mystic and the Physicist*
Turnstone, 1974
Meek, George W. (ed) *Healers and the Healing Process*
Quest Books, 1977
Tester, Morris *The Healing Touch* Barrie & Jenkins, 1970
Turner, Gordon *A Time to Heal* Corgi, 1975
Turner, Gordon *An Outline of Spiritual Healing* Psychic
Press

HOMOEOPATHY

Clarke, John H. *The Prescriber*. First published in the
1890s, 9th revised edition 1972
Nash, E. B. *Leaders in Homoeopathic Therapeutics*
Health Science Press, 1979
Roberts, Herbert A. *The Principles and Art of Cure by
Homoeopathy* Health Science Press, 1936, 5th imp
1976
Sharma, C. H. *A Manual of Homoeopathy and Natural
Medicine* Turnstone Press, 1975
Tyler, M. L. *Homoeopathic Drug Pictures* Health Science
Press, 1942
Wheeler, C. E. and Kenyon, J. D. *An Introduction to the
Principles and Practice of Homoeopathy* Health
Science Press, 1971

HYPNOSIS

Blythe, Peter *Hypnotism: Its Power and Practice* Arthur
Barker, 1971
Blythe, Peter *Self-Hypnotism: Its Potential and Practice*
Arthur Barker, 1976
Kroger, William S. *Clinical and Experimental Hypnosis*
J. B. Lippincott, Philadelphia, 1963

IMPACT THERAPY

Tracey, John B. *The Handbook of Impact Therapy* Pinhoe,
Exeter, 1967, revised ed, 1970

IRIS DIAGNOSIS

Jensen, Dr Bernard *The Science and Practice of Iridology*
1948
Kriege, Theodor *Fundamental Basis of Irisdiagnosis*
L. N. Fowler, 1969

KIRLIAN PHOTOGRAPHY
Dakin, H. S. *High-Voltage Photography* Washington Street Center, San Francisco, 1975
Kripner, S. and Rubin, D. *The Energies of Consciousness* Interface, 1975
Snellgrove, Brian *The Diagnostic Possibilities of Kirlian Photography* London, 1979

LAKHOVSKY OSCILLATORY COILS
Copen, Bruce *Radio-Biology Therapy* Dane Hill, Sussex, 1976
Lakhovsky, Georges *The Secret of Life* Heinemann, 1939

LÜSCHER COLOUR TEST
Lüscher, M. (trans Scott, I.) *The Lüscher Colour Test* Jonathan Cape, 1970

MANIPULATIVE THERAPY
Beard, Gertrude and Wood, Elizabeth C. *Massage, Principles and Techniques* W. B. Saunders, Eastbourne, 1964
Serizawa, Katsusuke *Massage: the Oriental Method* Japan Publications, San Francisco, 1972
Tidy, N. M. (ed J. Wade) *Massage and Remedial Exercises* John Wright, Bristol, 1932, last reprint 1976

MEDICAL HERBALISM
Schauenberg, P. and Paris, F. *Guide to Medical Plants* Lutterworth Press, 1977
Flück, Hans *Medicinal Plants* W. Foulsham, 1976

MEDICAL RADIESTHESIA
Mermet, Abbé *The Principles and Practice of Radiesthesia* Watkins & Robinson
Richards, Dr Guyon *The Chain of Life* Health Science Press, 1954
Westlake, Aubrey T. *The Pattern of Health* Shambhala, Berkeley and London, 1973
Wethered, Vernon D. *The Practice of Medical Radiesthesia* L. N. Fowler, 1967

MEDITATION
Guenther, H. V. and Trumpa, C. *Dawn of Tantra* Shambala, 1975
Lutyens, Mary (ed) *The Second Penguin Krishnamurti Reader* 1973
Naranjo, Claudio and Ornstein, Robert E. *The Psychology of Meditation* Allen & Unwin, 1972
Rajneesh, Bhagwan Shree *Meditation: the Art of Ecstasy* 1976
Russell, Peter *The TM Technique* Routledge, 1977
Tulku, Tarthang (ed) *Reflections of Mind* Dharma Publishing, 1975

MUSIC THERAPY
Nordoff, Paul and Robbins, Clive *Therapy in Music for Handicapped Children* Gollancz, 1971

NATUROPATHY
Barker, J. Ellis *Good Health and Happiness* Homoeopathic Publishing Co, 1927, reprinted 1947
Benjamin, Harry *Everybody's Guide to Nature Cure* Thorsons, 1961
Bircher-Benner, M. *The Prevention of Incurable Disease* James Clarke, 1959
Ledermann, E. K. *Natural Therapy* Watts & Co, 1953
Lindlahr, Henry *The Practice of Nature Cure* 28th edition, 2nd Indian reprint, Poona, 1954
Lindlahr, Henry *Philosophy of Natural Therapeutics*
reprinted by Maidstone Osteopathic Clinic, 1975
Newman Turner, R. *Naturopathic First Aid* Thorsons, 1969
Shelton, Herbert M. *An Introduction to Natural Hygiene* Natural Hygiene Press, Chicago, 1922, 3rd edition 1963
Warmbrand, Max *Encyclopedia of Natural Health* (2 vols) Souvenir Press, 1964

THE NEW PRIMAL THERAPIES
Broder, M. S. *An Eclectic Approach to Primal Therapy* 1974 Available from the author at 517 South 22nd Street, Philadelphia, PA 19146
Freundlich, David *An Historical Perspective of Primal Therapy* Available from the author at 304 West 105th Street, New York, NY 10025
Janov, Arthur *The Primal Scream* Doubleday, 1970
Swartley, William *Primal Integration* Centre for the Whole Person, Mays Landing, New Jersey, 1975

NUTRITION
Abehsera, Michel *Cooking for Life* Avon, 1976
Benjamin, Harry *Your Diet in Health and Disease* Health for All Publishing Co, 1931, Thorsons reprint 1978
Bircher, Ruth *Eating Your Way to Health: the Bircher-Benner Approach to Nutrition* Faber, 1961
Carque, Otto *Vital Facts About Food* Natural Brands, LA, 1933, 10th impression 1940
Chapman, J. B. *Dr Schuessler's Biochemistry* New Era Laboratories, revised edition 1973
Dickey, Laurence (ed) *Clinical Ecology* Charles C. Thomas, Springfield, Illinois
Dinshah, Freya *The Vegan Kitchen* American Vegan Society, New Jersey, 1965, 6th impression 1970
Ehret, Arnold *Mucusless Diet Healing System* Ehret Publishing Co, Beaumont, California
Hawkins, David and Pauling, Linus (eds) *Orthomolecular Psychiatry: Treatment of Schizophrenia* W. H. Freeman, 1973
Hoffer, Abram and Osmond, Humphrey *How to Live with Schizophrenia* Johnson Publications
Lief, Stanley *How to Eat for Health* Health for All Publishing Co, 1933, Thorsons reprint 1978
Lindlahr, Victor *You Are What You Eat* Newcastle Publishing Co, USA, 1971
McCance, R. A. and Widdowson, E. M. *The Chemical Composition of Foods* HMSO, 1946, 4th impression 1978
Mackarness, Richard *Not All in the Mind* Pan Books, 1976
Ohsawa, Lima *The Art of Just Cooking* Autumn Press, Tokyo, 1974
Quick, Vivien and Clifford *Everywoman's Wholefood Cookbook* Thorsons, 1976
Randolph, Theron G. *Human Ecology and Susceptibility to the Chemical Environment* Charles C. Thomas, Springfield, Illinois, 1962
Shelton, Herbert M. *Fasting for Renewal of Life* Natural Hygiene Press, Chicago, 1974
Vegetarian Society Leaflets: *Slimplan, Just for One, Dayplan* etc
Whitehouse, Geoffrey T. *Why Health Foods?* Newman Turner Publications, 1968

ORGONE THERAPY
Boadella, David *Wilhelm Reich: the evolution of his work* Vision Press, 1973
Boadella, David (ed) *In the Wake of Reich* Coventure, London, 1976
Mann, Edward *Orgone, Reich and Eros* Simon & Schuster, 1973

Raknes, Ola *Wilhelm Reich and Orgonomy* St Martin's Press, 1970

Reich, Wilhelm *The Discovery of the Orgone* Part I: *The Function of the Orgasm* Orgone Institute Press, New York, 1942 Part II: *The Cancer Biopathy* Orgone Institute Press, 1948. Part I reprinted by Panther Books, 1966; Part II by Vision Press, 1973

ORIENTAL DIAGNOSIS
Kushi, Michio *Introduction to Oriental Diagnosis* Sunwheel Publications, 1978

ORIENTAL MEDICINE
Kushi, Michio *Book of Macrobiotics: The Way of Life for Health, Happiness and Freedom* Japan Publications, New York and Tokyo, 1977

Lavier, J. *Points of Chinese Acupuncture* Health Science Press, 1965

Lawson-Wood, D. and J. *First Aid at Your Fingertips* Health Science Press, 1963

Masunaga, Shizuto *Zen Shiatsu* Japan Publications, New York and Tokyo, 1978

Muramoto, Naboru *Healing Ourselves* New York: Avon, London: Dempsey/Cassell, 1973

Ohashi, Wataru *Do It Yourself Shiatsu* Allen & Unwin, 1977

Ohsawa, George *Acupuncture and the Philosophy of the Far East* Boston, Mass, 1973

Sakurazawa, Nyoiti (George Ohsawa) *Macrobiotics* London: Tandem Books. Published in the US as *You Are All Sanpaku*, New York: University Books

Stiskin, Nahum *The Looking Glass God* Autumn Press, Tokyo, 1971

Veith, I. (trans) *The Yellow Emperor's Classic of Internal Medicine* University of California Press, 1966

Wu, Wei-P'ing *Chinese Acupuncture* Health Science Press, 1962

OSTEOPATHY
Fryette, Harrison H. *Principles of Osteopathic Technic* Academy of Applied Osteopathy, Carmel, California 1954

Proby, Jocelyn *A Short Essay on Osteopathy* Osteopathic Institute of Applied Technique, Maidstone, 1955

Stoddard, Alan *Manual of Osteopathic Practice* Hutchinson, 1969

Stoddard, Alan *Manual of Osteopathic Technique* Hutchinson, 1959

PSIONIC MEDICINE
Reyner, J. H., Lawrence, G., Upton, C. *Psionic Medicine* Routledge, 1974

Westlake, Aubrey T. *The Origins and History of Psionic Medicine* Psionic Medical Society, 1977

PSYCHIC SURGERY
Fuller, John G. *Arigó – Surgeon of the Rusty Knife* Panther, 1977

Sharman, Harold *The Wonder Healers of the Philippines* Psychic Press, 1967

PSYCHODRAMA
Blatner, Howard *Acting-In: Practical Application of Psychodramatic Methods* Springer Books, New York, 1973

Moreno, J. D. *Psychodrama Vols 1, 2 and 3.* Beacon House Press, New York, 1946, revised edition, 1964

PSYCHOSYNTHESIS
Assagioli, R. *The Act of Will* Wildwood House, 1974

Assagioli, R. *Psychosynthesis: A Manual of Principles and Techniques* Viking Press, 1971

PYRAMID ENERGY
Kerrell, Bill and Goggin, Kathy *The Guide to Pyramid Energy* Pyramid U, Inc., 1975

Schul, Bill and Pettit, Ed *The Secret Power of Pyramids* Coronet, 1975

RADIONICS
Day, Langston and de la Warr, George *Matter in the Making* Vincent Stuart, 1956

Day, Langston and de la Warr, George *New Worlds Beyond the Atom* Vincent Stuart, 1956

Russell, Edward W. *Report on Radionics* Neville Spearman, 1973

Tansley, David V. *Dimensions of Radionics* Health Science Press, 1977

Tansley, David V. *Radionics – Interface with the Ether Fields* Health Science Press, 1975

Tansley, David V. *Radionics and the Subtle Anatomy of Man* Health Science Press, 1972

REFLEXOLOGY
Ingham, Eunice D. *Stories the Feet Can Tell* Ingham Publishing, Rochester, New York, 1938, reprinted 1976

Ingham, Eunice D. *Stories the Feet Have Told* Ingham Publishing, Rochester, New York, 1951, reprinted 1959

ROLFING
Rolfing: The Integration of Human Structures Rolf Institute, 1976

Gallwey, Timothy *The Inner Game of Tennis* Random House, 1974

Johnson, Don *The Protean Body* Harper Colophon Books, 1977

SENSITIVITY TRAINING
Blumberg, A. and Golembiewski, R. T. *Learning and Change in Groups* Penguin, 1976

Lakin, M. *Interpersonal Encounter: theory and practice in sensitivity training* McGraw-Hill, 1972

TOUCH FOR HEALTH
Thie, J. F. and Marks, M. *Touch for Health: a new approach to restoring our natural energies* De Vorss & Co, Los Angeles, 1973

TRANSACTIONAL ANALYSIS
Berne, Eric *Games People Play* Penguin 1968

VITA FLORUM
Wielkopolska, E. Bellhouse *Vita Florum and the Master Science* Vita Florum Trust, 1977

YOGA
Asrani, U. A. *Yoga Unveiled* Motolal Banarsidas, Delhi, 1977

Hewitt, James *Yoga and Vitality* Barrie & Jenkins, 1977

Kirschner, M. J. *Yoga for Health and Vitality* Allen & Unwin, 1977

Oki, Masahiro *Healing Yourself Through Okido Yoga* Japan Publications, 1977

Ramacharaka *Science of Breath* L. N. Fowler, 11th impression 1975

Sivananda, Swami *Science of Pranayama* Divine Life Society, Shivanandanagar, UP, India, 1975

Yesudian, S. and Haich, E. *Yoga and Health* Allen & Unwin, 1976

Foreword

One of the contributors to this encyclopedia says that most people keep their cars in a better state than they keep themselves. This is a disturbing observation, but one could lead on to a broader one and say that a great deal of modern life is bad for health. We travel in crowded trains, breathe polluted air, dash out for hurried meals, eat 'convenience' foods which are often processed and over-refined. We submit to work pressures and social demands which are excessive. And then some part of us begins to break down. When the discomfort becomes intolerable we go to our doctors and ask for help. We want to be fixed up quickly so that we can return to that complicated life. And so come the prescriptions for sedatives, stimulants, tranquillizers, 'pain killers' and megadoses of vitamins. We may be told to take things easily for a while, but that is no kind of an answer.

This book is concerned with health, not simply as an absence of disease, but as a positive state of mental and physical well-being. Increasingly over the past few years, interest has been gathering and concern expressed about the nature of our health systems and as a result some of the barriers between 'conventional' and 'unconventional' medicine are beginning to come down. If one were to define the difference, it would probably still be true to say that conventional medicine is directed towards man as a system of levers, chemical reactions, tubes and pumps, whereas the natural therapists look at the whole man, who has a body, but also a mind and a spirit.

Holistic medicine has a new ring to it, and yet it has ancient origins in both Eastern and Western philosophy. It was probably first revived in modern times by Hahnemann, the founder of homoeopathy, and later expressed by Dr Edward Bach, when he said ''treat the patient and not the disease''. A concern with stress reduction is common to all alternative therapies, and a healthy body is less prone to psychological and physical stress. As a start, therefore, we should contrive to breathe some fresh air, take some normal exercise and feed ourselves intelligently. And we should listen to the constant stream of informational signals that flow in and out of our bodies and respond to them.

Health is a state of harmony between our physical, mental and spiritual states. If our energy channels get blocked, we become sick. We all have the power to heal ourselves, both at the pragmatic and intuitive levels, but sometimes we need help. This is where healing , relaxation and meditation prove their worth. As another of our contributors has said : ''we do not relate to one another as piles of protein but energetically as one spiritual being to another''.

It is not the intention of this book to suggest that all of conventional medicine is wrong, or that unconventional therapies can necessarily provide all the answers. The two systems should be complementary. But there are very many resources available to us, some well established over the years, others newer and less familiar. We have tried to gather together as many of them as seemed useful and to present them without bias. If as a result some good new doors are opened to its readers, the book will have done its job.

All of the therapies have been presented by practitioners of those therapies. I am grateful to each of them for the sympathy and enthusiasm with which they have approached the project. The book would not have been possible at all without the support and guidance of the six members of the Editorial Board. Their broad knowledge and generosity and concern sustained the publication and its editor at every stage.

A.H.

Oriental Medicine

"IN OLDEN TIMES, those people who understood the Tao (the Way of Nature) patterned themselves upon the Yin and the Yang (the two fundamental forces in Nature) and they lived in harmony. There was temperance in eating and drinking. Their hours of rising and retiring were regular and not disorderly and wild. By these means the ancients kept their bodies united with their souls, so as to fulfil their allotted span completely, measuring unto a hundred years before they passed."

The above passage from the Yellow Emperor's classic of internal medicine, the *Nei Ching*, gives us a clear picture of the spirit of Oriental medicine. This rich tradition is firmly based on the understanding that humanity is very much a part of the natural environment, and that health can only be achieved if man actively acknowledges this fundamental fact. Conversely, sickness is the direct result of an inability to live in accordance with the Laws of Nature. Although nowadays most public interest in Oriental medicine is concentrated on such areas as acupuncture and herbal medicine, it is important to realize that it is in the field of prevention and self-help that the Far East has the most to offer.

The philosophical base of Oriental medicine is Taoism (the Way of Life), a school of thought whose roots stem back to prehistoric times. The major contribution of Taoist thought is its philosophy of universal dialectics. Some of the main principles of this philosophy are that:

1. All phenomena exist within infinite space.
2. All phenomena are interrelated.
3. All phenomena are relative.
4. Everything has energy or vibration.
5. Everything is in a constant state of change.

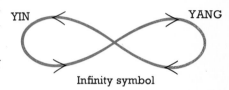

Infinity symbol

Yin and Yang

According to Taoist belief, the activating force of all phenomena is the movement of energy between two poles. These two poles, or extremes, are known as the yin and the yang. It is interesting to note that this cosmic view corresponds very closely with the dialectic model used by many modern physicists.

In order to understand Oriental medicine, it is necessary to come to terms with the principles of yin and yang. Yin and yang should not be thought of as entities, but rather as tendencies in the movement of energy. Between these two extremes there is constant movement. It is the varying combinations of these two tendencies which give all things their distinctive character. Yin is the term used for the tendency towards expansion or centrifugality; yang is the tendency towards contraction or centripetality. When the contracting force reaches its limit it changes direction and begins to expand, and vice versa. This constant flux between the two extremes can be observed in all things – from the smallest molecule to the pulsation of the galaxies. Within the human body we can perceive this in the rhythm of the heart and lungs and also in the peristaltic waves of the intestines. Often the transition from yin to yang takes place in a spirallic manner. This can be observed in the development of the human form from the spirallic formation of the embryo to the structure of muscle and bone.

On the right are some illustrations showing the dynamics of the way yin and yang operate.

The ancient Chinese and Japanese symbolized yin as the force of Earth (centrifugal energy emanating from the planet) and yang as the force of Heaven (centripetal energy acting on the planet from outside). These terms, Earth and Heaven, are used in place of yin and yang in many writings.

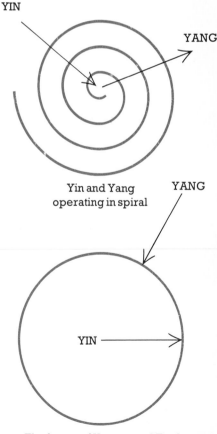

Yin and Yang operating in spiral

The forces of Heaven and Earth

Oriental Medicine

Chi or Ki Energy

The vehicle through which yin and yang operate in all things was called *chi* by the Chinese and *ki* by the Japanese. This term denotes the dynamic, subtle energy present in all things. Everything has ki, be it mineral, vegetable, animal or human, but the rate and quality of vibration varies in different phenomena. When a person is healthy, they resonate with the vibration of their environment, i.e. their ki is in harmony with that of their surroundings. Oriental medicine aims at maximizing the harmonious flow of ki in the body. The diagram below shows the relationship of ki to other phenomena.

We take in ki in its more dense forms in the food and drink we consume each day. It is through the regulation of food and drink that we can harmonize the energy in the vegetable and mineral kingdoms. If this is done, then we become more sensitive to the movement of ki in its more refined state, which enriches our lives with sensitivity, judgment and harmony. This is not to be regarded as mysticism but as a practical desire to fulfil the human potential. The regulation of food in this regard is usually referred to as macrobiotics, which is covered in another section.

The regulation of food and drink is usually combined with certain activities. This generally means just physical work but in some cases the individual's constitution or character may not allow for this. In these cases, many forms of meditation or exercise can be used, often together in the form of T'ai Chi Ch'uan. If diet and activity are not in balance then stress and/or stagnation arise, the circulation of blood and body fluid is impaired and toxic conditions or degeneration begin. In the state of sickness, the flow of the more refined ki in the body is affected. In this state, adjustments must be made in the individual's life-style. In some cases where imbalances arise, massage, moxibustion or acupuncture are used to restore balance.

The true goal of Oriental medicine is that each person learns the dynamics involved in maintaining good health. In the Far East, the traditional function of the 'superior doctor' was to help people to reach that goal. He was an educator, teaching people the proper way of life. The second category of medicine was what we would term preventive medicine. This involved teaching, as well as simple treatment, and was the province of the common doctor. The lowest classification was that of the 'inferior doctor' who dealt with the person's symptoms. These distinctions illustrate the truly great gap that exists between modern and traditional medicine. Oriental medicine, as well as other traditional approaches to healing, makes the point that the individual should take personal responsibility for his own sickness. The doctor can only assist in the healing process, the most important work being done by the sick person by adjusting his life-style.

If the individual is to accept responsibility for his or her own health, then it is important that he understands the dynamics involved in the development of sickness; through this he can come to an understanding of the various steps he needs to take in order to restore his health.

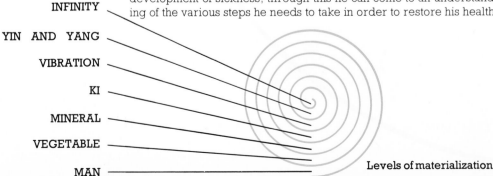

INFINITY
YIN AND YANG
VIBRATION
KI
MINERAL
VEGETABLE
MAN

Levels of materialization

Oriental Medicine

Yin and Yang Organs

The ki which nourishes the various organs has different qualities or characteristics and the organs are grouped into pairs. These pairs are made up of a yin organ and a yang organ which have a complementary relationship. In terms of structure, the organs can be classified as follows:

YANG ORGANS	YIN ORGANS
dense, blood-filled organs of regulation	*hollow, organs of absorption and discharge*
heart	small intestine
liver	gall bladder
kidney	urinary bladder
spleen	stomach
lungs	large intestine

Note: some classifications will be listed differently because the ki of the organ rather than its structure is used to define its quality. Thus the structure and function of the organs are different i.e. a structurally yang organ is animated by yin ki and vice versa.

The movement from yin to yang and back again gives us the picture of an ever-changing universe with no beginning and no end. In this universe the only constant is change, and all understanding comes from an understanding of this process of change. The Japanese philosopher, Nyoiti Sakurazawa, known in the West as George Ohsawa, outlined the laws governing change as follows:

THE UNIQUE PRINCIPLE

Seven Principles of the Order of the Universe

1. All things are differentiated apparatus of One Infinity.
2. Everything changes.
3. All antagonisms are complementary.
4. There is nothing identical.
5. What has a front has a back.
6. The bigger the front, the bigger the back.
7. What has a beginning has an end.

Twelve Theorems of the Unifying Principle

1. One Infinity differentiates itself into Yin and Yang which are the poles that come into operation when the infinite centrifugally arrives at the geometric point of bifurcation.
2. Yin and Yang result continuously from the infinite centrifugality.
3. Yin is centrifugal. Yang is centripetal. Yin and Yang together produce energy and all phenomena.
4. Yin attracts Yang. Yang attracts Yin.
5. Yin repels Yang. Yang repels Yin.
6. The force of attraction and repulsion is proportional to the difference of the Yin and Yang components. Yin and Yang combined in varying proportions produce energy and all phenomena.
7. All phenomena are ephemeral, constantly changing their constitution of Yin and Yang components.
8. Nothing is solely Yin or solely Yang. Everything involves polarity.
9. There is nothing neuter. Either Yin or Yang is in excess in every occurrence.
10. Large Yin attracts small Yang. Large Yang attracts small Yin.
11. At the extremes, Yin produces Yang and Yang produces Yin.
12. All physical forms and objects are Yang at the centre and Yin at the surface.

Oriental Medicine

The Five Elements

The five elements theory is fundamental to understanding the more specialist practices of acupuncture, moxibustion and herbal medicine. This theory is an extension of yin and yang, describing the character of various combinations of yin and yang forces. The word element, which is commonly used, should more accurately be transformations. The terms used – fire, soil, metal, water and wood – do not refer directly to the substances themselves but rather to the energy expressed in their formation. These transformations are seen as operating in a cycle as shown below.

Each of these qualities is associated with certain structural and functional aspects of the body. Sickness shows its cause by the location and character of the symptoms, (*see* section on Oriental diagnosis), which can be corrected through the proper food or herbs, the stimulation of chi through the use of needles (acupuncture), heat (moxa), pressure (shiatsu) or exercise to stimulate the particular energy which is lacking or to drain energy that is in excess.

In the past ten to fifteen years public interest in Oriental medicine has grown steadily in the West. Acupuncture, shiatsu massage, herbal medicine and macrobiotics are now practised in most countries of Europe and in North America. This interest has drawn the attention of many people in the medical professions to explore the ways that this traditional approach to sickness can be used in the West. It also provides a great opportunity for social unification through the application of this ancient intuitive art.

William Tara

The creative cycle of the five elements. Clockwise from top: fire, earth, metal, water, and wood.

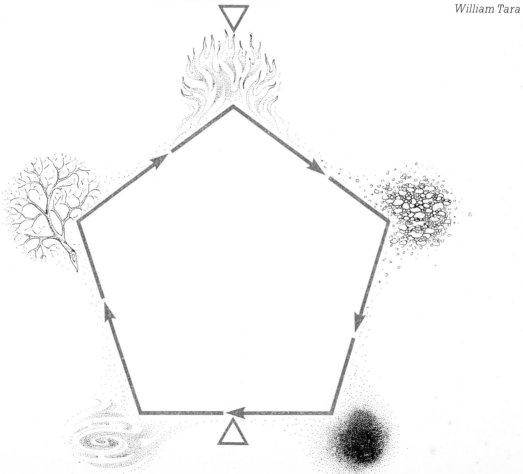

Ayurvedic Medicine

HISTORY

Ayurveda is a Sanskrit word meaning 'Laws of Health' and is one of the four *Vedas*, or Hindu sacred texts. The name is associated with Indian traditional medicine, a science which first appeared three thousand years ago. Because no historical records exist of the period, little is known of its origins, and what has been handed down to contemporary Ayurvedic practitioners has been modified by contact with foreign systems and by the changing values which resulted from India's contact with foreign cultures.

Many of Ayurveda's most extraordinary practices such as vaccination, anaesthesis by inhalation, and dietetics have been practised in the West only in the last hundred years or so, but the most profound and significant notions are cosmological in nature and these have been neglected or their importance ignored. These are the doctrine of the whole man, including all his physical, psychological and spiritual attributes, and the theory of *Tridosha*, or three elements, air, water and fire. Fundamental to the Ayurveda is the belief that the human being must be considered as a single existent, without separation of body, psyche and soul. Medicine based on this premise is made possible through the Tridosha.

Four main periods or stages can be distinguished, which are:

1. The Vedic period, in which the theory of the three elements of material existence – air, fire and water – were related to human life.

2. The period of original research and the classical authors.

3. The period of documentation. This was when the tantras, or symbolic diagrams were composed and the siddhas or chemist-physicians appeared. Ayurvedic medicine was then at its zenith and treatises were composed on paediatrics, obstetrics, gynaecology, caesarian section and surgery (including lithotomy and rhinoplasty), which are considered to be recent advances. Evidence points to knowledge of bacteriology, immunology and methods of preventive medicine, and isolation of persons suffering from infectious diseases.

4. The period of stagnation or recompilation. By this time the medicine of the ancient Aryans had begun to have a strong influence in other centres of culture, notably the Arabian and Egyptian. In the early middle ages there was a strong cultural interchange between the Arabian and Greek civilizations particularly in the field of medicine, and the term *unani* – from Aryan word for Greece – now represents that sector of Indian medicine which derives from this source.

Possibly as a consequence of contact with Western civilizations, a prejudice developed against the dissection of cadavers, and this led to a breakdown of anatomical and surgical research. In general, during the middle ages, the ancient notions of Ayurvedic cosmology diminished in importance and the emphasis fell on the mechanical means of healing, and many remarkably advanced practices were developed, such as trepanning, and the use of the ultraviolet components of the sun's rays. What has remained unchanged throughout the history of Ayurveda, is the Tridosha.

With the sweeping changes which accompanied the birth of the British Empire, Western medicine replaced Ayurveda as the most widely practised system in India. Since 1945 a resurgence has taken place in the study and research of those systems which were peculiar to pre-Empire India, and particularly Ayurveda with its essentially Hindu foundations. Today, many colleges and universities offer degree courses in Ayurveda and these are recognized for registration in India and so have independent status. In Russia and China, the system has been adopted and made the subject of extensive research programmes. In India itself, Ayurveda is once more an effective part of the medical system in hospitals, colleges, schools and villages.

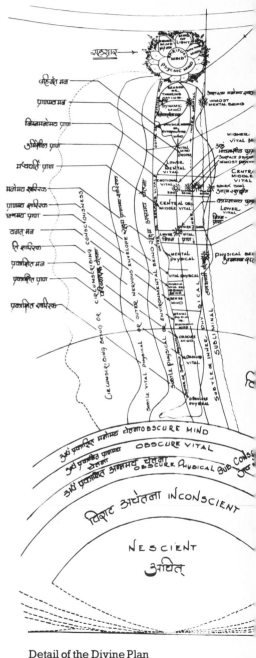

Detail of the Divine Plan prepared for the Aurobindo Ashram by Amidhar Bhatt depicting the planes, parts and entities of the total consciousness.

Ayurvedic Medicine

AYURVEDIC PRACTICE
Training

As in all modern medical systems, Ayurvedic physicians have always been instructed in colleges and training schools, and, as is the practice in schools throughout Asia, lessons are learnt by recitation and repetition, as opposed to the Western penchant for the written word.

The training of Ayurvedic physicians covers *kaya*, the body, *shalya* or surgery, *shalakya* or ear, nose and throat, mouth and eye diseases, *bhuta vidya* or materia medica and sensitivities of the body, *kumara* or the study of youth (obstetrics, paediatrics, etc), *agada* or toxicology and the effects on the body of poisonous drugs, *rasa yana* or diet, and *vajakarana* or semen, aphrodisiacs and sex.

The physician is selected for his qualities of *vidhya* or knowledge, *tarka* or logic and wisdom, *smriti* or memory, *tatparata* or adaptability and *krita* or practical skill. He is trained to treat the patient individually, as a whole and considering what is curable and what is not.

The physician's role is ideally defined by Charaka, one of the foremost Ayurvedic physicians: "One need not be ashamed because one is not conversant with the names of all possible diseases, for all diseases are not definitely recognized by name. There is no end of medical science. Skilfulness in practice should be acquired from others without any feeling of humility. Unto men of intelligence the whole world acts as a teacher, unto men devoid of intelligence the entire world appears as hostile. Hence the wise should listen to the counsels even of an opponent, if they are instructive and praiseworthy, calculated to promote health and life and well suited to the conditions of the people".

Diagnosis

From the beginning, the physician examined the human being on all levels in terms of the Tridosha, or three elements, air, water and fire. All areas of human function are located in one or other of three *doshas* or cosmic forces. The doshas are in turn divided into two aspects, named *purusha* and *prakriti*, or the matter and the essence. So *kaph*, or the moon, corresponds to the elements of earth and water, *vayu*, or wind, to air and ether, and *pitta*, or sun, to fire and earth. When used in connection with human life, the terms purusha denotes the physical life of man and his conscious state, prakriti his unmanifested self and his subconscious, or his spirit. Prakriti comprises three parts which are: *mahat*, or that part of man which unites him with the cosmic individual, or his God-given essence; *ahamkara*, or man's self-will, and the expression of his psychosomatic states; and *abhimana* or man's true pride, the state of awareness of a will greater than his own and of which he is part, and thus reconciling *mahat* and *ahamkara*. The physician's approach to prakriti is through five tanmantras, or essence types: *akash* – ether, *vayu* – air, *teja* – fire, *aap* – water, and *prithvi* – earth.

That part of man which is defined as purusha, or material existence, is divided into three *gunas*, *satvika* or state of self-contentment, balanced, rational behaviour, *rajas* or pre-eminently positive man, but lacking equilibrium, and *tamas*, which is negative man, angry fiery impatient, on the one hand, and passive, irresolute and lacking initiative on the other. The physician's first task is to identify these by observing the patient's behaviour and attitudes.

More specific analysis is divided into four main *indriyas* or sciences, thus:

Gnanendriyas, or senses that provide information for the logical apparatus; sight, touch, taste, smell, hearing and the reproductive or sex sense.

Ayurvedic Medicine

Karmendriyas, or organs that are controlled by the senses: the tongue, the arms, the legs, the anus, the reproductive organs.

Shrotas or channels which were divided into

the internal:	and the external:
(1) veins	(1) eyes
(2) arteries	(2) ears
(3) lymphatic system	(3) mouth
(4) intestines	(4) nostrils
(5) liver	(5) breasts
	(6) vagina

Manas, or mental desires, lusts and aversions.

On the basis of this information, the physician considers twelve *pranas*, or vital aspects. Five are vital substances which correspond in the body to the five *tanmantras: agni* or temperature, *soma* or physical alertness, *vayu* or breath, flatus and wind, *satva* or the minerals of the body and *rajas*, *tamas* and *atmas* which form a single tanmantra and correspond respectively to positive emotions, negative emotions and individual character or personality. Seven *dhatus* or incoming forces are: *rasa* or food, *rakta* or blood, *mamsa* or bones, *meda* or fat and perspiration, *asthi* or marrow, *majya* or viscidity – now known as 'packed cell volume' – and *shukra* or movements creating satisfaction.

As a result of man's daily activities, he eliminates certain waste products or *malas:* urine, faeces, sweat.

Finally, the physician's diagnosis takes into account the patient's age, nationality, life and family circumstances.

Therapy

The Tridosha is the key to the physician's approach to his patient; firstly in diagnosis as has been described, and then in his therapy. The functions of the body are divided into three areas according to the characteristics of the three doshas.

To *vayu*, belong all functions connected to air, the respiratory and sound-producing apparatus, the digestive tract, the bladder, the testes and organs whose function is to retain substances, as well as wind and flatus. Movement of matter within the body-contraction, expansion, upward, and downward, were held to be properties of vayu.

Pitta, or sun, which implies the elements of fire and earth, is related to the liver, the spleen, the heart and the eyes, which are connected in the following way: when food is taken into the body through the mouth, chewed, mixed with saliva – the element water – and descends to the stomach where the action of the gastric secretions produces heat – the element fire – the resulting concentration is called pitta, a term which denotes, in this case, the bile. This transparent, hot and concentrated liquid produces in the liver and the spleen the bright red blood cells or haemoglobin. The heart, in turn receiving this substance through the veins, pumps it throughout the system, and maintains the flow, not allowing it to remain in the same place which would result in ulcers and other disorders. Thus pitta, or fire, causes vayu-inhaled air and kaph-water from the alimentary tract to be circulated throughout the body. The heart is the one point in which all three forces are equally dominant, and it activates and pacifies the entire circulatory system.

Kaph, or the moon, in the same way that it influences the ebb and flow of the tides, controls the ebb and flow of moisture in the body. The secretions of the skull maintain the efficient working of the brain, the salivary juices stimulate taste and appetite, the cardiac fluid maintains the correct temperature of the heart, the foamy gastric juices control the digestion and the fluid within the joints and articulations result in balanced posture and movement. All these functions and their effects on man's behaviour are the properties of kaph.

Ayurvedic Medicine

The physician's task is to maintain the balance of the three forces within the body and, since the same three types are identifiable in foods, minerals and natural remedies, choosing the correct remedy for a particular condition is a logical process. For example, the condition commonly known as asthma is one in which the Ayurvedic physician would observe that the element air was excessively dominant; he would therefore prescribe a diet which excludes any vayu foods, such as rice and spices, and would use a remedy which would stimulate the other two elements. Clearly in the case of a chronic condition, the physician would begin by prescribing a diet before a medicine, on the assumption that the milder the remedy, the less the danger from undesirable side-effects. Such a diet would be minutely prepared with due regard to the patient's individual susceptibilities and seasonal and climatic variations.

Surgery was already a highly developed science in the early days of Ayurveda, but the removal of an organ was only effected if it had become entirely morbid and was considered a threat to the proper function of the rest of the body. Wounds sustained in battle were treated surgically but otherwise surgery was mainly cosmetic and it is known that cataracts were removed and rhinoplasties performed.

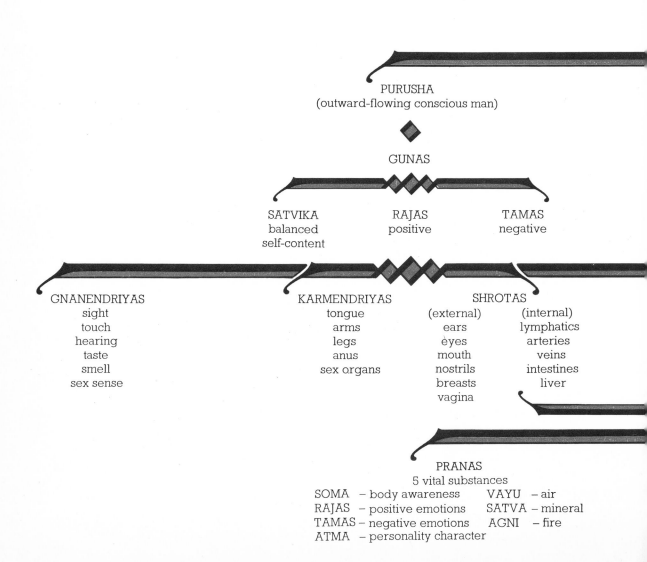

PURUSHA
(outward-flowing conscious man)

GUNAS

SATVIKA	RAJAS	TAMAS
balanced	positive	negative
self-content		

GNANENDRIYAS	KARMENDRIYAS	SHROTAS	
sight	tongue	(external)	(internal)
touch	arms	ears	lymphatics
hearing	legs	eyes	arteries
taste	anus	mouth	veins
smell	sex organs	nostrils	intestines
sex sense		breasts	liver
		vagina	

PRANAS
5 vital substances

SOMA	– body awareness	VAYU	– air
RAJAS	– positive emotions	SATVA	– mineral
TAMAS	– negative emotions	AGNI	– fire
ATMA	– personality character		

Ayurvedic Medicine

Unlike Western systems of medicine, Ayurveda has always been based on a positive interaction between the physician and his patient. An understanding of the need to strive for spiritual self-development is taken for granted and in this respect the physician combines the role of spiritual guide. The patient understands that his obligation is to direct himself towards purity and to overcome the mechanical, *tamassic* instincts which are more proper to the life of animals than to man.

The physician advises the patient, not only on the appearance of specific symptoms, but also in times of good health and is responsible for the patient's diet, the regulation of his personal habits, the choice of marital partner, and sexual behaviour. Insofar as the patient's own religious faith shares the same roots as the physician's art, physical and spiritual well-being are indivisible. This is in marked contrast to the relationship between a Western doctor and his patient, where the patient is the passive recipient of the practitioner's treatment, often ignoring his obligation to strive for his own physical well-being.

C. H. Sharma

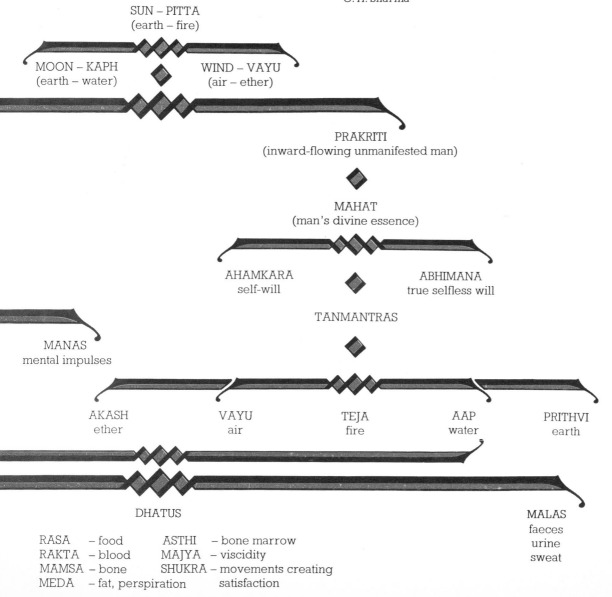

SUN – PITTA
(earth – fire)

MOON – KAPH
(earth – water)

WIND – VAYU
(air – ether)

PRAKRITI
(inward-flowing unmanifested man)

MAHAT
(man's divine essence)

AHAMKARA
self-will

ABHIMANA
true selfless will

TANMANTRAS

MANAS
mental impulses

| AKASH | VAYU | TEJA | AAP | PRITHVI |
| ether | air | fire | water | earth |

DHATUS

MALAS
faeces
urine
sweat

RASA – food ASTHI – bone marrow
RAKTA – blood MAJYA – viscidity
MAMSA – bone SHUKRA – movements creating
MEDA – fat, perspiration satisfaction

Homoeopathy

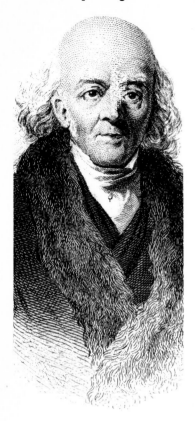

Samuel Christian
Hahnemann, 1755–1843.

HISTORY

Homoeopathy is the name given to a system of medicine which was discovered at the end of the 18th century by Samuel Christian Hahnemann. Hahnemann was born in Meissen, Saxonia in 1745 and studied medicine at Leipzig and Vienna, settling in the former city in 1789. The following year, he embarked upon a translation of W. Cullen's *Materia Medica* and was struck by the fact, hitherto given little significance, that the symptoms produced by quinine on a healthy body, were similar to the symptoms it was used to alleviate. From this he formulated the principle "similia, similibus curantur – like is healed by like" and published the theory in a paper in 1796.

Further researches led Hahnemann to the theory of potentization of substances, and this established him as the great founder of homoeopathy. He practised his system in Leipzig until 1821 when the antagonism of rival interests forced him to leave Leipzig, and until 1835 he served as personal physician to the Grand Duke of Anhalt–Kothen. By the time of his death in 1843 he had published four major works on medicine and laid down certain rules for the preparation and prescribing of remedies, which are followed by homoeopaths to the present day. Much of the philosophical side of Hahnemann's writing is derived from earlier medical thinkers such as Hippocrates, and Paracelsus (1490–1541) and his significance as a revolutionary lies mainly in his practical researches.

It is interesting to note that in 1798 Edward Jenner published his findings concerning the relationship between smallpox and cowpox, hence inaugurating the science of vaccination. It is clear that the principle of vaccination differs from the principle of homoeopathy in the action of the dose which is materially greater and serves to establish benign antibodies. Otherwise the principles are similar.

Since the days of Hahnemann, homoeopathy has been developed in all parts of the world and many researchers have published provings. Several major *materia medica*, or pharmacopoeia have been compiled and repertories or analyses of symptoms in relation to remedies, published.

Homoeopathy has never received official or public recognition in any Western country, although it is not generally known that members of the English Royal Family have been homoeopathic patients. The system has always been regarded as unorthodox and been practised privately. In most major Western countries there are distinguished and long-established societies of homoeopaths.

THEORY
Diseases and Remedies

One of Hahnemann's tenets was that disease itself is a non entity, and cannot be something to be purged out by 'cupping', or mechanically removed from the patient's body. In his *Organon de Rationallen Heilkunst* (1810) he defines disease as "an aberration from the state of health". Unlike Sydenham, who in the 18th century compiled a compendium of symptoms and diseases, he maintained that the range of morbid states is infinite; therefore the remedies which correspond most nearly to such 'aberrations', are infinite in number. Since the first days of homoeopathy, physicians have been making 'provings' of remedies, that is, dosing healthy men and women with substances and documenting the effect. New remedies are constantly being added to the homoeopathic pharmacopoeia.

Potency of Remedies

Hahnemann's most astonishing discovery was that the effect of a remedy is inversely proportional to its substance. To make a remedy

Homoeopathy

according to rules laid down by Hahnemann, a grain is taken of a certain substance, added to ten parts of a neutral substance such as pure alcohol, water or sugar, and shaken in a calculated way. The resulting mixture is called potency 1. When one part of the mixture is added to ten further parts of the neutral base and mixed the result is called potency 2. Each time the process is repeated the potency increases by one, up to 100,000. Homoeopaths therefore work on the principle that the smaller the material of the remedy is present in the dose, the more potent is its effect.

However, we can observe if the operation is performed six times – potency 6 – that one part in a million remains. In the case of one widely used remedy, *Natrum Muriaticum*, or common salt, a single molecule weighs 10^{-24} milligrams. It follows that at a potency of 30, not a single molecule of the original salt is likely to remain the dose. Hahnemann's discovery therefore was that the power of a substance is not in the material but in its pattern, and the further removed the material becomes the greater the power of the pattern. This is the greatest stumbling block to acceptance by conventionally educated men and women, who in our present society are trained to think that power is measurable by its quantity or volume.

Action of Remedies

While it is fundamental to homoeopathy that any diagnosis and therapy must concern the whole body as a single organism, it is also held that morbid or unhealthy cells only will respond to the remedy, because their resistance is lower and because the vital pattern of the cells will correspond to the essential pattern of the remedy itself. For this reason, and because of the lack of material substance in a homoeopathic remedy, there is little danger of harmful side effects, or ill effects in the event of a remedy being erroneously prescribed.

Because provings of remedies are carried out so exhaustively, it is possible for the experienced therapist to identify the minutest symptoms and attribute them to a specific remedy. For example, *Apis Mellifera*, the remedy made from the honey bee is associated with fussy, fidgety behaviour, a 'busy bee'.

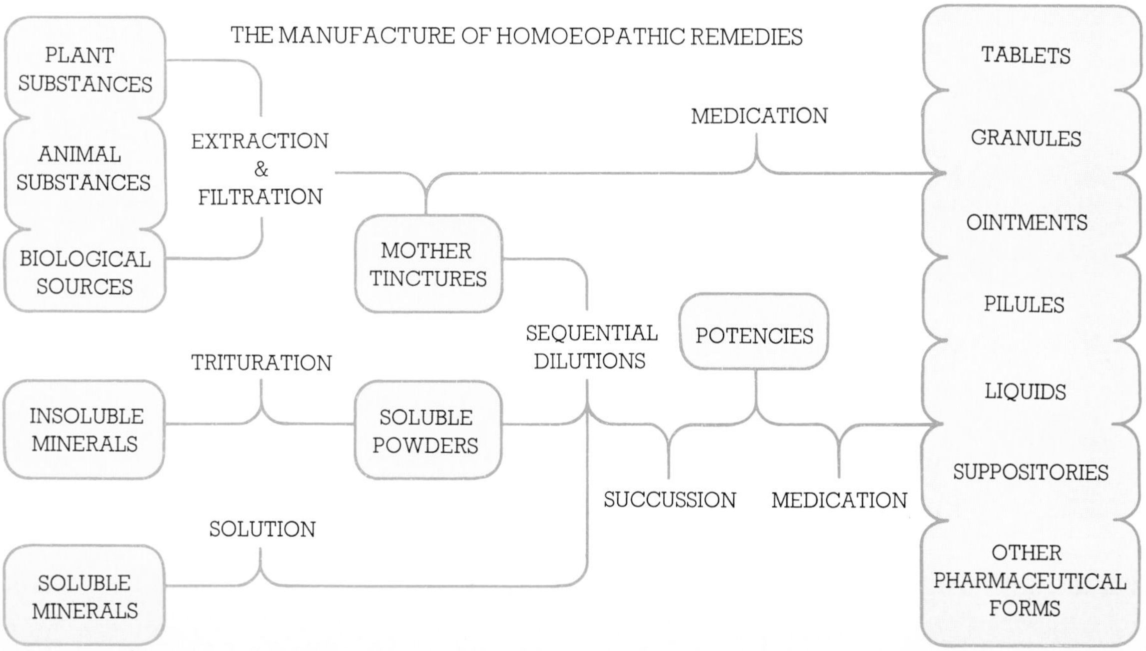

THE MANUFACTURE OF HOMOEOPATHIC REMEDIES

PLANT SUBSTANCES

ANIMAL SUBSTANCES

BIOLOGICAL SOURCES

EXTRACTION & FILTRATION

MOTHER TINCTURES

TRITURATION

INSOLUBLE MINERALS

SOLUBLE POWDERS

SOLUTION

SOLUBLE MINERALS

SEQUENTIAL DILUTIONS

POTENCIES

SUCCUSSION

MEDICATION

MEDICATION

TABLETS

GRANULES

OINTMENTS

PILULES

LIQUIDS

SUPPOSITORIES

OTHER PHARMACEUTICAL FORMS

Homoeopathy

Homoeopathic medicines are almost entirely prepared initially from fresh material whether this is from plant, animal or other biological sources. The fresh material, since it is only available at certain times of the year, is first extracted with alcohol and the resulting mixture of solids and liquid filtered to give the 'mother tincture', which can then be stored for later use or used directly as a medicament.

The various potencies of the medicines are produced by successive dilutions of the mother tincture. The equivalent of 99 drops of specially purified alcohol is dispensed from an automatic pipette into a vial and one drop of the mother tincture added to produce the required dilution.

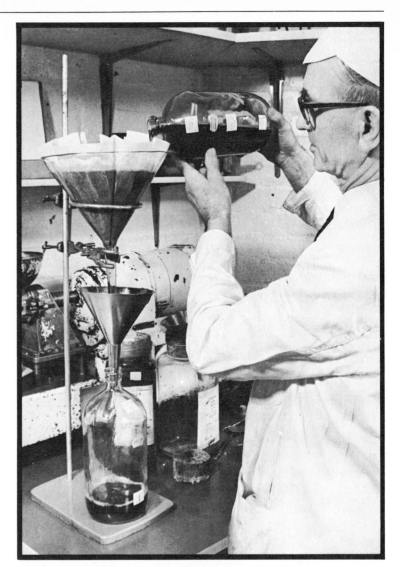

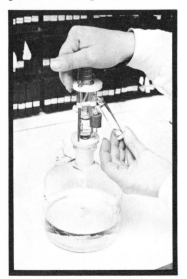

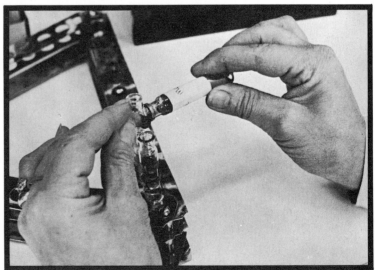

Homoeopathy

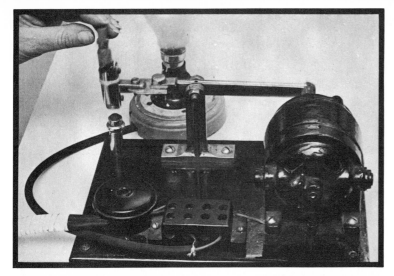

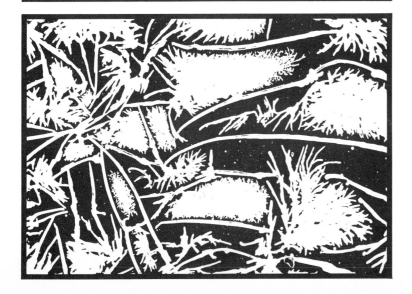

The diluted mother tincture is now rapidly shaken or 'succussed' on this special purpose-built machine. This is probably the single most important stage in the preparation of homoeopathic medicines – as well as one of the least understood. It is believed that the 'energy' associated with each plant, animal organ etc is transferred to the solution by succussion.

A small amount of the final, succussed dilution is now added to tablets which are made from four parts lactose to one part sucrose. The amount of solution that comes into contact with each tablet is unimportant as long as each tablet receives some of the energy contained in the solution.

A solution of potassium chromate allowed to crystallize will show random crystal formation. If, however, homoeopathic mother tincture is first mixed with the solution, then the resulting crystals show organized dendritic growth, with the growths exhibited being different for each remedy. The crystal growth shown here under the microscope, resulted from the addition of Calendula mother tincture to the chromate solution.

Homoeopathy

The Physician

According to Hahnemann's laws laid down in the *Organon* of 1810, the first and only duty of the homoeopath is to effect healing by the quickest, most reliable and most permanent means available to him. The physician's knowledge must cover four areas: (1) *disease;* that is etiology, bacteriology, pathology, prognosis and diagnosis, using every means available to him. (2) *Medicinal power;* he must be acquainted as fully as possible with toxicology and the pathogenesy of drugs. (3) *Pharmaco-therapy;* he must be able to relate his knowledge of the patient to that of the medication available to him. Here lies the greatest demand made on the physician's skill and experience, for, as we have noted, the symptoms and the remedies are infinite. (4) The physician must be capable of foreseeing barriers between the patient and good health and know how best to reduce them. This is distinct from the other three areas in that it may be unconnected with any of them and only the physician's individual perspicacity can serve him.

Hahnemann was insistent that it is no part of the physician's responsibility to administer palliatives. However, it was accepted that the patient's attitude to his own condition was of the utmost importance and the physician must help him to feel 'right in himself'.

Disease is considered in the patient in two forms: acute and chronic. In acute conditions, the body falters but can regain balance with time, therapeutic conditions and perhaps the support of a homoeopathic remedy. It may also be the recurrence of a past symptom. In chronic conditions, the vital forces and reactive powers of the body have been profoundly disturbed. In homoeopathic language this is called a miasm or miasmatic disorder, that is to say that the patient's condition is consistent with whichever type of infection to which he is peculiarly prone. Homoeopathy distinguishes five miasms of infectious types: psychotic, syphilitic, psoric, cancernic and tuberculinic. For each patient it is possible, as a result of meticulous observation, to identify one particular area of disorder. A chronic condition may be seen as a series, or group of acute conditions. The homoeopath, when called to treat an acute condition, will observe its progress or recurrence while waiting for a chronic condition to reveal itself.

Having identified the patient's miasm and chronic state, where applicable, the homoeopath can then go on to associate him with one or other remedy which is especially appropriate to him physically and temperamentally. This is known as the patient's constitutional remedy.

For prescribing a remedy, the homoeopath follows a certain procedure. Having established the symptom picture he has recourse to his materia medica and his repertory. The term repertorizing is used to describe the process of selecting a remedy according to symptoms.

Here homoeopaths differ from their orthodox colleagues in using a single remedy only, instead of a drug which may be composed of as many as twenty different chemical substances, as though diseases resulted solely from infection and the body could be used as a receptacle for counteractive drugs, much like a laboratory test tube.

The physician has at his disposal remedies ranging from potencies 3 to 100,000 and provings to show the effective life of each remedy within the body. The duration of action of a remedy is usually up to sixty days but in its bearing upon subsequently prescribed remedies, the effect may last for years. The physician's task is to choose the minimum potency in the smallest dose which will result in a cure.

By making himself familiar with the patient's type and constitution and by noting the minutest variation from the norm, both in pathology and according to the patient's own testimony, the homoeopath can detect the presence of an acute condition before it becomes sufficiently advanced to have any lasting effect.

Homoeopathy

Homoeopathy and Allopathy

In 1842 Hahnemann introduced the term 'allopathy' to mean the curing of a diseased action by the introduction of another of a different kind, yet not necessarily diseased. Because the allopathic drug is prescribed not on the basis of its pathical relationship to the condition under treatment, its induction to the body simply adds a synthetic condition to the already diseased organism, and increases its burden. This is the antithesis of homoeopathy and was wholly unacceptable to Hahnemann.

Homoeopathy, throughout its history has always been regarded by allopaths as a symbol of dissension from what might be called orthodox medicine. This is perhaps because no researcher has been able to explain the unquestionable power of potentized remedies; a homoeopathic pill, pillule or granule, under chemical analysis shows only the presence of the base substance. More significant, perhaps, is the fact that palliatives are given only secondary importance, that cathartics such as aspirin are unknown in homoeopathy, and that the patient must actively co-operate with his doctor. In short, homoeopathy is not as 'easy' as orthodox medicine. This is a definite disadvantage insofar as most people desire nothing but a ready state of comfort, regardless of whether this derives from good health. The homoeopath cannot simply 'make the pain go away'.

As a system of medicine, homoeopathy has always taken into account the interdependency of the patient and his social, domestic, geographical and industrial conditions, and also the occult factors. Hahnemann said, over 150 years ago, that the physician in curing, derives assistance from a knowledge of facts connected with the history of a case of chronic disease, more particularly the character of the patient's mind and temperament, his occupation, his mode of living and daily habits. Empirical science, on which orthodox medicine is based, cannot accept that which cannot be measured or proven, refuses to take into consideration factors such as whether the patient feels better in the morning or evening, whether the right side is worse than the left and many other phenomena which all know to exist.

Homoeopathy has been derogatorily described as being founded on symptomatology. While it is true that the homoeopath's concern with symptoms is considerably more detailed than most of his allopathic colleagues, it must also be noted that in all Western countries, homoeopaths must receive the full orthodox training and be registered with their national medical association in order to practise. Therefore it would be true to assert the superiority of homoeopaths over allopaths since they combine both orthodox and homoeopathic training.

Homoeopathy Today

The true significance of homoeopathy today can be seen parodied by the growing problems which we face as a result of environmental pollution. Unable to prove to his own satisfaction the long-term effects of such a policy, empirical 20th-century man is content wantonly to exhaust his natural resources, burn irreplaceable hydro-carbons and indiscriminately dispose of waste matter, harmless or otherwise. This is the result of his placing the highest importance on ready comfort. In the same way allopathic doctors are content to prescribe palliatives, antibiotics and steroids, filling the patient's body arbitrarily with powerful foreign substances, on the simple provable assertion that the beneficial effects outweigh the harmful.

Furthermore, it can be observed that homoeopathic remedies are found in nature and so are much better suited to an epoch which foresees the inevitable breakdown of a society based on the petro-chemical industry.

C. H. Sharma

Homoeopathy

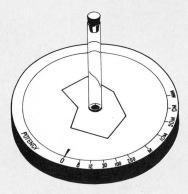

In his early experiments, Rae placed a vial containing purified water or sac lac, in the centre of the pattern card. When the pattern was correctly aligned with the earth's magnetic field, an almost infinite potency remedy resulted. By turning the card to produce various degrees of misalignment with the magnetic field, remedies of differing potencies could be produced.

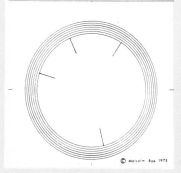

THERIDION CURASSAVICUM

© Malcolm Rae 1975

The first magneto-geometric cards were made by measuring the potency of a homoeopathic remedy at various degrees of alignment to the earth's magnetic field, plotting the result on circular graph paper and joining the points to form the pattern. Rae later found that it was unnecessary to join the points on the graph paper, the simple indication of their position being sufficient, as in this typical card.

The Rae Potency Simulator, named after its creator Malcolm Rae, of London, is perhaps the most radical advance in homoeopathy since Hahnemann advanced the theory and practice of homoeopathy. Simply described, the Simulator enables the preparation of homoeopathic remedies without recourse to the biological materials – plant, animal or inorganic – from which these remedies are normally prepared.

Rae's discoveries took place in the 1960s while he was investigating radiesthetic methods of measuring homoeopathic potency. The usual method is to place the remedy at one end of a 100 cm rule and then to dowse along the rule with a pendulum until a point is reached where the pendulum swings exactly at right angles to the rule; this gives a relative potency figure. It occurred to Rae that this balance point might be a 'boundary' between the remedy's local energy field and a component of the earth's magnetic field. This was to some extent verified when he took measurements with the rule and remedy oriented at varying angles to the earth's magnetic field, and found that the readings with the pendulum differed.

Rae then made a series of measurements for different homoeopathic remedies. The results for each were plotted on polar (circular) graph paper and the adjacent points linked to give a geometric pattern on the paper. He found that each remedy had its own unique pattern, whose size varied with potency.

Rae's first thought was whether the reverse was true – that the interaction of a pattern with the earth's magnetic field would create a replica of that remedy. Again his theory was borne out experimentally – this time with unexpected results. The resulting 'magneto-geometric' preparation was found to possess extremely high potency.

These early experiments were relatively simple: a cylindrical glass vial containing purified water or a mixture of sucrose and lactose (sac lac), was placed in the centre of the pattern for a particular homoeopathic remedy, which was then aligned in the direction from which the original measurements were taken. After ten minutes or so, the vial was found to contain an almost infinite potency replica of that particular remedy.

In the following years, Rae refined both the geometric cards and the potency simulator itself, which became a small, compact, portable instrument capable of producing remedies in a range of potencies. More importantly, it was found that the remedies so produced were as effective in treating illness as were traditionally prepared remedies.

Prepared from information supplied by Malcolm Rae

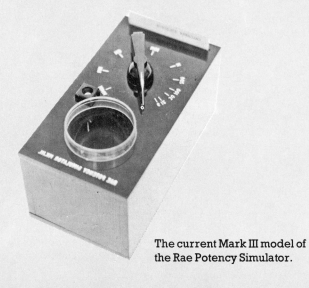

The current Mark III model of the Rae Potency Simulator.

Anthroposophical Medicine

The term anthroposophical medicine indicates an approach based on, and inspired by, the work and teaching of Rudolf Steiner (1861–1925).

Anthroposophy and Modern Scientific Medicine

Anthroposophical medicine is practised only by doctors who have previously acquired recognized medical qualifications and experience. It is thus regarded not as an alternative, but an extension of mainstream Western scientific medicine. In saying this one must remember that many of the assumptions underlying modern medical practice are based on the theories of 19th-century physics. Since that time, however, physics, and other more fundamental sciences, have moved on, and many basic assumptions, such as the mechanical nature of the universe, have been overthrown. Yet the implications of these developments for the teaching and practice of medicine have not always been fully acknowledged.

The empirical school of philosophy, which has gained increasing dominance since the 17th century, regards as knowledge only that which can be experienced through the senses. This fundamental assumption of modern science is taken so much for granted that it is hardly ever questioned and, when faced with the problem of studying aspects of the world that cannot essentially be weighed or measured, scientists tend to reduce them to the level of tools at their disposal. The irony of the present situation is that, while great efforts are being made to reduce such phenomena as individual self-consciousness and feelings to the level of physics and chemistry, equally great efforts are being made to demonstrate how 'animal-like' plants are (through methods of biofeedback) and how 'human' animals are (through the comparative study of human and animal behaviour).

Rudolf Steiner's Approach to the World

While for modern Western man the world of the senses is the primary reality, Rudolf Steiner approached life from the opposite direction. As a child, his primary experience was of the world of Being behind the sense world. At the same time, he was painfully aware of the fact that he did not share this experience with other people. Thus it became an existential need for him to find a bridge. The first opportunity of finding such a bridge came to him at the age of nine from a book on geometry He came to feel that knowledge of the spiritual world was something to be grasped in the same way as a geometrical concept, the truth and reality of which was experienced inwardly, rather than through external observation. From then on he made it his life task to establish the nature of the relationship between the spiritual and physical world, and to communicate the results of his research in a language which could be understood by ordinary people.

In order to create a solid foundation for this work, he studied philosophy, mathematics and natural science. If he was to make any contribution to the cultural life of the West, he had to experience for himself the limited extent to which the image of the world built up by that science conveyed the truth.

At the age of twenty-one, Steiner was invited to edit Goethe's scientific works. Goethe had been aware of the great contribution, as well as the limitations, of the reductionist approach to nature, for "while life can be broken into its elements, it cannot be reconstructed out of them and revitalized". In his *Metamorphosis of the Plant* he endeavoured to lay the foundations for a new science of organic nature. As a result of these studies, Steiner published his own thoughts on the new organic science. In this work he does something that Goethe always avoided – he reflects on his own thinking. Only in this way could he prove that Goethe's method of studying nature was scientific.

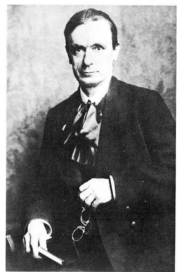

Rudolf Steiner.

Anthroposophical Medicine

Steiner's Theory of Knowledge

In 1894 Steiner published *The Philosophy of Freedom*, his standard work on the theory of knowledge. Essentially, it embodies everything that he was to develop later in anthroposophy. His aim was to create a science of the mind by the rigorous method of natural science, his search embracing both the natural and the supernatural world. In this book, Steiner sets out to refute the notion, firmly held since Kant, that there are ultimate limits to man's capacity for knowledge. Kant says that we can only have sense perceptions, which are essentially subjective, but that we can never reach reality. Steiner points out that reality meets us, as it were, split into two parts – one being the sense perception and the other the concept, or thought. Man, by his own inner activity, has to bring the two together if he is to get in touch with reality. This fact of the separation of percept and concept is the true basis of human freedom. The experience of the world does not come to us pre-determined and ready-made. Only one part comes to us through our senses. If we have no concept to bring to it, we cannot experience anything.

Steiner stresses that the thinking which man has to bring to his sense preceptions must not itself be bound up with the sense world; it must be sense-free. By perception, Steiner does not mean merely sense perception. Our feelings, too, are organs of perception, just like our eyes and ears. The seeker after knowledge needs to look at what he has subjectively observed in the same objective way as he does at information furnished by the scientific apparatus that he uses in his experiments. From a certain point of view, progress in knowledge is essentially linked to the training, refinement and extension of the powers of observation. But observation of the world at every level of physical, mental and spiritual life still does not constitute knowledge. Knowledge comes only with the intervention of thought, purged of all subjective and non-spiritual elements.

In making us aware of the fact that in every act of cognition we ourselves have to become active, and that in reality there is no such thing as passive objectivity, Steiner challenges us to take responsibility for that which takes place at the moment of cognition. We can no longer persuade ourselves that because certain objective facts exist, we have no choice of action.

This has far-reaching implications for the practice of medicine, where there is a growing tendency to replace true observation, judgement and conscious decision by tests, diagnostic tools and statistics. We have to realize that the synthesis of observation and conception does not come about by itself, but that it is the result of the mental activity of the thinker. Only if the thought process is undisturbed by wishes, instincts, impulses or passions can it be said to be free. "A free being is one who can will what he himself believes to be right."

The Development of Anthroposophy

Using the opportunities which life offered to lecture and to write, Steiner entered into the cultural debate of his day, while at the same time formulating the results of his spiritual investigations in such works as *Theosophy* (1904), *Knowledge of Higher Worlds. How is it achieved?* (1904), *Cosmic Memory* (1904), and *Occult Science – An Outline* (1910). In 1907 he wrote *The Education of the Child in the Light of Anthroposophy*. During the years 1910–16 Steiner's main contribution was towards the renewal of the arts; he wrote four mystery dramas, gave indications for a new art of movement, called eurythmy, which was later also developed as a form of therapy, and he gave a new impulse to the arts of drama, speech, music, painting, sculpture and architecture. In 1919 the first Waldorf school was founded at Stuttgart.

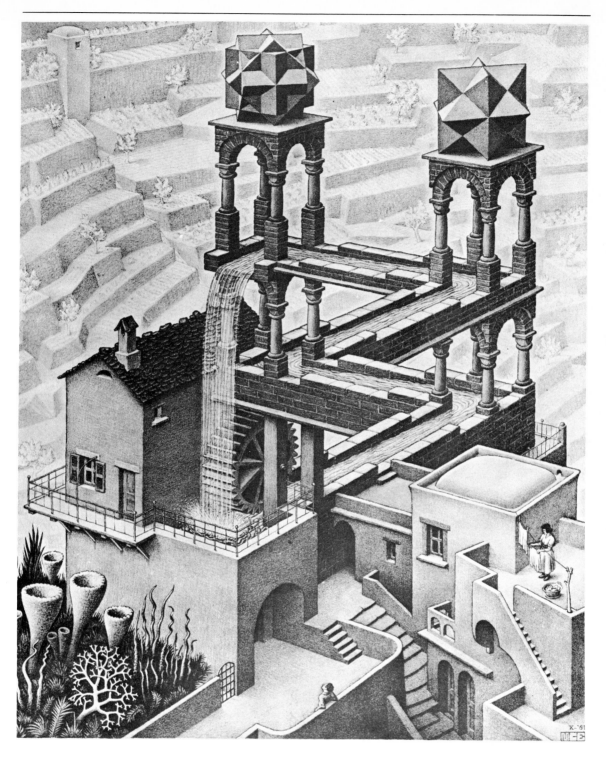

Waterfall by M. C. Escher. (Escher Foundation, Haags Gemeentemuseum, The Hague.) We can bring two concepts to this percept, one arising spontaneously from the painting (water flows upwards as well as down) and the other arising from previous experience (water can never flow upwards), making us look at the painting more closely.

Anthroposophical Medicine

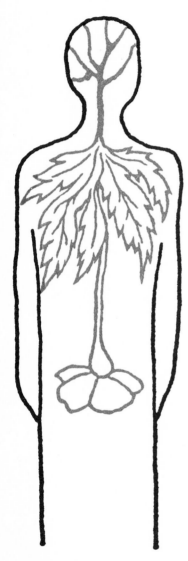

Both the human organism and the plant have a three-fold nature. From the point of view of medicine as well as nutrition, their relationship is an inverse one, the cool head forces being related to the roots of the plant, the warm metabolic forces to the flower, and the leaves to the rhythmic system in man.

The Beginnings of Anthroposophical Medicine

Soon after 1919, Rudolf Steiner was asked whether there was any contribution that he could make to the art of healing. With a few carefully-chosen exceptions, he admitted only doctors and medical students to the courses on therapeutics that he conducted in 1920–24.

In his book *Von Seelenrätseln (Riddles of the Soul)* (1917), he had traced the relationship between the functioning of the mind and physical processes. This was now applied to physiology. He gave an account which represents a radical departure from the commonly-held view that all the functions of the human mind and soul are centred in the brain. Steiner describes the dynamics of the healthy human organism as the result of three more or less autonomous, yet interacting, and to some extent interpenetrating, systems of organs:

1. The system of nerves and senses, extending throughout the body, but with its main activity focused in the head, providing the physical basis for sense perceptions and thinking.

2. The system of metabolism and limbs, which provides the physiological basis for the life of will.

3. The rhythmic system of circulation and respiration, which is the physiological basis of the life of feeling.

The essential difference between these three systems lies in the fact that the activity of the nervous system, being concentrated in the head, is point centred, while the metabolic system has a more peripheral, expanded quality. Brain and nerve cells are highly specialized, and are continually dying throughout life, whereas the cells in the metabolic pole tend to retain an active, regenerative capacity. The nerve-sense pole can also be described as the cool pole which is always at rest, whereas the metabolism is accompanied by warmth and movement. Steiner pointed to what he called "a continuous death process of nerve cells", indicating that consciousness arises as a result of the continuing release of organic life from matter. This polarity underlies an anthroposophical understanding both of physiology and pathology and provides a fundamental classification of illnesses into those in which there is an over-activity of the metabolic pole (inflammatory conditions) and those in which there is a preponderence of the nerve-sense pole (degenerative conditions and tumours). The blood continuously moves through these two poles of the human organism. The cold and the warm streams come together in the heart, which acts as a sense organ for that which lives as subtle dynamics in our thinking and our will. Through this picture of the human body a new understanding of the interrelation between the spirit, soul and body can be developed.

The Anthroposophical Approach to Illness and Healing

If we know that we possess consciousness only at the expense of a continuous death process in our physical body, while our feeling life always has the tendency to cause disease, and if at the same time we regard the human being as a being of spirit as well as of body and soul, which, moreover, is in a process of continuous development and evolution, it is impossible to aim for a life totally free from illness.

While the anthroposophical physician will always strive for the healing of an illness, that healing can never be a mere elimination of the illness. The illness itself is seen as a process by which the individual can achieve greater freedom and wholeness, and it is the task of the doctor to guide that process in the most fruitful way.

With our thinking we experience that which has come about in the past, and with our will we create the future. In our feelings we experience ourselves in relation to that which is and that which is to come. It is very helpful to look at any illness from this point of view.

Anthroposophical Medicine

Practical Developments

Rudolf Steiner never played the part of a doctor or healer, but always worked through qualified doctors. Yet everyone who knew him during the final period of his life was amazed at his detailed knowledge of medicine. His main collaborator in the medical field was Frau Dr Ita Wegman (1876–1943), a Dutch physician. With her he wrote his only textbook especially designed for a particular profession – *Fundamentals of Therapy*. To test Rudolf Steiner's indications in practice, Dr Wegman founded a clinic in Arlesheim, near Basle. When Rudolf Steiner founded the School of Spiritual Science at the Goetheanum in Dornach, Dr Wegman became the leader of the medical section.

Since Steiner's death, interest in this approach to medicine has grown, and in Europe there are now more than a thousand doctors practising anthroposophical medicine, while probably about two thousand medical practioners are using remedies developed according to anthroposophical principles.

Rudolf Steiner gave many indications for the preparation of specific remedies, using substances from the mineral, plant and animal kingdoms, which are often homoeopathically potentized or otherwise prepared in a special way. The activities of these medicines is not to be understood primarily in terms of the chemistry of their active ingredients. The remedies are manufactured mainly by two anthroposophical pharmaceutical firms, Weleda AG, with its main factories in Arlesheim and Schwäbisch Gmünd (South Germany) and branches in many countries including Britain, and Wala Heilmittelbetriebe, with its factory near Stuttgart.

The *Verein für Krebsforschung* (Cancer Research Association) is working on a treatment for cancer prepared in a special way from different species of mistletoe *(viscum album)* according to indications given by Rudolf Steiner. This medicament, which has been given the name of Iscador, actually stimulates the immunological system of the body. Although this remedy has had a measure of success, much further research is needed. In Germany, a number of other groups of anthroposophical doctors and scientists are pursuing independent lines of research on the development of a cancer remedy from mistletoe.

In Germany, two large anthroposophical hospitals were opened in the early 1970s, one in the Ruhr and one near Stuttgart, both of which provide the services of a general hospital for the surrounding community. There are also at least ten smaller hospitals or clinics based on anthroposophical medicine, including one psychiatric hospital.

In the English-speaking world, growth has been more gradual, partly due to the fact that most of the fundamental literature was for a long time only available in the German language. The English-speaking world has, however, seen a much stronger development in the care and treatment of mentally handicapped and emotionally disturbed children according to anthroposophical principles, the success of which has received general recognition. There are thirty-two such schools in the English-speaking world, quite apart from the Rudolf Steiner or Waldorf schools for normal children. Probably anthroposophists were the first to found village communities for handicapped adults. There are many Camphill Village Communities, but it is not usually realized that their therapeutic approach is complemented by an anthroposophical approach to medicine.

Both in the USA and in Britain, there is at present an upsurge of interest in this form of medicine among the new generation of doctors and medical students. They are organizing regular conferences and workshops for the purpose of their own training and as an introduction to interested enquirers.

James A. Dyson
Carlotta Hollmann

Oriental Diagnosis

In Western medicine, diagnosis is the classification of symptoms which have presented themselves. Oriental diagnosis is the study of biological change. The practitioner can often spot a change as it develops, before there is any pain or discomfort. If the simple and practical basis of this art is not understood it can appear to be divination. The most basic rule of Oriental diagnosis is that inside and outside are one. Any condition of stress or imbalance effects the total functioning of the body and is expressed in some trait, attitude or physical sign which is perceivable if we know what to look for. The ancient author of the *Nei-Ching*, the classic of Chinese medicine, states, "By observing myself I know about others, and their diseases are revealed to me, and by observing the external symptoms one gathers knowledge about internal disturbances".

Every individual is a walking history of their development and condition. The strengths and weaknesses of our parents, the environment we were raised in and the food we eat are all expressed in our total being. Our posture, the colour of our skin and the tone of our voice are nothing more than an externalization of the condition of our blood, organs, nervous system and skeletal structure. Since no sickness develops spontaneously, the real art of the experienced practitioner is to recognize the signs indicating a particular set of changes and to bring about harmony before the sickness has a chance to develop.

Usually more than one method of diagnosis is used out of the many approaches. The four most commonly used forms of diagnosis are:

Bo-Shin. The art of diagnosis by observation (posture, skin colour, eyes, bone structure and habits).

Bun-Shin. The art of diagnosis by sounds (tone, pitch and tempo of voice).

Mon-Shin. The art of diagnosis through questioning.

Setsu-Shin. The art of diagnosis by touch (skin texture, pulses and the use of diagnostic points on the acupuncture meridians).

Bo-Shin, the Art of Seeing

Just as a plant reflects the soil, weather and strength of seed in its growth, so a human reflects its nutrition, environment and parents. There are two main categories in Bo-Shin, seeing constitution and seeing condition. Constitution is a reflection of our development in the womb. This aspect of Bo-Shin uses the features of the face, bone structure and general characteristics. The embryo is a spirallic structure, the main influence governing its growth is the food which is eaten by the mother. If foods which have a yin or yang effect (*see* the section on macrobiotic diet) are taken in excess this is reflected in the features of the face and in the bone structure. We can understand this mechanism by seeing the development of the embryo during the first eight weeks. As is shown in the illustration left, the face is formed by a contracting force.

It is easy to see the contracting force which is working in the formation of the features. Remember that happening simultaneously with this contraction and simplification of the facial features (yang) is the expansion and diversification (yin) of the internal organs. It is the simultaneous development of these parts that gives us an indication as to why certain facial features reflect or have a direct relationship with certain organs. In the figure left we can see that the embryo is layered. These layers are: (a) the digestive tract, the realm of Earth, our internal soil out of which we grow, (b) the circulatory system, the realm of Man, our blood being a reflection of the way we use that which we take in, (c) the nervous system, or realm of Heaven, the seat of Judgment. The drawing shows the areas of the face which represent these systems.

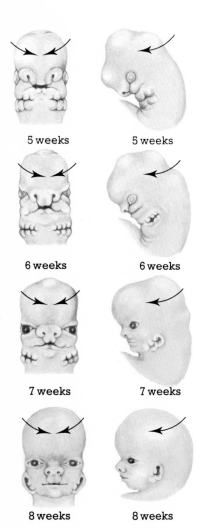

5 weeks 5 weeks

6 weeks 6 weeks

7 weeks 7 weeks

8 weeks 8 weeks

Stages in the development of the face in the embryo.

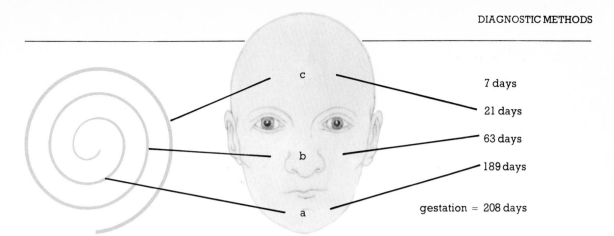

7 days

21 days

63 days

189 days

gestation = 208 days

The areas of the face and the main periods of development during pregnancy.

The general shape of the head can give us a clue as to the constitution of the person in question. A square, wide jaw with a smaller crown is an indication of an aggressive and active person. The opposite structure, a weak jaw with a wide crown, is an indication of a more thoughtful and passive person.

The eyebrows correspond to the life line in the palm. Short and sparse eyebrows show a weak constitution and a tendency to become sick easily. Long and full eyebrows are the sign of a strong constitution. The angle of the eyebrows is also important. Eyebrows which slant abruptly towards the centre are the sign of a family with much meat eating and a tendency toward anger. Eyebrows with a gentle slope down toward the outside are the sign of a relatively more vegetable quality food, and are generally found on those with a more peaceful disposition. Do this experiment: draw two faces and put each type of eyebrow on them and see the difference. In the first illustration we can see that the structure of these features is governed by the force with which the contracting pressure is operating. If the force is weak, then the face becomes more yin, that is the eyes are wider apart, the eyebrows are weaker and the mouth is wider. If the yang force is very strong, then the eyes are closer together, the eyebrows are pinched towards the middle and the mouth is tighter. The extreme in either case is not good. We could say that a perfect face is one where the forces of yin and yang are in harmony, with a minimal domination of one over the other.

The most important factor governing the strength or weakness of this force is the diet of the mother. If the diet contains too much meat or salt (yang), then the contraction is too violent. If the diet is yin, with sugar, drugs, or too many fruits, then the force is weak, producing the above results. By her eating habits the mother is controlling the appearance of her baby at this early stage. A balance should be made which provides a proper tension between the forces of yin and yang so that development happens smoothly and evenly.

The construction of the nose and ears is also an indicator of constitution. The length of the nose from the surface of the face is governed somewhat by the structure of the teeth. People who come from an ethnic background of vegetable eating tend to have a more protruding set of top incisors (yin). This allows the nose to lie flatter against the face, since the nose is supported by an outgrowth of the jaw bone above the incisors. In races with a long history of meat eating there is a more vertical or slightly inward slant to the teeth, which pushes the nose forward. These are illustrated right.

Although there are racial characteristics which involve the development of large families of people, these guidelines can still be used within these groups since no two faces are the same, and each reflects a unique growth pattern.

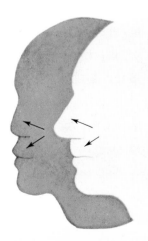

The drawing on the left shows a person with yin eating habits. On the right is a yang face.

Oriental Diagnosis

The placement of the ear on the head reflects this contracting force with an abundance of yang force causing the ears to be set fairly high on the head and more pointed, and more yin causing the ears to be low on the head and protruding. All the above points have to do with the constitution and can give us an indication of the relative strengths and weaknesses of an individual. But they are very general, and in order to see a person's present condition we must look at the face in more detail.

Each individual feature on the face is the mirror of an organ or system. The skeletal structure of the face can tell us something of the inherent strengths and weaknesses. The colour of the skin and the swelling of various features give us a clear indication of the condition of the various organs.

The mouth is the gateway to the digestive system, and shows us the condition of the stomach and the intestines. The introduction of large amounts of yin foods into the diet (sugar, drugs, tropical fruits) and over-eating has caused our intestines to become swollen. This swelling is revealed in the pendulous lower lip we see so much now. It is interesting that this sign of sickness has become accepted to the point where it is considered sensual in models and pop stars. If the intestines are strong, the mouth will become tighter and the lower lip will reduce its size. Cracks and sores on the lower lip indicate fissures and ulceration in the colon and intestine, while those on the upper lip indicate problems with the stomach. The mouth should be closed while breathing. If the mouth must be kept open to breathe, this indicates an over-consumption of dairy products which cause the sinuses to become filled. Doctors are now saying that infants in Britain are drinking too much milk and are suffering from obesity. Look at the babies in prams with their mouths open to breathe. This is a result of excess dairy foods.

The nose is the mirror of the heart. A swollen red nose is the sign of a weak heart. This can often be observed among those who eat too much meat and who drink heavily. These people are often stricken with heart attacks without warning, and yet probably see themselves in the mirror every day. The redness is caused by a swelling and rupturing of the blood vessels under the skin, a message that the circulatory system is being taxed.

The areas directly below the eyes tell us the present condition of the kidneys. Swelling, bags and dark discolouration are all signs of weak kidneys. If bags are under your eyes, then the condition is serious and has existed for some time. If the condition is treated by giving the kidneys a rest and not drinking too much liquid, avoiding sugar, alcohol, cold drinks, and other foods which put a stress on the kidneys, the condition will improve and the bags will disappear. The discolouration under the eyes is caused by the same factors, but less developed. People who have this discolouration and bags are often tired and easily exhausted. This is because of the connection of the kidneys with the adrenal glands. When the kidneys are damaged, the adrenals cease to function correctly and we have no energy.

Diagram of the eye, showing areas in the white and the iris which correspond to the various organs.

1. SMALL BRAIN
2. LARGE BRAIN
3. FACE
4. THROAT
5. TOP
6. UPPER ⎫
7. MIDDLE ⎬ SPINE
8. LOWER ⎭
9. SEX
10. BLADDER
11. INTESTINES
12. DUODENUM
13. STOMACH
14. LUNGS
15. NECK
16. HEART
17. LIVER PANCREAS
18. KIDNEYS

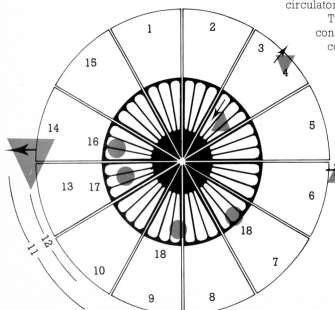

The eyes have been called the mirror of the soul, and can tell us much about the condition of the whole body. The diagram shows the white of the eyes divided into various areas which represent parts of the body. Discolouration, spots and 'blood-shot' lines indicate trouble in the corresponding organs. These discolourations can be listed in terms of the seriousness of the condition. Dark lines (blue, purple or brown) indicate a very serious condition of stagnation. Yellow spots are less serious, but can often indicate stones or calcification, and red lines indicate a developing weakness. The white of the eye should be clear, and if there is a yellow cast to the whole area, this indicates trouble with the liver or spleen.

Another means of diagnosis using the eye is the presence of a *sanpaku* condition. In Japanese sanpaku means 'Three Whites'. This is a condition where the eye has rolled back in the head. When a person with this condition is facing straight ahead and relaxed, it is possible to see white on three sides of the iris. This condition is serious in that it indicates a swelling of the eyeball, which means that there is an excess of liquid in the cranial cavity. If this condition persists, the person is unable to make proper decisions and is destined to serious trouble and death. George Ohsawa, in William Dufty's book *You are all sanpaku*, points out that many people who commit suicide or are killed (such as Americans, John and Robert Kennedy and Martin Luther King) have this condition. Three sets of eyes are shown right.

Sometimes we notice a vertical line between the eyebrows, directly above the bridge of the nose. This is a sign of a weak liver, and is found on people who are often angry.

Facial colour is important. In Oriental medicine each of the primary viscera has a corresponding colour. Trouble with the liver is indicated by a greenish colour. The colour red dominant in the complexion indicates a weak heart, the colour yellow the spleen, and if there is dark discolouration it indicates problems with the kidneys. Persons with bad lungs have a chalky white complexion.

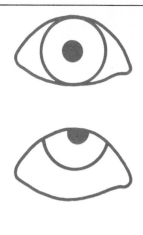

The top eye is healthy and centred. The centre eye is sanpaku, caused by too much yin. The bottom eye is sanpaku, caused by too much yang. The bottom type is caused by meat eating, and is found in people who tend to be violent.

Bun-Shin, the Art of Hearing

Different aspects of the voice are used for diagnosis in Bun-Shin. Certain characteristics of the voice can be classified into yin and yang:

YANG	YIN
High	Low
Fast	Slow
Loud	Soft
Sharp	Soft
Dry	Wet
Clear	Unclear
Penetrating	Flat
Tense	Loose
Regular	Irregular

The practitioner listens to the voice and by hearing the various qualities can judge the general condition of the sick person.

As an example, a person with a high, fast voice shows an excessive amount of yang energy. If a person drinks too much liquid then the voice has a characteristic sound as if the person's throat is watery.

By listening to the sound of the voice we can also judge the way a person uses his or her energy. If the person is constipated or has problems with the organs of discharge, then the expression of the voice will be restrained and the rhythm irregular and tense.

The resonance of the voice also tells the possible location of stagnation in the body. Different sounds resonate in different parts of the body. If we can hear the sounds which are vibrating and those which are missing we can have an insight into the persons condition.

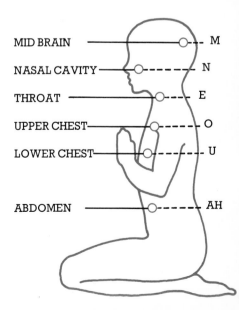

MID BRAIN — M
NASAL CAVITY — N
THROAT — E
UPPER CHEST — O
LOWER CHEST — U
ABDOMEN — AH

The basic sounds and the areas which they resonate.

Oriental Diagnosis

Mon-Shin, the Art of Questioning

The questioning in Oriental diagnosis serves two purposes, first to have the sick person's own insight into their problem and to receive relevant background information and secondly to gain insight into their character. There is no separation between physical and psychological problems in Oriental medicine. A person's emotional state and attitudes are an indication of the deeper physical symptoms. The ruling emotions and the organs involved are listed below.

ORGAN	IN SICKNESS	IN HEALTH
heart/small intestines	hysteria	happiness
lungs/large intestines	depression	positive
spleen/stomach	suspicion	trust
kidney/bladder	fear	courage
liver/gall bladder	anger	peacefulness

It is the art of the practitioner to be able to judge the mixture of these emotions and to understand which of the emotions and attitudes is the one which is foremost and to understand the combinations which are usually involved. By doing this he can judge the organs which are weak and strong.

Setsu-Shin, Diagnosis through Touch

The most common form of Setsu-Shin is the taking of the pulses. Oriental diagnosis recognizes three pulses on each wrist, each of which can be taken on the surface or by pressing deeply. The pulses and the corresponding organs are as follows:

RIGHT HAND	Number 1	Deep	Lungs
		Surface	Large intestine
	Number 2	Deep	Spleen and pancreas
		Surface	Stomach
	Number 3	Deep	Heat governor
		Surface	Triple heater
LEFT HAND	Number 1	Deep	Heart
		Surface	Small intestine
	Number 2	Deep	Liver
		Surface	Gall bladder
	Number 3	Deep	Kidneys
		Surface	Bladder

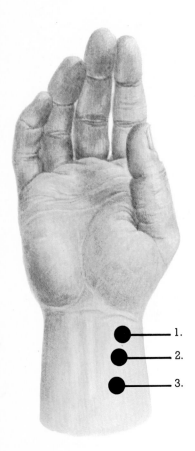

The location of the pulses.

After practice, it is possible to feel the subtle differences in the rhythm of the pulses at these locations and thus the health of the organs which they represent, but the development of this skill can take many years.

Another form of Setsu-Shin is the use of the acupuncture diagnosis points. Using certain points on the acupuncture meridians, the practitioner can judge the condition of the associated organ. If the points are firmly pressed and there is pain or discomfort, then the Chi of that organ is not flowing well and the organ is in a state of imbalance. A point you can test for yourself is the intersection of the bones of the thumb and the first finger. This area is a place for judging the condition of the large intestine. If firm pressure here causes discomfort, then the condition of the intestines is not good. There are hundreds of these points on the body which are used for diagnosis as well as treatment.

William Tara

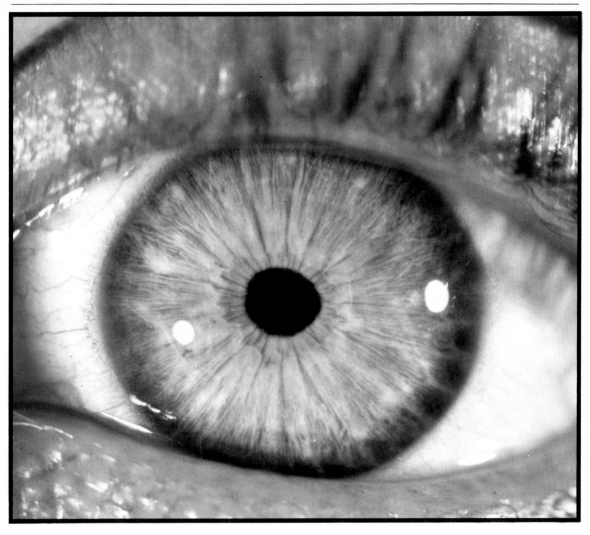

Iris Diagnosis

Iris Diagnosis, or Iridology, as it is also called, is the diagnosis of disease based on observations of the iris. Medical observation of the eye is as ancient as medicine itself, references being found in the works of Hippocrates and Philippus. In 1670, Meyens published his *Chiromatica Medica* in which he discusses signs in the iris and their relation to disease.

Modern iris diagnosis owes its origins to the Hungarian doctor, Ignatz von Peczely, who published his findings in 1881. Von Peczely determined that markings in the iris could be related to organic disease and that by localizing these markings one could relate the disease to a specific organ. Most important of all the early iris diagnosticians was Pastor Felks (1856–1926) during whose lifetime the most significant advances occurred.

For the purposes of accurate recording and diagnosis when examining the iris, an agreed system for the division of the iris must be adopted. It is normal to divide the iris into radial and circular divisions:

Radial division. The most suitable radial division of the iris is into minutes, 1–60, corresponding to the normal clock face.

Circular division. Starting from the pupil to the outer border, the iris is divided by concentric rings into three equal major zones, each subdivided into two minor zones.

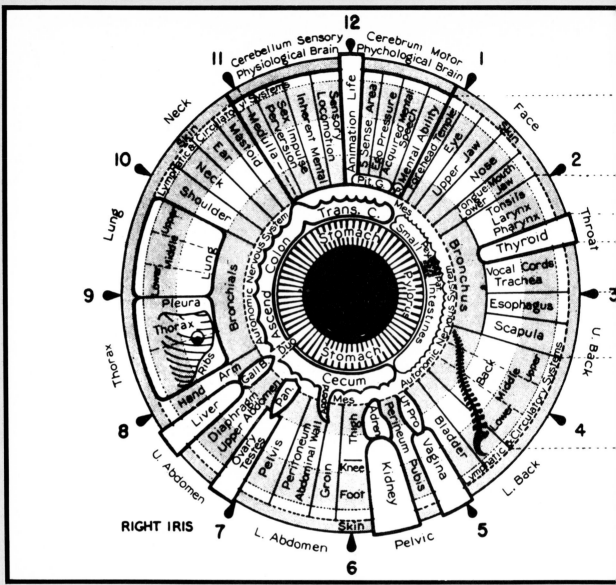

Diagnostic iridology chart developed by Dr Bernard Jensen.

As will be seen, these zones represent specific systems, but it is now necessary to define exactly the position of the individual organs. This is done by dividing the iris into one half, quarter, eighth and sixteen segments by drawing lines from the outer border of the iris to the pupil. Hence the iris is divided into ninety-six small components by a combination of radial, circular and segmental sections. It is now possible, using this system to record findings and to know that these observations will be repeatable by other workers using the same system.

The first major zone contains organs of digestion. The first minor zone contains the stomach and the second minor zone the intestines. The second major zone contains organs of transport and utilization and elimination through the kidneys. The third minor zone shows the blood and lymph vessels and the fourth minor zone the muscular system. The third major zone contains organs for body support and utilization, the fifth minor zone containing the skeletal system and the sixth minor zone, the skin.

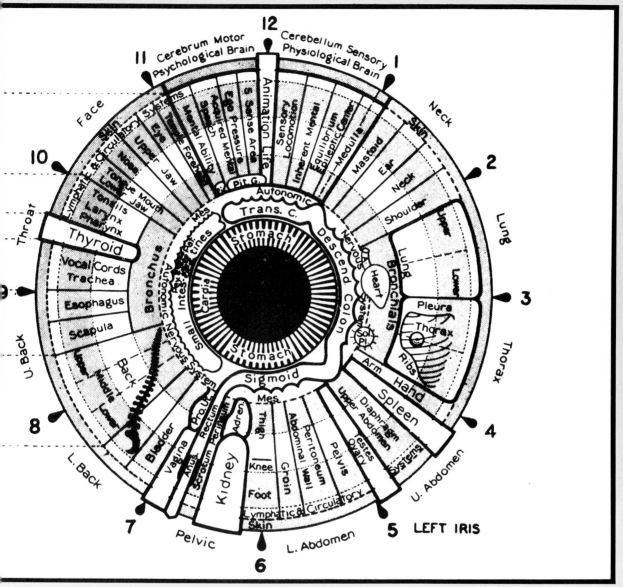

Iris Diagnosis

The three basic colours of the iris are blue, grey and brown. The appearance of local 'toxin-flecks' as dark-coloured areas of pigment are occasionally noted in blue or grey eyes. The change from blue to brown can sometimes occur in one eye or even in part of one eye. Changes in the iris colour following organic diseases are significant.

The examination of the iris should be done with the pupil contracted using a strong light source and a magnifying lense. Recent developments have made available binocular microscopes with built-in cameras linked to closed circuit video machines. This arrangement allows an image to be frozen on the screen and examined at length without discomfort to the patient.

There are three basic iris-signs: unnatural colourings; white, dark and black signs as dots or radiating lines; circular or contraction rings. White signs represent inflammation and over-stimulation, while dark signs indicate under-stimulation and reduced function. Black signs represent a loss of substance and coloured signs or toxin-flecks are dependent upon the type of pigment deposited.

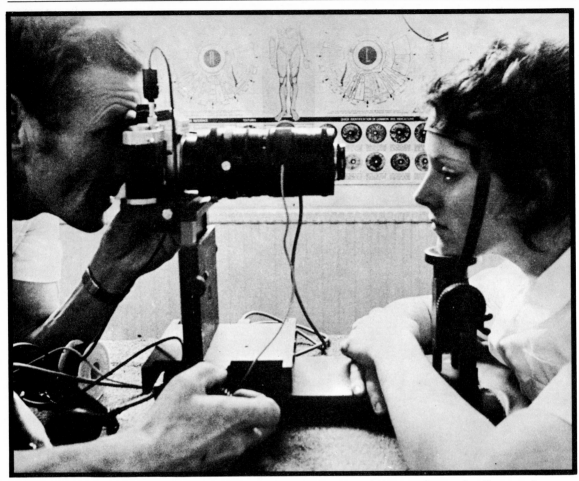

Photographing a patient's iris.

Here are a few examples of diseases that can be diagnosed:

Diseases of the liver. The liver is situated between 37 and 40 minutes in the sixth minor zone of the right iris. Hence white or yellow clouds or wisps in this area indicate inflammatory states of the liver.

The heart. Signs are seen in the second major zone between 10 and 15 minutes in the left iris and 45 and 50 minutes in the right iris. Cardiac valve lesions for example, show as one to three black spots in the heart area lying in the upper part of this region.

The kidneys. These show their signs in the right iris at 28 to 30 minutes and in the left iris at 30 to 32 minutes in the fourth and fifth minor zones. If there are signs in both kidneys it is an indication that the system is showing functional insufficiency. Kidney disease normally affects only one kidney as with nephritis. Small white areas, wisps or clouds are found in the kidney area. These become yellow as the condition becomes chronic.

Disorders of the spine. These may be seen in the right iris at 15 to 22 minutes and the left iris at 37 to 45 minutes in the fifth minor zone. White signs indicate inflammation whereas white lines running outward from the iris wreath indicate damage to the intervertebral discs.

Although iris diagnosis is by no means a new science, it has gained little acceptance in the world of orthodox medicine. It is in essence a simple procedure which any practitioner with keen powers of observation can put to good use. Iris diagnosis provides the open-minded with a quick, safe and effective extra string to his diagnostic bow.

Michael van Straten

Tongue Diagnosis

A very simple method of self-diagnosis for vitamin B deficiencies can be performed by an examination of your tongue. Normal tongues are an even, red colour; smooth, but not shiny and without cracks, fissures or indentations. A prolonged lack of the B vitamins (there are several, in fact), causes the taste buds to clump together, forming grooves and ridges. This is called a geographic tongue.

The accompanying chart provides a description of the various tongue conditions and their associated deficiencies. It is as well to be aware that there is probably no such condition as a deficiency of a single B vitamin, for all these vitamins are too closely related. If you find you have a deficiency of one B vitamin and supplement your diet with this one alone, then you may soon have a deficiency in another B vitamin. It is wiser to use a complete B vitamin instead.

TONGUE SYMPTOM	VITAMIN B FACTOR DEFICIENT	IMPORTANCE OF B FACTORS AND RESULTS OF DEFICIENCY
Scarred tongue	Vitamin B1 (thiamine)	Controls the release of energy from body carbohydrates. Deficiency leads to depression and irritability, and stunts the growth of children
Purplish or magenta tongue	Vitamin B2 (riboflavine)	Helps the body to obtain energy from food. Deficiency checks growth and leads to cracks and sores on the skin
Brilliant red tongue, as well as sore gums and inflammation of the mouth, tongue and throat	Vitamin B3 (niacin; nicotinic acid)	Is a further link in the food-energy chain along with riboflavine. Deficiency results in similar symptoms to riboflavine deficiency with additional digestive and mental disturbances
Burning sensations in the mouth	Vitamin B6 (pyridoxine)	Essential to the normal functioning of the nerves and for good skin condition
Enlarged and beefy tongue	Vitamin B5 (pantothenic acid)	Aids the body's metabolism of carbohydrates. Helps build resistance to infection. Insomnia and irritability can result from deficiency
Smooth, shiny tongue, as well as ulcerated lips, sore mouth and throat, inflamed oesophagus	Vitamin B12 (cyanacobalamin) and folic acid	B12 and folic acid are important for the development of red blood cells and are necessary for growth. Deficiency of B12 can result in pernicious anaemia. Without folic acid, cells cannot divide
Coating of fuzzy debris	Indicates putrefaction in the intestines	
Fissures and cracks in the tongue	Severe overall Vitamin B deficiency	

Applied Kinesiology

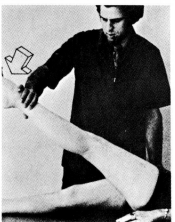

In this picture, the *fascia lata* is being tested. This is the muscle which helps to flex or bend the thigh, draw it away from the body sideways, and keep it turned in. The patient lies face upwards with the leg raised to 45° and slightly to the side. The therapist exerts pressure against the outside of the leg to push the leg down and in. If the muscle is weak, this indicates intestinal problems of constipation, spastic colon, colitis or diarrhoea. It can be remedied by nutritional supplementation.

Applied Kinesiology uses a system of simple muscle-testing procedures to tap the innate intelligence of the body in order to assess the energy levels of the life forces which control the body. In 1965, Dr George Goodheart, a respected chiropractor in the United States, discovered that the tests used in kinesiology to determine relative muscle strength and tone over the range of movement of the joints, could also reveal the balance of energy in each of the body's systems – the stomach, lungs, intestines, etc.

Further research led him to identify the relationship between each specific muscle group, the particular organs and the meridians of acupuncture. It is now possible to check for imbalances and improper compensations in the body which are caused by undue stress, using practical muscle stress tests which give instantaneous indications of where the problems lie.

Goodheart's original research is now being expanded, and more investigations are being carried out by many of his fellow chiropractors, hundreds of whom are finding applied kinesiology of inestimable value in their practices as a diagnostic aid. It is a fast and reliable way to discern where structural imbalances lie, to assess dietary deficiencies and allergies, to detect organ dysfunctions, and even determine the extent to which psychological factors are involved.

Once imbalances in the energy distribution have been identified by muscle testing, any treatment considered appropriate may be carried out, and the effects monitored by repeating the muscle tests and comparing the results before and after. It is often found that a number of therapies are necessary to obtain optimum balance, as almost all disease and ill health has its roots in several causative factors, the mind, the food we eat, the way the body is used. All need to be taken into consideration. Tests also reveal how effective the treatment has been, how often treatment is required, and even the dosage of any medication or dietary supplement that the body needs.

For the general public interested in preventive health care, a special basic course has been designed by Goodheart and some of his colleagues called 'Touch for Health'.

Brian H. Butler

Psychic Diagnosis

In psychic diagnosis, the human mind is the diagnostic tool which, under certain conditions, can attune itself to the mind of another person. This attunement requires total relaxation, leading to an altered state of consciousness, total caring for another human being and total love. When we are sufficiently attuned to diagnosis we are attuned enough to do the healing also.

With the evolution of consciousness, man became aware of himself and of others – and was able to experience all the fields of energy which surrounded him. His physical senses extended to other realms – to other levels of consciousness – thus he was able to 'feel', to 'see', to 'hear', and to 'sense' in another, a non-physical reality. With the development of intellect, this ability to tune in to other levels of consciousness began to disappear. However, in unsophisticated societies, the ability still exists and is the only method of diagnosis available. In our industrialized society we have lost contact with our inner awareness and rely on our physical senses alone – on our logical, rational reasoning. This causes a conflict because, not being in contact with our inner awareness which 'knows' what is wrong with us, we have to rely on others to diagnose our problems.

Some people are born with the ability to experience their inner awareness and to express it in a variety of ways. A few examples will help in understanding what takes place. Some sensitives are clair-

Psychic Diagnosis

voyant – that is, they can 'see' into a patient, almost as if they are reading an X-ray plate. Others are clair-audient because they can 'hear' a voice which tells them what is wrong. The late Arigó in Brazil was an outstanding example of this kind of psychic; others, such as the late Edgar Cayce and Paul Solomon in the United States fall into a deep trance-like state and answer questions put to them which provide remarkable, unusual and very accurate diagnoses. Still another manifestation is that of George Chapman in England who falls into a trance state and is taken over completely by a spirit guide who speaks through him to the patient and describes the symptoms and the cause of illness, suggesting what can be done to help or heal that individual. Ronald Beesley practises another method. He 'sees' the aura of individuals, whether mental, emotional or spiritual, and diagnoses past, present and even future problems which may not yet be manifested on the physical body.

The presence of the patient is not always essential; diagnosis can be carried out by psychometry. Many healers have the ability to tune in to the vibrations of the patient by holding in their hand a photograph, a letter, or some personal article belonging to the patient. All matter vibrates, and on these natural vibrations are superimposed the vibrations of the individual. The psychometrist uses any one of the above objects to tune in to the vibration of the patient. Bertha Harris is one of the most gifted psychometrists in England.

These are the born sensitives, whose natural ability becomes even greater over the years. There are others, however, who develop this sensitivity later in life as a result of some traumatic experience, such as an accident or a severe illness. In fact, anyone can develop the ability – it is latent in all of us. Different methods of developing sensitivity are available, but tremendous dedication and years of practice are required before realiable results can be assured. What is not generally realized is that in every one of us, in circumstances of great need, the rational, intellectual mind withdraws – our consciousness makes a quantum jump to another level where we act without realizing what we are doing – and love and caring take over.

The manner in which psychic diagnosis is manifested, varies from country to country and depends on belief systems, social and economic factors and on the individuals concerned. In China, for example, practitioners of acupuncture use pulse diagnosis, and astrologers are much in demand; both these practices depend on the sensitivity of the individual concerned. In the Philippines, most forms of psychic diagnosis are used. An unusual method is to place a sheet of white paper over the patient and coat it with oil. Where a problem exists, the oil does not mark the paper.

A method which is growing in popularity in the West today is to attune to the patient and, using sensitivity and telepathy, to 'become' the other person – to feel their pains and experience their problems and worries. This intuitive method is very effective.

It is important to realize that sensitives are only able to tune in to certain aspects of an individual. This attunement depends on their innate ability, their background and their life experiences. Their effectiveness varies from day to day. To obtain a complete and realiable diagnosis of an individual, a team of sensitives is needed. This method is practised by the Spiritists in São Paolo, Brazil.

Psychic diagnosis can be extremely accurate, requires only a few minutes and can produce excellent results – even in cases where every form of medical diagnosis has been tried and failed to provide an answer. The underlying causes of problems can be located, so the procedure can be very rewarding for both patient and sensitive.

Marika McCausland

The Aura

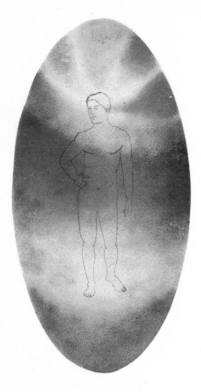

The Human Aura (from *Man Visible and Invisible* by C. W. Leadbetter). Viewed through a Kilner screen, this is how the aura might appear.

Aura theory postulates that every object is enveloped in a field of magnetic energy which acts as a medium for the interplay of other energies present in its immediate environment. This magnetic energy field, or MEF, is composed of seven rays related to the glands of the endocrine system. The harmony and balance of every individual and the degree and quality of each of these can be ascertained by observing the aura either subjectively, as some sensitives are capable of doing, or objectively using a special type of glass called a Kilner screen. The screen, which was developed in the 1920s by the British scientist Walter J. Kilner, sensitizes the vision and makes it possible to see the aura. More recently, the development of Kirlian photography has provided a second method of viewing the aura.

Every animate and inanimate substance, provided its function is not impaired, has an aura, which exists because of the life force inherent in the natural constituents of its form. This life force, whether from mineral, vegetable, animal or human sources, creates a common auric realm or plane, which is a storehouse of pure, untapped energy. On this plane the mineral and vegetable kingdoms are constantly engaged, through their own channels of communication, in transferring their particular life force to the more subtle natures of animals and humans. Thus the aura depicts the sum total of all these qualities and presents a complete and whole picture of the subject.

The aura is seen as a colourful, stratified, oval emanation surrounding the subject. Its appearance, shape and size whether bright, opaque or dull, determines among other things the state of health.

The MEF that surrounds material objects has four basic characteristics to its nature which can be represented by the word AURA: A – Attraction, U – Unison, R – Repulsion, A – Activation. These natural characteristics allow the aura to be interpreted for a variety of purposes, principally diagnosis and prognosis.

The MEF can also be used for other purposes, for instance psychometry, where information can be elicited about people, places and events, by interpreting the auric field of an object by touch and sensing. This rapport can often be extended to the deeper insights of clairvoyance.

An alternative method of judging the mental and physical health of a person is by means of an auragraph, a kind of blueprint of the whole person. An auragraph relies on the interpretation of what are known as the auric bodies or vehicles which are associated with the various types of tissue in the physical body. The four principal vehicles and their functions are, in ascending order of quality:

1. The Etheric or Vital Body which controls and unifies the cosmic or life energy pouring into the physical body.

2. The Astral or Emotional Body which registers the feelings, desires or sensory faculties of the individual.

3. The Mental Body which reacts to the thoughts generated or received by the individual.

4. The Causal Body which retains all the potential of the individual for his future development.

Each of these auric bodies has a counterpart in the glands and organs of the physical body. A trained sensitive can draw an auragraph either by viewing the person directly or by holding an object that has been touched by that person. When properly evaluated, the auragraph helps us to know ourselves and to understand something of the effect we are having on others. With this knowledge of human radiation, we can stimulate our natural forces in a positive way and in so doing diminish the more negative aspects of our being, which in turn assists in maintaining a good state of health.

Karl Francis

The Aura

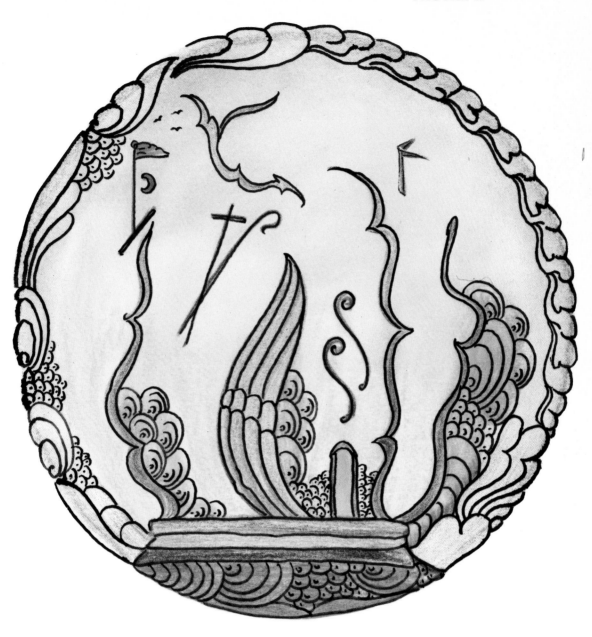

The auragraph, shown here, is a symbolic drawing of the quantity and quality of the seven rays of the human magnetic energy field (MEF), as well as the different frequencies of the rays for each individual. Auragraphs can be drawn by trained sensitives either by direct viewing of the aura or by handling an object that has been touched by the person who wishes to have an auragraph drawn. The skilled sensitive can use the patterns and colours of the auragraph to diagnose not only a person's mental and spiritual state, but also physical illness.

There are seven colours in the aura spectrum. Of the primary colours, red symbolizes life, yellow the intellect, and blue, inspiration. The secondary colours are orange, relating to energy, green to harmony, indigo to intuition and violet to spirituality, wisdom and the highest point of man's evolving consciousness.

Kirlian Photography

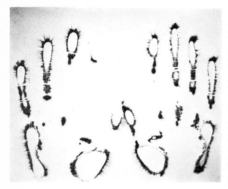

A Kirlian photograph of the left and right hands. Both the hands and the feet record and reflect changes in the mental and physical state of the individual. The information captured depends on the area photographed and the equipment used, as well as the characteristics and duration of the high frequency field used during the exposure.

The left hand and foot correspond with the right side of the brain and monitor the intuitive aspect of the psyche. The right hand and foot correspond with the left brain and with the logical, thinking part of the mind. For psychological purposes, a Kirlian photograph of the whole hand gives a more complete picture of mental state than one fingertip. Psychological changes are not reflected equally in all fingers. Psychological factors influence the following:

1. Balance of energy between the left and right hands.

2. The comparative strengths of each finger.

3. The length of the streamers.

4. The strength and continuity of the inner corona.

5. The presence or absence of large circular masses of energy.

Kirlian photography, named after the Russian husband and wife team Semyon and Valentina Kirlian who developed the method, is a technique of high-voltage photography which is being researched as both a physiological and psychological diagnostic tool. The Kirlians originated the technique in the 1940s after Semyon, during the course of some high-frequency research, noticed a spark jumping from an electrode on his equipment across to a patient lying close by. He decided to place a photographic plate between the electrode and the patient's hands. The developed plate showed a kind of luminescence which followed the contours of the fingers; furthermore, what appeared to be streams of energy could be seen flowing from the fingertips. Semyon then further refined his equipment to enable continuous monitoring of this luminescence. The result, as Semyon described it, was "the most fantastic scene they had ever witnessed. The hand was transformed into a display of lights, flares, sparks and twinkling effects in a constant movement of glorious colour. Some lights appeared to be moving, while others pulsated; parts of the hand showed cloudy patches, but the whole appeared as a firework display with the physical hand seen dimly in the background. The impression was of a giant computer screen constantly adjusting to a read-out."

Over ten years of further experimenting, the Kirlians became convinced this 'inner body' reflected the state of well-being or otherwise of the physical body. Their breakthrough came when they photographed two apparently identical leaves, one of which gave the expected aura, while the other appeared dull and lifeless. The donor of the leaves then explained that the first leaf was from a healthy plant, whereas the other was from a contaminated plant. It appeared from this experiment that the Kirlian method could predict that disease or death was imminent. Eventually the Kirlians came to realize that this second 'inner body', the aura, is a whole unified organism in itself, manifesting its own electromagnetic field, and in addition is the basis of biological energy fields. This second body is also found in plant as well as animal life.

While the Kirlians were the first to stir widespread interest in electrophotography and to develop new techniques and apparatus design, early variations of the method had been described by Nicola Tesla in the United States in 1891 and subsequently by other researchers in France, Czechoslovakia and the Soviet Union. In the field of aura research, Dr Walter Kilner at St Thomas's Hospital in London developed a special screen for viewing the aura in the 1930s.

The study of Kirlian photography has only recently spread to the United States and Europe. One of the leading researchers in the United States is Dr Thelma Moss of the School of Medicine at the University of California. In answer to criticism that the phenomena observed with Kirlian photography is simply due to physiological variations at the surface of the skin, Dr Moss has demonstrated that there is no correlation between the observed corona and variations in skin temperature, peripheral vascular changes or sweating. She has found, however, apparent correlations with psychological states – states of relaxation produced by hypnosis, meditation and acupuncture are characterized by wider and more brilliant coronas, while states of tension and emotional excitement result in a contracted corona with a red blotch on the fingertip sometimes appearing.

Photographs taken of healers while healing show a much wider corona than when they are at rest; fingertips of patients reveal increased corona activity after they have been healed. Acupuncture points show up clearly as blobs of energy on the skin which vary in size with different diseases, a discovery which offers enormous possibilities for studying the mechanisms involved in acupuncture as well as providing a useful means of diagnosis.

Kirlian photography may well prove useful in psychiatry as well. Two American doctors, Dr Michael Shacter and Dr David Sheinkin of Ponoma, New York State, have demonstrated an almost total lack of fingertip corona in a patient undergoing a schizphrenic episode. It may be possible to predict the onset of such episodes by monitoring changes in the fingertip corona.

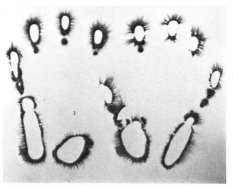

There are literally hundreds of applications of Kirlian photography. Here are just a few:

1. Measuring the life force in seeds and plants.

2. Detecting illness before physical symptoms appear.

3. For use in conjunction with other therapies such as acupuncture, homoeopathy and healing, to evaluate the effectiveness of the treatments.

4. For a wide variety of psychological purposes in industry and commerce, and for staff selection.

5. To investigate the residual toxic effects of drug addiction.

6. To evaluate the effect of parental conflict on children.

7. To assess psychological compatability between two people.

8. To evaluate the ability of a therapist to activate the self-healing process in a patient.

Brian Snellgrove

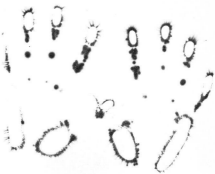

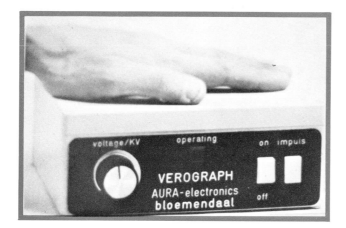

A simple, commercially available device for producing the Kirlian effect. The equipment generates a high frequency field which is delivered to an aluminium plate on the top of the device. Over this plate is placed a sheet of protective plastic. A piece of film or photographic paper is placed between the object being photographed and the plastic sheet. The voltages used range between 16,000 and 32,000 volts. The author has found that 22,000 volts and an exposure time of two seconds is sufficient for most purposes.

After exposure, the paper or film is developed in the normal way. The author uses soft (Grade One) paper. The equipment generates small quantities of ozone during operation and should not be used for long periods without suitable ventilation. Home-made devices can be dangerous.

Physical factors such as temperature, pressure and humidity have no direct effect on the picture. Exerting extra pressure on the object to be photographed will often result in a weaker aura as the energy body withdraws.

A Kirlian photograph of a patient before (top) and after (above) a psychotherapy session. The general effect of the session was to bring into the open the creative energies of the patient and give him more self-confidence. A break-up in the middle finger of the right hand however, shows that certain problems have been brought to the surface and need to be discussed before healing can be said to have taken place.

Kirlian photographs are invaluable in establishing the exact benefits of a healing or counselling session. An unchanged aura means that the basic problems are not being touched, or that the therapist is not right for the patient, or vice versa. Sometimes a successful session shows a weaker aura afterwards indicating that an emotional problem has surfaced and has to be faced by the patient before a breakthrough to creativity can be made. Kirlian photography can be used by psychoanalysts to keep a record of their patients' progress.

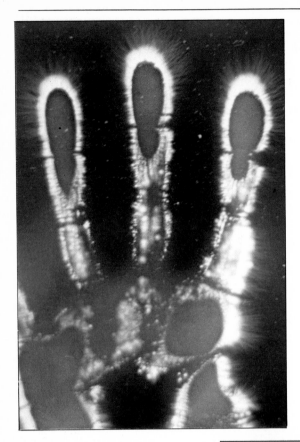

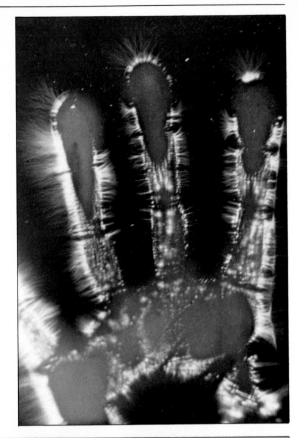

Above

The effect of thought on the aura. This example shows the effect of healing thoughts which are being sent to two other people. The first person (left) is a warm, lovable person, while the second (right) has many unsolved problems. This last fact, unknown by the sender at the time of making the photographs, affects and influences the aura of the hand.

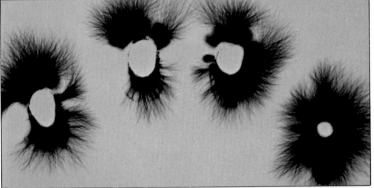

Right

Two examples of the subtlety of configuration obtainable from the fingertips. On the left the subject is 'tuning in' to another person, a friend with problems. On the right, the subject is sending healing to a sick child. The aura of the child is therefore influencing hand of the healer. In this case the child is very withdrawn, which shows in the cut-off lines emanating from the fingertips.

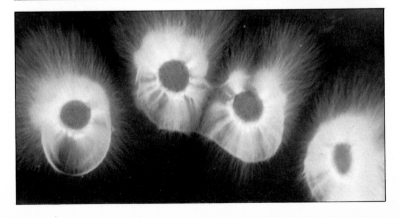

Right
Thumb print photograph by Thelma Moss of a person showing the symptoms of influenza. This is an example of warning signs starting to show before the physical disease has manifested itself.

Below
A person's strengths and weaknesses can be seen from a very early age on Kirlian photographs. The top photograph is an example of a well-balanced one year old child, showing strong radiations and regular inner coronas. Below is an example of two children of separated parents, exhibiting an irregular aura.

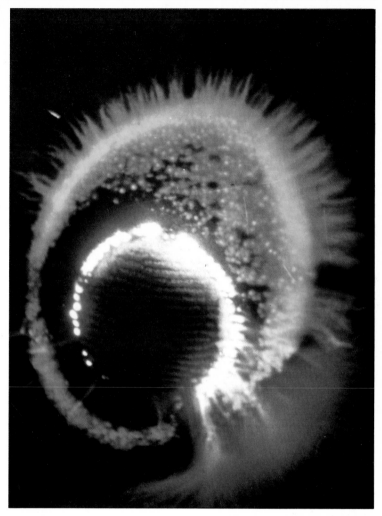

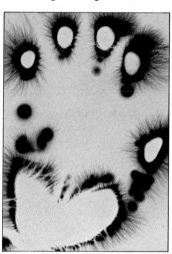

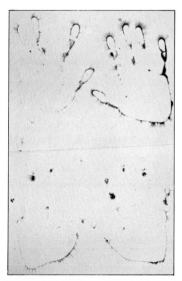

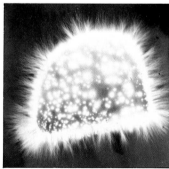

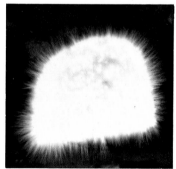

Above
A small piece of whole-wheat bread before (left) and after (right) being touched by a healer. These photographs appear to show the ability of the human aura to influence the energy fields of food without, necessarily, the intention to do so. The energy specks within the left-hand photograph of the bread correspond to the individual grains of wheat, the grains of the right-hand bread are not visible because the energy fields of each grain have increased so much that they now overlap.

Biorhythms

Biorhythms, or the rhythms of life, are the three biological rhythms concerned with variations in physical, emotional and intellectual capacities. They were originally put on a scientific observational basis by two doctors at the turn of the century. One was Dr Wilhelm Fleiss, a physician, who later became President of the German Academy of Sciences, and the other Hermann Swoboda, an Austrian, who later became a professor of psychology at the University of Vienna.

The discovery arose from their independent observations of regular variations in, or recurrence of, particular physical or psychological symptoms in large numbers in their patients. Both came to the conclusion that certain physical symptoms had a 23-day cycle, and some emotional symptoms a 28-day cycle. They then took the cycles for an individual and, looking to see at what point they originated, discovered that the cycles originated on the day of birth.

The intellectual cycle was discovered in the 1920s by Alfred Teltscher, an Austrian doctor of engineering. Following the discovery of Fleiss and Swoboda, Teltscher decided to observe the intellectual performance of his students in Innsbruck and, having collated and analysed his data, he found a regular cycle of 33 days.

The earliest attempted application of biorhythms was by the Swiss, shortly before the Second World War, when they wished to increase efficiency and lower the accident rate in industry.

In 1956, Dr Kichinosuke Tatai, concerned with the enormous traffic accident problem in Japan, took up the Swiss work again. The Japanese have claimed remarkable success for accident prevention schemes based on biorhythmic forecasting, and the writer has spoken to a Japanese insurance broker who told him that he now arranges reduced premiums for firms who operate transport safety schemes based on biorhythms.

Biorhythm theory has only been examined again on a scientific basis since 1973. The results of this work have been to confirm the existence of the cycles, but it has also thrown some doubts on the rather simplified explanation of the effect of these cycles on everyday life which were originally proposed.

The most satisfactory explanation of how biorhythms affect everyday life is to regard each biorhythmic cycle as being a variation in the energy available to the individual. The active phase of each cycle indicates a good supply of energy, and the passive phase, a less plentiful supply. The days separating these phases are best looked upon as unstable, or changeover days, when the energy supply can switch backwards and forwards between active and passive, depending upon the external stimulus. This idea accommodates the observations that results of stress on these days can produce 'good' performances as often as 'bad' ones. The cross-over day between active and passive days are known as critical days. On these days the rhythms become unstable and erratic; extra care is therefore needed at this time.

Biorhythms thus provide a pattern of our reactions. Every individual has various ways of reacting to particular situations and biorhythms provide a map of these variations in our behaviour. Displayed on a chart over a twelve-month period, it is possible to see the pattern of biorhythmic energies spread out. We can then more easily relate the pattern of energies to our behaviour pattern.

Modern biorhythmic theory states that while a number of reactions to stress situations can be standard, the overall pattern of an individual's behaviour is unique. A person's reactions to the biorhythmic variation of energies obviously depends on whether they are of an intellectual, emotional or physical type, or whether they dig ditches or write symphonies. But whatever they do, provided they are working to near capacity, their pattern of behaviour is linked to their biorhythms.

On June 5th 1968, the day that he assassinated Robert F. Kennedy, Sirhan was intellectually critical and low in both his emotional and physical rhythms.

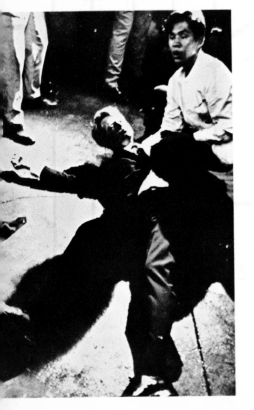

Biorhythms

As a simple example, if each biorhythm is in an active phase, extroverts find this good, for they can use all this energy in pursuing their normal goals, and still have some to spare. On the other hand, there are introverts who do not like these periods a bit. They feel restless, irritable and sometimes depressed, because their life-style is not orientated to spending all that energy. The result of piling up too much energy can be as uncomfortable as overspending.

By getting to know the relationship between our biorhythmic pattern and our behaviour pattern we can learn to compensate for the unwanted variations that are due to the biorhythmic effect.

For example, a young professional golfer having studied his bio-calendar for the past year, announced that he had discovered his pattern and now knew what to watch for, and how to improve his performance.

His personal pattern showed that he performed best in tournaments when he was in the passive phase of his physical cycle. This, he now realized, was due to the fact that when he had a good supply of physical energy, he was trying too hard to hit the ball, rather than just swinging.

Michael McDonald

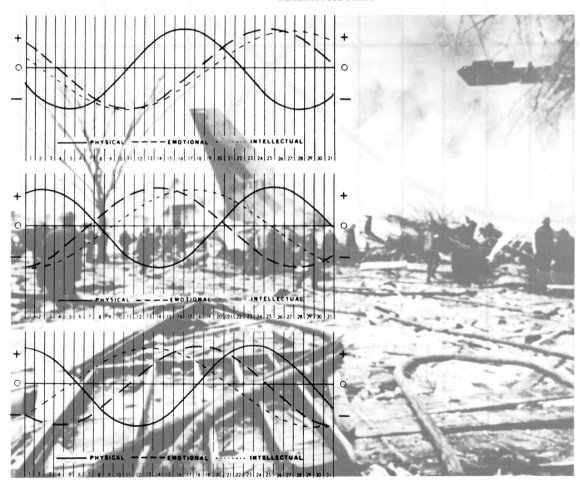

On December 8th 1972, a United Airlines flight crashed in Chicago. The cause of the crash was later found to be due to pilot error. On that day, the captain was low in all three rhythms, the co-pilot had a double critical in the physical and intellectual rhythms, and the flight engineer was low emotionally and physically.

The Lüscher Colour Test

The Lüscher Colour Test was introduced as a method of personality testing some twenty years ago by Dr Max Lüscher, Professor of Psychology at Basle University. The test is based on the theory that a person's preference for certain colours and dislike of others is indicative of an existing state of mind, of glandular balance, or both.

The origins of this colour significance lie far back in man's history, when his daily life was governed by two factors – night/darkness and day/light. The colours associated with these two environments are dark blue and yellow, and even the body's automatic responses are linked with these – dark blue with low metabolic rate and glandular activity, and yellow with an increase in the metabolic rate and glandular secretion providing energy to hunt and forage during the day. Also, in these primitive environments man was either hunting or being hunted much of the time. The actions of attack have universally evolved as being associated with the colour red, while defence (even if it involves 'attack') is associated with green. Experiments have confirmed these associations; a person exposed to pure red for a period of time becomes stimulated, and the blood pressure, respiration rate and heartbeat all increase. Exposure to dark blue has the opposite effect.

The full Lüscher test employs seventy-three colour patches, consisting of twenty-five different hues and shapes, requiring forty-three

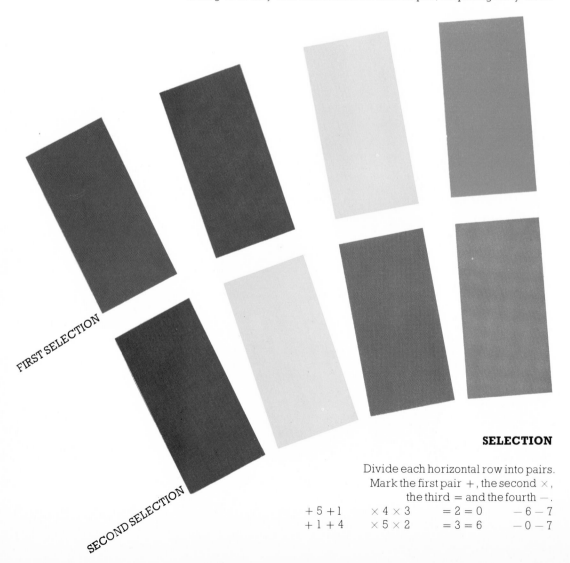

FIRST SELECTION

SECOND SELECTION

SELECTION

Divide each horizontal row into pairs.
Mark the first pair +, the second ×,
the third = and the fourth −.

| + 5 + 1 | × 4 × 3 | = 2 = 0 | − 6 − 7 |
| + 1 + 4 | × 5 × 2 | = 3 = 6 | − 0 − 7 |

different selections to relate. The 'short' test uses eight colours and this version can be highly instructive for identifying areas of psychological and physical stress, providing an early warning of the approach of many ailments.

Dark blue, yellow, red and green are the four 'psychological primaries'. The auxiliary colours of the short test are violet (a mixture of blue and red), brown (a mixture of yellow-red and black), grey (which is neutral and lies halfway between light and dark) and black (which is the blanking out of colour).

The method of self-administering the test is to place the eight colour cards in a semi-circle in front of you and decide which colour you like best, without associating the colour with anything extraneous, such as wallpaper, cars or clothing. This card is then turned over and a further selection made from the remaining colours. The process is repeated until all the cards are face down. The whole test is then undertaken a second time, trying not to relate, positively or negatively, to the previous selection. The resulting two rows of colours are then used to provide the interpretation. Each colour card corresponds to a number and the sequence of numbers is interpreted according to a table of psychological and physical diagnostic statements.

The Lüscher Colour Test

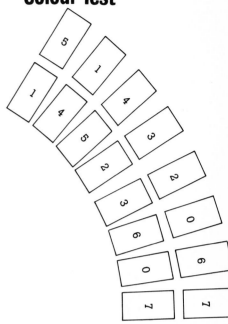

Each pair of numbers has a different interpretation (for example — 6 — 7 indicates a desire to control one's own destiny) and the sum of the pairs makes up the total diagnosis.

Acupuncture

In China, thousands of years ago, it was noted that soldiers wounded by arrows sometimes recovered from illnesses which had afflicted them for many years. The idea evolved that, by penetrating the skin at certain points, diseases were, apparently, cured. It was observed that the size of the wound did not matter, but only its location and depth. The Chinese then began to copy the effects of the arrow, puncturing the skin with needles.

Writings on acupuncture go back 4,500 years when thirty-four books were published known as the *Nei Ching*. This collection took over 1,500 years to complete, the final chapter being written about 3,000 years ago. Traditional Chinese medicine still adheres largely to the wisdom contained in these works and includes acupuncture, diet, manipulation and massage, hydrotherapy, herbalism, sun and air therapy and exercise.

In the *Shi Ji* (Historical Records) by Szuma Chien, a historian of the Han Dynasty (206 BC–AD 220), an account is given in *Biographies of Pien Chueh and Tsang Kung* on how Pien Chueh, a renowned doctor, brought a patient out of coma by applying acupuncture needles. Pien Chueh was in the State of Kuo, when he heard that the prince had lost consciousness that morning. Death was suspected. Pien Chueh hurried to the palace, where funeral preparations were under way. Pien Chueh carefully examined the patient and diagnosed coma. He then administered acupuncture. The prince was soon able to sit up. Pien Chueh then prescribed herb drinks for twenty days and the prince completely recovered.

The earliest recorded acupuncture needles were of stone, described as 'stone piercers' or 'stone borers'. A doctor named Yu Fu treated patients with stone needles. In the *Stan Hai Jing*, (Book of Mountains and Seas), written over two thousand years ago, a passage reads: "In the Kaoshih Mountains are rich deposits of jade, underlaid with stone suitable for making needles". In the *Canon of Medicine* is written: "In the eastern region all . . . abscesses are best treated with a small sharp-edged stone flake or needle". By neolithic times, the Chinese were using needles of bone and bamboo. When metal was discovered, needles made of various metals were introduced. Succeeding dynasties saw the development of iron, silver and other alloys, with the use of acupuncture needles made of these materials. Today, the acupuncturist uses needles made from processed stainless steel.

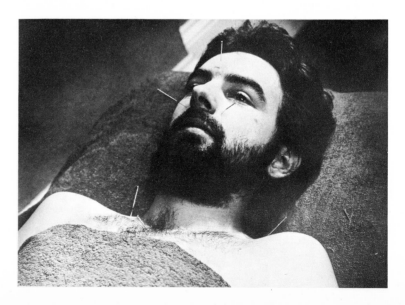

Treatment of a sinus problem with acupuncture.

Acupuncture

Originally it was thought that it was the metal itself which cured disease. Later it was established that it was not the metal which produced the effect, but the method of application. It became known that certain points on the skin affected and controlled certain organs in the body and by the use of needles these organs i.e. the liver, heart, intestines, gall bladder etc., could be affected and if diseased, healed.

The theory behind acupuncture is that there exist in the body dual flows of energy called yin and yang, contained within an overall conception of energy known as the Ch'i or life force. These are expressed in everything in the universe, day and night, elasticity and contractability, hot and cold, life and death, etc. Everything has its force of opposition, but this opposition by its very existence is itself complementary. Yang tends to stimulate, to contract, and is the positive principle, while yin tends to sedate, to expand and is the negative principle. Health is dependent on the equilibrium of yin and yang, firstly within the body and secondly within the entire universe. They must be protected and kept in equilibrium, for otherwise disease will develop. The Chinese discovered that this 'vital energy' (yin and yang) circulates in the body along 'meridians' similarly to the blood, nerve and lymphatic circuits. The flow along the meridians may be detected in the living body by electronic and other means. These paths of vital energy (Ch'i) disappear at death.

There are twenty-six main circuits or meridians, each associated with a different body function or organ. The state of these meridians can be assessed at the two radial pulses felt on the forearm just above the wrist. The condition of yin and yang and the state of the various systems in the body, can be estimated before any signs and symptoms become apparent. Traditionally there are about 800 acupuncture points, but new ones are continually being discovered. In diseased conditions, there is a breakdown of this process and the energy flows are unbalanced. Often, certain of the points become painful when pressed and these are associated with the condition which is developing. In order to treat the illness, it is necessary to rectify any imbalance in the energy flow. By piercing the skin at certain points, the energy flow is stimulated or sedated; its balance is altered within the body so as to restore the functioning equilibrium in the organism.

The traditional acupuncturist will assess the condition of the meridians by feeling the pulses at the radial artery. In disease, the pulses become disturbed and a wide variety of differing tensions – hardness, fullness, quietness, over- and under-activity can be felt. An experienced acupuncturist can distinguish hundreds of different variations in the pulses. Hence he will know which meridians need to be balanced and, by using one of the many systems of treatment, he will know exactly which acupoints to needle. Once the exact points have been located, needles are inserted in the skin to varying depths according to the point and condition being treated. They are left in place for various lengths of time ranging from a few seconds to several minutes. In some conditions, very special minute needles may be left in for two to three weeks. The operation is almost painless and dramatic reduction of disease syndromes often follows.

Conditions which can be successfully treated include migraine, headaches, ulcers and digestive troubles, lumbago, arthritis, fibrositis, neuritis, sciatica, rheumatism, dermatitis, exzema, psoriasis and other skin conditions, high blood pressure, depressions and anxiety states, asthma and bronchitis and many others.

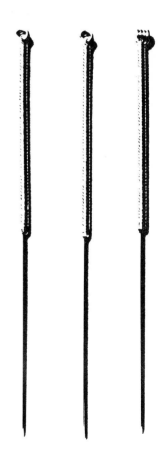

Standard stainless steel Chinese acupuncture needles.

Acupuncture

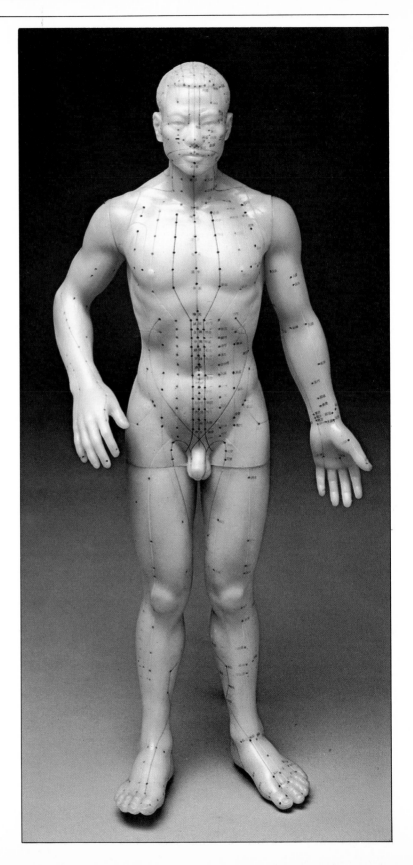

The twenty-six principal meridians or ducts which carry the *ch'i* energy are divided into twelve identical pairs plus two – the front and back midline meridians. In these photographs of a Chinese acupuncture teaching model, the front and back midlines are those down the exact centre of the torso; each side of the midline lie the twelve main meridians. For instance, the meridian immediately either side of the front midline is the kidney meridian, while the next one, moving outward from the midline is the stomach meridian.

The acupuncture points occur where the meridians emerge at the surface of the body, and like the meridians, each acupuncture point is paired, its companion point being located in a mirror-image position on the body. Recently a Korean researcher, Kim Bong-han, claimed to have discovered the existence of additional meridians.

Acupuncture

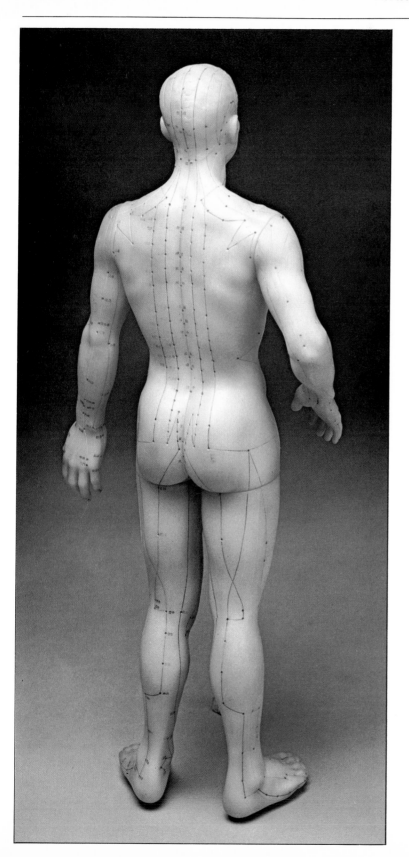

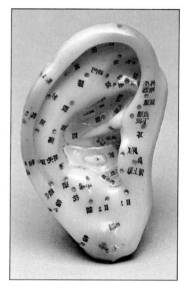

A Chinese acupuncture training model of the ear, showing the distribution of some of the known points. Many of the points in the ear are useful for the rapid alleviation of pain, and, in recent years several points have been used for inducing acupuncture anaesthesia. Various surgical operations have been performed using only ear acupuncture points to achieve anaesthesia, including eye operations, appendectomies and gynaecological operations. *(See also overleaf).*

Acupuncture

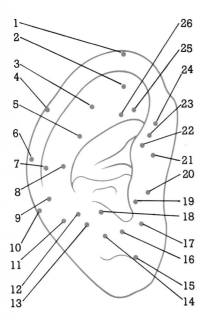

1. top
2. ankle
3. knee joint
4. helix 2
5. abdomen
6. helix 3
7. shoulder joints
8. chest
9. helix 4
10. clavicle
11. cervical vertebrae
12. neck
13. back of head
14. forehead
15. eye
16. eye 2
17. eye 1
18. special asthma point
19. kidney
20. nose
21. external ear
22. descending colon
23. urinary tract
24. external genitals
25. hip joint
26. buttock

A Korean Professor, Kim Bong Han, has demonstrated photographically the existance of the meridians as a separate physiological system. He has also shown that the meridians contain DNA and RNA – two substances basic to life and reproduction. His work, documented with histological, pathological and photographic evidence is now available in English.

One of the most important advances has been the introduction of electro-acupuncture. Here a meter records the reduced skin resistance over the acupoints. A photoelectric cell indicates to the practitioner when he is over these points. The states of yin and yang are assessed by electro-acupuncture and the treatment is applied prophylactically and therapeutically, according to the state of the Ch'i imbalance.

The use of acupuncture anaesthesia began in 1958, when it was used to relieve post-operative pain; success led to the idea of extending its use to replace anaesthetic drugs in surgical operations. That same year, acupuncture anaesthesia was introduced successfully for tonsillectomy. The patients reported feeling no pain during operations and, as a bonus, they had none of the undesirable after effects connected with drug anaesthesia. The technique was then extended to tooth extraction, thyroidectomy and herniotomy. After much further experimental work and clinical practice, the Chinese acupuncturists made public their discoveries, and after 1959 major surgery was undertaken on the neck, chest, limbs, abdomen and brain. As the patients are fully conscious throughout the operation, they can cooperate and respond to the surgeon's questions and directions. Clinical practice has shown the method to be safe, simple and non-conductive to physiological disorders.

Many hospitals in China now use acupuncture anaesthesia extensively for patients of all ages. It has proved successful in more than a hundred types of major and minor operations, including cardiac surgery under extra-corporeal circulation. As the technique has advanced, the number of points used has been reduced. For example, whereas originally more than eighty points were used in pneumonectomy, now four, three or even only two are sufficient.

In China today, over a million doctors practise acupuncture. In Japan there are 60,000 practitioners and throughout the East the total approaches three million. It is used in hospitals in France and Germany where this treatment can be obtained under national health schemes. In Russia, it is taught in several universities. There are now over 10,000 practitioners in Europe alone and its use is spreading dynamically throughout the West, especially in the United States where it is finding wide acceptance. Indeed, there is hardly a country in the world where its efficacy is not being recognized.

As practitioners combine traditional Chinese methods with modern Western techniques, many more advances are being made. There is little doubt that within a decade acupuncture will become one of the most important diagnostic and therapeutic methods in medicine, provided always that it is combined with other treatments and not used as a panacea.

Sidney Rose-Neil

Reflexology

The study of reflexology massage to the feet is claiming much public attention now that interest in alternative medicine has caught the imagination of people at large. Reflexology, sometimes known as zone therapy, is used as a means of bringing the body back to a state of balance. All disease is a manifestation of maladjustment somewhere in the intricate working of the body mechanism. The body is a composite whole and every part must be in harmony for the organism to be in a state of good health.

The origin of the reflex method is obscure. It is said that it came from China to the West and may have existed side by side with acupuncture. Again, it is known to have been used by the natives of Kenya, and also by some American Indian tribes.

At the beginning of this century it was called zone therapy by one Dr Fitzgerald in America who used it as a form of anaesthesia to render the patient insensible to pain when performing small operations, and to ease childbirth. Dr George Starr White, Dr Bowers and Dr and Mrs Riley also pioneered this work, developing their own methods. Many variations occurred. Miss Eunice D. Ingham, who trained under Dr Jo Riley, brought the work of reflexology before the American public. She toured every state, holding seminars for those who wished to learn how to use the therapy.

As a method of reflex massage the Eunice Ingham technique stands supreme. It presents a clear and concise set of reflexes which, if correctly worked upon, will bring fantastic results. Only the hands are used to massage the reflexes, which are present in the feet and which link up with all parts of the body. Whenever an organ is out of order, the corresponding reflex in the feet will be very tender upon pressure. The discomfort will vary according to the severity of the condition and the success of the treatment depends upon the skill with which it is applied. The fundamental principle is one of releasing tension and encouraging the full blood supply to areas in distress. Reflexology also stimulates the subtle energy flow to bring about the revitalizing of the whole organism.

In the hands of a trained practitioner, reflexology may be used as a speedy and very accurate method of diagnosis and to give a valuable assessment of the patient's condition. A practitioner is guided in his work not only by the reflexes, but by the ten zones which divide the body longitudinally on either side of the medial line. The hands have the same reflexes at the feet and can be used as a means of treatment if the feet cannot be worked upon. Also, there are the cross reflexes linking shoulder and hip, elbow and knee, hands and feet. These are of great value in difficult cases.

Working as a reflexologist is a fascinating experience. The person to be treated may arrive in a jaded condition, but as the massage is given and the tension released, so the whole appearance changes and the face will show a glow of returning vitality. Of course the age and condition of the person being treated affects the speed of the recovery. If the trouble has been some time in manifestation, the replacement of weak and diseased cells is a gradual process.

People of all ages benefit from reflex massage. It may be given to a baby or a very old person. A gentle stroking movement on the sole of the foot is sufficient for a baby. Older children require a lighter massage than adults. In cases of very elderly people with failing circulation, great help may be given and where acro-cyanosis (blueness of the extremities) is present, a remarkable change takes place. The hands and the feet return to a natural colour after a few treatments.

Trained students of reflexology have a first-aid kit in their hands to be used, whenever needed, for the rest of their lives.

Doreen E. Bayly

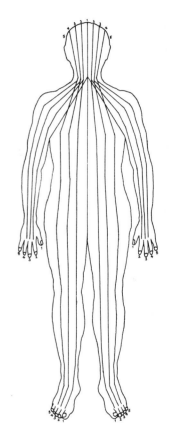

The ten zones in reflexology.

Reflexology

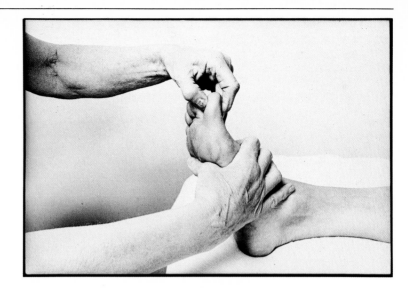

This picture illustrates massage of the right big toe, the reflex to the pituitary gland. This is always the first point to be attended to in a treatment. The pituitary gland is the most important of our endocrine glands, controlling all glandular functions.

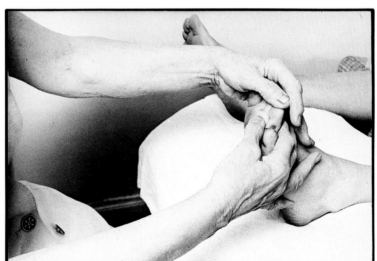

The eye reflex is situated in the pad immediately below the junction of the second and third toe.

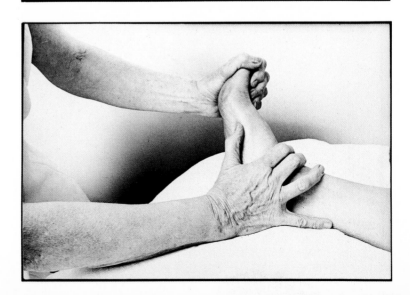

The spinal reflex follows the arch of the foot. Here the therapist is working on the 12th thoracic vertebra.

Reflexology

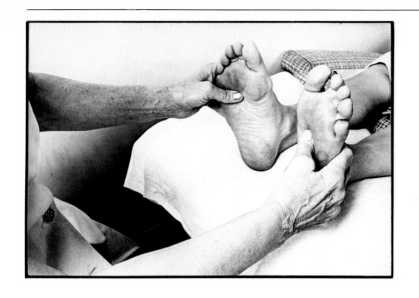

Relaxing exercise for the solar plexus. The therapist massages the reflex point while the patient breathes in unison. The resulting relaxation of the diaphragm enables the lungs to expand more fully, thereby increasing the intake of oxygen.

REFLEXOLOGY CHART
The Eunice Ingham Method · Chart produced by Doreen E. Bayly

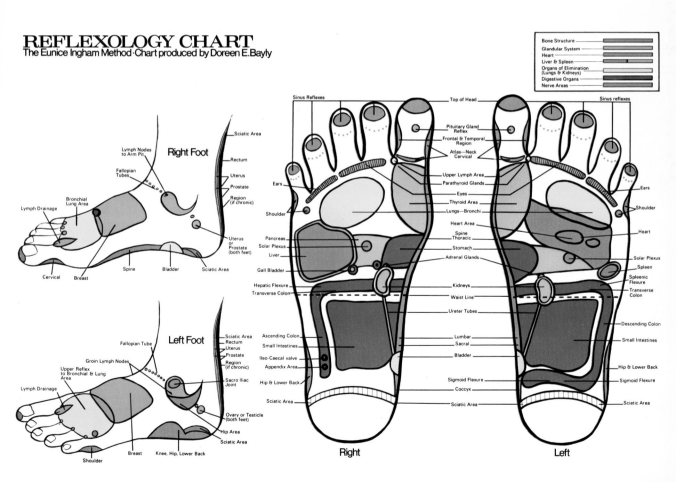

Legend:
- Bone Structure
- Glandular System
- Heart
- Liver & Spleen
- Organs of Elimination (Lungs & Kidneys)
- Digestive Organs
- Nerve Areas

Right Foot
- Sciatic Area
- Lymph Nodes to Arm Pit
- Rectum
- Fallopian Tubes
- Uterus
- Prostate
- Bronchial Lung Area
- Region (if chronic)
- Lymph Drainage
- Uterus or Prostate (both feet)
- Cervical
- Breast
- Spine
- Bladder
- Sciatic Area

Left Foot
- Fallopian Tube
- Sciatic Area
- Rectum
- Uterus
- Prostate
- Groin Lymph Nodes
- Region (if chronic)
- Upper Reflex to Bronchial & Lung Area
- Sacro Iliac Joint
- Lymph Drainage
- Ovary or Testicle (both feet)
- Hip Area
- Sciatic Area
- Shoulder
- Breast
- Knee, Hip, Lower Back

Right / Left (soles)
- Sinus Reflexes
- Top of Head
- Sinus reflexes
- Pituitary Gland Reflex
- Frontal & Temporal Region
- Atlas—Neck Cervical
- Upper Lymph Area
- Parathyroid Glands
- Eyes
- Thyroid Area
- Lungs—Bronchi
- Heart Area
- Spine Thoracic
- Stomach
- Adrenal Glands
- Kidneys
- Waist Line
- Ureter Tubes
- Ears
- Shoulder
- Ears
- Shoulder
- Heart
- Solar Plexus
- Spleen
- Splenic Flexure
- Transverse Colon
- Descending Colon
- Small Intestines
- Hip & Lower Back
- Sigmoid Flexure
- Coccyx
- Sciatic Area
- Pancreas
- Solar Plexus
- Liver
- Gall Bladder
- Hepatic Flexure
- Transverse Colon
- Ascending Colon
- Small Intestines
- Ileo-Caecal valve
- Appendix Area
- Hip & Lower Back
- Lumbar
- Sacral
- Bladder
- Sigmoid Flexure
- Sciatic Area

Shiatsu

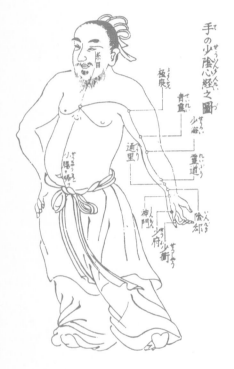

Shiatsu, in Japanese, means 'finger pressure'. The various techniques used in shiatsu massage almost all involve firm pressure to various points and areas on the skin, known as meridian paths or the *tsubo*, or pressure points. Most of these points are the same as the points used in acupuncture, hence shiatsu is often referred to as acupressure massage. Both arts are based on the same philosophy of medicine and are aimed at promoting better health by stimulating the flow of 'Chi' or 'Ki' energy.

Shiatsu has been used as a simple home treatment in the Orient for centuries, where it was practised by family members on one another. It is a simple and direct approach to massage which can be used to vitalize when a person is tired or to give relief from pain in times of sickness. Since its introduction to the West, and especially in the past ten years, shiatsu has been learned by thousands of people who practise in the home.

Although an advanced practitioner of shiatsu can treat specific illnesses and stimulate individual organs in the body through using the appropriate tsubo, the beginner can have much success by using a general body massage such as outlined here. For the exact location of the tsubo and the paths of the acupuncture medidians, there are many books on shiatsu and acupuncture which can be of aid. There are also many centres in major cities where shiatsu is taught.

Like any massage, shiatsu cannot be thought of as a 'cure' for disease divorced from proper diet, activity and attitude. Shiatsu can be a tool for us to understand more about ourselves since we are using our own innate healing power when we are practising it. All people have this ability, but it is seldom exercised. When we are not feeling well, we instinctively place our hand over the pain. When a child has been hurt a simple caress from its mother can sooth the pain. Shiatsu is simply amplifying this process by using the hands in areas where the body's energy or ki is flowing the strongest.

Ki Energy

Ki energy has been recognized for ages, whether it is referred to as Kundalini, Chi, Electro-Magnetic energy, Orgone or the will of God. It circulates through the body through defined pathways just like the blood, lymph or nerve impulses. These pathways were charted by early physicians in India, China and Japan thousands of years before the Christian era. The accuracy of these charts can now be validated using equipment to measure the electrical resistance on the surface of the skin.

Sensitivity is an obvious help in giving shiatsu. A person giving a massage should be in good health, active and have a positive outlook. Sensitivity to feeling the ki of a person comes with practice in massage and a proper life-style.

The flow of ki through the body is a continuous process. It vitalizes the body, together with the food we eat, the water we drink and the air we breathe. When the body is well nourished, active and flexible, the ki moves well. If the body is stiff, inactive and over-fed, the movement of ki is impaired and we feel heavy and ill at ease. The function of shiatsu, as well as acupuncture, is to stimulate the ki. In this sense, it is a symptomatic treatment unless the sick person also adjusts their life and eliminates the basic cause of the illness.

All the organs can be classified into yin and yang as to their form and structure. The solid organs are the more yang and the hollow organs are the more yin. The flow of ki through the organs is antagonistic to the form and structure. This means that the ki is yin for the yang organs and vice versa.

Shiatsu

YIN	YANG
Large intestine	Lung
Gall bladder	Liver
Stomach	Spleen/Pancreas
Urinary bladder	Kidney
Small intestine	Heart

To remember the flow of ki from the organs, picture a human form with the arms extended up and out. In this position the flow of ki from the hollow organs (yin) is toward the earth (yang) and the flow of ki through the solid organs (yang) is toward heaven (yin).

The life process within the body is a beautiful drama of spirallic movement. From the earliest stages of development we can see the spirallic unfolding of the embryo. This spirallic movement is imprinted on us, in the spirallic growth pattern of the hair on the head, the whorls at the fingertips, the spirallic structure of the muscles of the heart and the other organs, the spirallic conch of the inner ear, in fact everywhere we look within the human form. This pattern is the 'ghost image' of the energies which created us.

The meridians mentioned above are the most common used in shiatsu. The best areas for treatment with shiatsu are:

LARGE INTESTINES
Along the upper outside surface of the arm and between the thumb and index finger in the fleshy part of the hand.

GALL BLADDER
Along the outside of the leg from the pelvis to the knee.

STOMACH
Just to the outside of the front ridge of the shin bone from the knee to the ankle.

URINARY BLADDER
In the middle of the back of the thigh and on both sides of the coccyx.

SMALL INTESTINE
Along the bottom inside surface of the arm from the little finger to the armpit.

LUNGS
Along the upper inside surface of the arm and beneath the clavicle on the upper chest.

LIVER
Under the fleshy part of the calf between the knee and ankle.

SPLEEN
Under the shin bone on the inside of the leg between the ankle and the knee.

KIDNEY
On the top inside surface of the calf on top of the muscle.

HEART
Along the bottom outside surface of the arm and the shoulder blades.

If pain is felt when working on the meridians, it indicates stagnation of ki in the corresponding organ. After several sessions of massage the pain decreases and the ki is moving once more.

The outline for massage which follows is a basic massage which you can practise. Exact technique can be learned from a teacher, or through your own experience.

Some General Principles for Shiatsu

1. The person giving the massage should be in good health, calm and responsive.

2. If the person receiving the massage is seated, their spine should be straight.

3. The room should be quiet and simple, with no distractions.

4. If clothing is worn it should be light weight, loose-fitting and made with natural fabrics (synthetics disturb ki flow).

5. Study the *Unique Principle of Yin and Yang* as applied to diet, diagnosis and medicine.

6. Use pressure appropriate to the person you are working on and don't use heavy pressure on the abdomen, face or behind the joints of the knees or elbows unless you have had instruction.

7. Use your intuition; massage is a natural art. You already know how to do it.

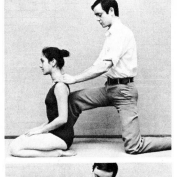

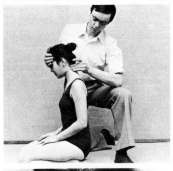

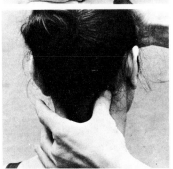

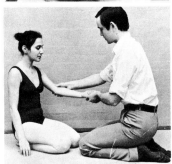

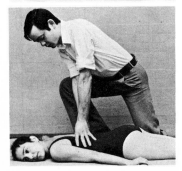

Outline for General Shiatsu Massage

1. To begin, have your partner sit facing away from you as in figure 1. He or she should be comfortable and have the spine straight with the arms down and relaxed. Grip the shoulders with both hands and begin to massage, kneading with the thumbs in a circular motion and pulling back and up with the fingers. This area corresponds with the small and large intestines and is often tense. Intestinal problems such as constipation and cramps can often be dealt with in this area.

2. Next, move to the neck as shown in figure 2. Meridians for the urinary bladder, gall bladder and intestines are all moving through this region. Placing the fingers as in figure 3, use a rotating motion pulling back and down the neck starting from the base of the skull. If the neck is very stiff, gently rotate the head first to the right and then the left. When massaging the neck, use your free hand to steady the head by placing it on the forehead. Headaches are easily dealt with by massaging this area. Two points used for eye strain and headaches behind the eyes can be located on either side of the tendons running parallel with the spine at the base of the skull. Tip the head back and give steady pressure at the base of the skull.

3. If you wish to massage the skull, this can be done from this position, seated behind your partner and using the tips of your fingers. Vigorous head massage is good in cases where there is tension in the face.

4. Now move into a position facing your partner as in figure 4. Working with the fingers and the thumb massage vigorously down the outside and inside of the arm, making sure to cover both the upper and lower surfaces. Massage well between the muscles and bones working down to the hands where you should massage the hands starting with the junction of the finger bones and the wrist. Rotate each finger gently and massage the palm.

5. Next, let your partner lie on the stomach as in figure 5 with the arms at the side. You are now prepared to work on the back. First give the back a general massage using the heels of the hands to soften up the muscles in the back. Massage well the area of the shoulder blades and the muscles in the small of the back. Then, rub along the sides of the spine with the edge of hand to stimulate ki flow and circulation of blood. The bladder meridian, which runs parallel to the spine, bi-laterally, contains some of the most important points in shiatsu. Their location in relation to the vertebrae are:

between the 2nd and 3rd thoracic vertebra	Lungs
between the 3rd and 4th thoracic vertebra	Lungs
between the 4th and 5th thoracic vertebra	Heart
between the 9th and 10th thoracic vertebra	Liver
between the 10th and 11th thoracic vertebra	Gall bladder
above the 1st lumbar vertebra	Spleen
above the 2nd lumbar vertebra	Stomach
above the 3rd lumbar vertebra	Intestines
above the 4th lumbar vertebra	Kidney

on either side of the sacrum lie the points for the bladder and sexual organs.

To stimulate these points, kneel as in figure 5 with the thumbs on either side of the spine as in figure 6. Starting at the top of the back, press slowly but firmly with the thumbs between each vertebra. Do not press with the muscles, but rather allow your weight to sink slowly onto the thumbs. Let the first series of movements down the spine be more light and, as you repeat the process, allow more weight to be used. Areas of pain indicate problems in the corresponding organs. Continue down the spine to the tip of the coccyx. If any areas are particularly painful, you can return to them and massage them with the thumbs using a circular motion. When using pressure, have your partner exhale as the pressure is increased using slow and deliberate movements.

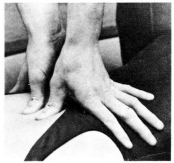

6. After finishing the back, move down to the buttocks and massage both sides using the heels of the hands. Massage in a circular motion following the contour of the buttocks massaging from the coccyx towards the outside and up again. This area is also connected to the intestine and is an effective area for massage in the case of constipation.

7. Now you are ready to massage the legs. The meridians for the liver, spleen and kidney run along the inside surface of the legs. The meridian for the bladder continues down the back centre of the leg and the meridians for the gall bladder and stomach run along the outside.

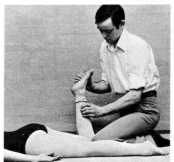

After relaxing the legs with a general massage using the heels of hand and the fingers, proceed to use the thumbs, as on the back, and apply firm pressure down the backs on the thigh and the calf, avoiding the soft area behind the knee. This medial line should be massaged several times. Next raise the bottom part of the leg as in figure 7 and massage the under-side of the calf on the inside of the leg as in the picture, starting at the knee and working down to the ankle. Next, massage up the inside of the shin bone from the ankle to the knee staying close to the bone. This should be done to both legs. When this is finished, give the bottoms of both feet strong stimulation with the thumbs and massage the top of the feet especially between the bones of the toes and the toes themselves.

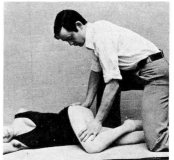

8. Now have your partner lie on the side as in figure 8 with the bottom leg straight and the upper leg bent at the knee. In this position, massage the thigh and then apply thumb pressure down the median line of the outside of the leg. Start at the pelvis and continue down to the knee and from there along the outside of the shin bone. This is the area of the gall bladder meridian. This area is good for general revitalizing and pains in the liver. In this position you can also apply pressure along the ridge on the top and outside of the shin bone, where the stomach meridian lies. This meridian can be used for cramps in the stomach or acid stomach.

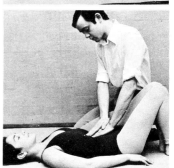

9. Now have your partner lie on the back as in figure 9, with the knees raised. In this position you can massage the abdomen. First use soft massage in a circular motion starting just above the pelvis on the right side and slowly massage up following the edge of the ribs up and around the abdomen and down the left side. Repeat this several times. Then use the fingers as in figure 10 and give slow even pressure following the same pattern. Do not apply full pressure, only continue until you meet resistance and then slowly release. Have your partner exhale as the pressure is applied as with the back. This massage is especially good for intestinal cramps, constipation, irregularity or wind.

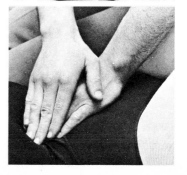

When you are finished, cover your partner with a blanket and allow them to relax.

William Tara

Moxibustion

In the period of the Southern and Northern Dynasties, Fan Yeh (398–446 AD), recorded in his *History of the Later Han Dynasty* several episodes about moxibustion. One doctor, known as Fue the Elder, popularized moxibustion and another section of the book records the work of Hua To, an ancient doctor who was skilled in moxibustion and often achieved results by puncturing only one or two points. The author recounts how Hua To treated Tsao Tsao (155–220 AD), statesman, strategist and poet of the Three Kingdoms period who it is said suffered from persistent headaches. When all else failed to give relief, Hua To cured him by applying moxibustion.

Moxibustion is a form of acupuncture, whereby heat is used. Mugwort *(Artemisia vulgaris)* is rolled into small cones which are placed, point upward, then lit, on specific acupuncture points. When the cone is burned almost to the skin, it is swiftly removed. The patient feels a pleasant sensation of warmth at the point. The procedure is not painful. The use of moxibustion follows similar rules to the use of needles, but to achieve slightly different results, particularly to stimulate the Ch'i energy, the body's life energy.

There are several other methods of using moxibustion. Sometimes, long, cigar-like sticks of mugwort are used. They are rolled into a cone about eight inches long and half an inch thick and covered with soft paper. They are lit at one end and the heated end applied to the skin surface for a short time until a feeling of warmth is experienced at the treated acupuncture point. The procedure is repeated at other points. In another form of moxibustion a special needle is used, which has a small cup-like structure at one end. The *Artemisia vulgaris* is placed on the end of the needle and lit. The heat runs down the needle, which has previously been inserted into the acupuncture point.

Acupuncture and moxibustion are usually used in combination. They complement each other and are considered as part of one total form of treatment.

Sidney Rose-Neil

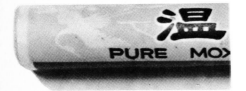

Moxibustion stick, prepared from dried, compressed *Artemisia vulgaris*.

Moxibustion of an acupuncture point on the hand. A small quantity of the herb *Artemisia vulgaris* is fashioned into a cone, placed on the acupuncture point and lit. The cone is allowed to smoulder until the patient begins to feel the heat, when the cone is quickly removed.

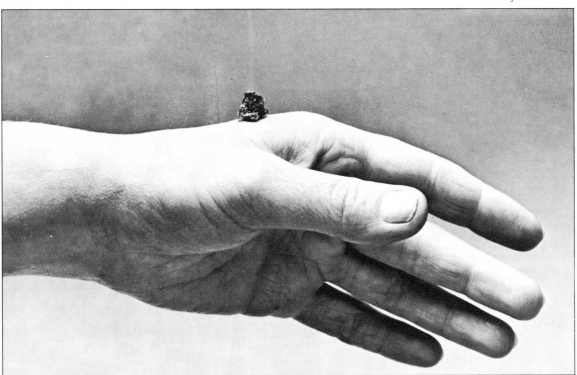

Osteopathy

The founder of osteopathy, Dr Andrew Taylor Still (1828–1917), was a physician from Missouri who first set about searching for a new approach to disease after being forced to watch three of his sons die from meningitis, knowing that all his medical knowledge and that of the medical world was powerless to help him. He claims to have studied for sixteen years before describing the new method of healing, which he called osteopathy, in 1876. Whilst his was the first proper description of a complete system of healing by manipulation, the concept is not original, as forms of manipulative therapy had been used in many parts of the world since the time of Hippocrates. Before his discoveries, Andrew Still himself practised bone setting, which was common in his time. But this was limited mostly to breaking down adhesions and re-aligning broken bones.

The first College of Osteopathy was established in Kirksville, Missouri, in 1897, and Still was helped by his sons and several other assistants who become famous as osteopaths in their own right. Not the least of these was J. Martin Littlejohn who came to England and established the first osteopathic school in the United Kingdom.

Dr Still died in 1917 at the age of 89, by which time he saw osteopathy recognized in every State in the USA. It now enjoys equivalent recognition to that of orthodox medicine. Such is the recognition, however, that it would appear that some American osteopaths prefer the relative ease of writing prescriptions to the more exacting work of osteopathic therapy.

The Basic Theory

Structure and function in the human body are completely interdependent – if the structure of the body becomes in any way altered or abnormal, then the function immediately alters as well. Primary alterations of function lead eventually to an alteration of structure. Looked at in this way, disease can be seen to be a perversion of either structure or function. The osteopath believes that through a very thorough understanding of the structure of the human body he can so influence it that normal functioning will return. Dr Still believed that abnormal structure influenced the circulation of the body, and from this came his axiom "The rule of the artery is supreme", meaning, of course, that where arterial blood supply was normal the bodily structure would function normally. At one time, some osteopaths believed that abnormalities in spinal structure caused the arteries to become pressed as they left the spine, whereas chiropractors thought that the nerves were being pressed. In point of fact neither was correct in their ideas of direct pressure.

However, it has been very thoroughly demonstrated that where spinal problems exist, biochemical changes occur which are capable of interfering with normal nerve transmission and normal circulation, and this can have a profound effect not only upon the muscles and skeleton but also upon the circulation and all organs of the body.

Osteopathy does not concern itself just with the spine, but with all parts of the body. A great deal of emphasis can be put upon the mobility of the rib cage and the thoracic and pelvic diaphragms in many respiratory and digestive problems. It is however to the spine that the osteopath pays greatest attention.

The vertebral column is composed of twenty-four movable segments which surround and protect the spinal cord, while at the same time allowing for the maximum possible movement. Weight is transmitted through the front of the spine via the cotton-reel shaped vertebral bodies, with flexibility being provided by the vertebral discs which are about one-third as thick as the bodies. Protective arches of bone pass backwards and surround the spinal cord with nerves

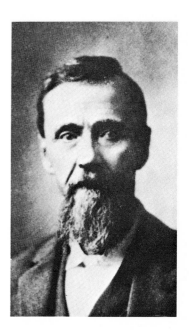

Andrew Still (1828–1917)

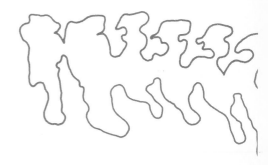

Osteopathy

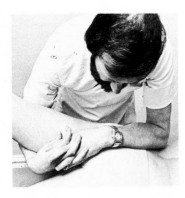

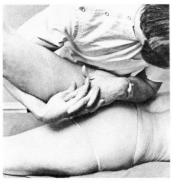

The leg is used as a lever in order to position the pelvis. A corrective thrust is then made with the upper part of the forearm moving the iliac bone forwards.

passing between adjacent arches to and from the cord. The vertebral arches have joints above and below which are not weight-bearing, but serve to guide movement, and if too great a movement is attempted, the joints will run up against each other producing a wedge which acts like a brake. If this wedging is too severe, the joints will lock and muscle spasm will hold them rigidly at this extreme of normal movement. The osteopath calls this an osteopathic lesion, while chiropractors call it a subluxation. The body now has to adapt to this abnormal situation, which it does by further shifting the spinal structures above and below, so that relative balance will occur. If the spinal lesion is not corrected, the altered balance will become permanent. Physiological changes at and around the spinal nerve exit and entrance can now influence the nerve, and abnormal function can, and often does, ensue. The cause however, of this spinal problem does not need to be local, for if any part of the body becomes disordered, sensory nerves which register pain, or position sense etc., send alarm impulses back to the spinal cord. These impulses may affect the motor nerves at the same spinal level, causing the small muscles at the back of the spine to contract. This contraction will cause small joints to become very close, and sometimes to lock. The area of the spine will become sensitive and the position of the vertebrae will be slightly altered, while their movement will be restricted to one direction. This can produce short- and long-term effects both locally and in some other parts of the body. Locally, there is initial spinal pain or soreness which may be quite mild, or so severe as to be crippling. If this situation is not corrected, the pain will often subside and the vertebrae above and below are able to take over the lost movement.

The reduced movement between two vertebrae however, can damage the disc between them, since it is entirely dependent upon motion for its nutrition and drainage. It has no blood supply and relies upon osmosis and diffusion, assisted by the increased and decreased pressures produced by spinal movements. Enzymes which give it strength can become deficient, and excessive wear can result. If a piece of cartilage chips away, or the central, more jelly-like substance oozes out through cracks, this can press directly upon a nerve or other highly sensitive structure. This is the 'slipped disc' which is extremely painful, but not nearly as common as was once implied by orthodox medicine. Another local result is spondylosis (spinal arthritis) which is so common as to be considered by orthodox practitioners to be almost inevitable in the elderly patient. However, it is by no means completely unavoidable. The local inflammatory changes around the injured joint can influence the autonomic nervous system which is responsible for controlling the function of all the organs, blood vessels, and some of the glands of the body. Abnormal impulses will cause faulty control of the organs as a direct result of structural derangements in the spine.

A basic controlling mechanism of the body is the endocrine system, a series of glands secreting hormones which control a great many functions of the body – the amount of growth, sexual characteristics, the balance of minerals in the body, sugar levels, the rate of metabolism and so on. It would appear that some of these functions can be influenced by manipulation of the spine. Whilst this area has not been fully studied, Parnell Bradbury and Dr Tee have described one physiological pathway in their book *The Mechanics of Healing*, and several others have been suggested in recent work at the Ecole Européenne d'Ostéopathie.

Of great interest to osteopaths is the effect of lesions in the upper cervical (neck) vertebrae upon the circulation of the brain, and there are many well-documented cases of conditions which were considered to be mental/emotional, being cured by pure manipulation. It is possible that they were due to insufficient oxygen supply to the frontal areas of the brain.

It should be emphasized that whilst Still described a system of manipulation, he never ignored other factors which might lead to ill health. For example, it would be ridiculous to perform manipulations on someone who had gross dietary deficiencies and expect them to get better. Since the structure of the body would be incapable of altering, the diet would have to be changed. Hydrotherapy might well be used as a temporary measure to help in the control of a fever. There are many links between osteopathy and nature cure, but unlike the pure naturopath, the osteopath does not believe that you can restore health without correcting anatomical derangements. If an osteopathic lesion is left unattended, the patient cannot recover completely.

The Examination

After taking a careful case history and finding out the present symptoms, past illnesses, accidents and so on, the osteopath proceeds to a physical examination. He first uses conventional diagnostic methods, after which he sets out to examine his patient as a whole; believing that the whole body is totally inter-acting, he does not restrict himself just to the area that the patient is suffering from, but will examine all the structures, taking them through active and passive movements to see how the body coordinates as well as palpating the joints and soft tissues. He then lays the patient on the couch and proceeds with a peculiarly osteopathic method of examination. It is in the technique of diagnosis and treatment that the osteopath varies from the chiropractor, the osteopathic diagnosis being dynamic whereas the chiropractic method is usually passive with the patient lying still.

The osteopath begins by moving each joint through its range of movement using the arms and legs as levers, and as he does so he probes, feels and attempts to reinstate general movement within restricted joints. If a joint is too restricted for this general approach, the osteopath will specifically open the joint by taking the patient through the movement that will open the joint whilst stabilizing the vertebrae below. In this way he is able to prize open a specific joint whilst the body is in motion, so minimizing the trauma to the body.

Again this differs from the chiropractic adjustment which is generally a direct thrust on to the vertebrae whilst the patient is lying on his face. As the joint opens, there is generally a fairly loud click which is very satisfying to the patient – the osteopath however, realizes that it is only useful if the right joint is opened, and so he relies on his sense of touch. It has recently been discovered that this click is due to the lubricating fluid in the joint momentarily changing from liquid to gas under negative pressure and producing a vacuum pop. This separation of joint surfaces allows the structures to glide immediately back into motion, relieving the vicious circle which maintains muscle spasm and local inflammation.

If the lesion was of recent origin, this manipulation will normally clear the problem, but where the condition is more long standing, the structural alterations which have occurred due to adaptation will frequently cause the condition to recur after a very short time – possibly hours or days – and in this case it requires a longer period of treatment in order to take the body back through its past adaptation.

The majority of patients will arrive with pain of a spinal nature, because the osteopath has built up a reputation for being able to deal with all types of spinal pain that do not respond to other forms of treatment. It is unfortunate that his great success with acute spinal problems has led the public to believe that this is the sole area of his work. A

Osteopathy

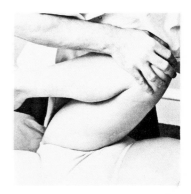

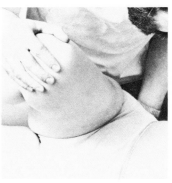

A general technique which helps restore movement to the whole of the lower spine. The flexed leg moves the lower spine and pelvis whilst the osteopath's hand is securing the vertebrae above.

Osteopathy

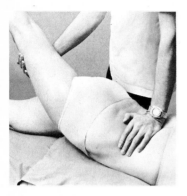

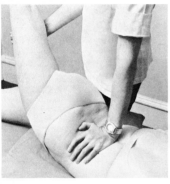

A specific technique to correct
an individual lesion in the
lower thoracic spine. The
corrective thrust is made upon
the vertebrae with the heel of
the hand. The use of the leg
helps to align the vertebrae and
enables the thrust to be quite
gentle.

competent osteopath should be capable of handling a very large range
of medical conditions and diseases without the use of drugs and sup-
pressive agents.

Of course some cases may be too far advanced before they reach
him and so require surgery or other forms of treatment, and where
this is the case the osteopath will advise appropriate treatment.

Types of Treatment

As osteopathy has developed, different forms of treatment have also
emerged. The most notable and distinct is cranial osteopathy which
was introduced this century by Dr W. G. Sutherland. This maintains
that the individual bones of the skull are in constant minute rhythmical
motion, and that each cranial bone is capable of becoming locked and
altering the mechanics of the skull. This, in turn, can influence the functions of the brain and hence the rest of the body.

A series of techniques has been devised in order to reinstate a
rhythmical motion into the cranial bones. Results can be, and often are,
impressive. Sutherland was at pains not to distinguish this from osteopathy as a whole, looking on it as only part of the total science.

Parnell Bradbury introduced another system which he called
'Spinology' in which he laid great emphasis on the application of the
minimum treatment possible. He would often give one specific adjustment and await results, the idea being that if a principal or primary
lesion is adjusted it will trigger the body to repair itself. He also postulated a chemical mediator which is released and produces a neuro-
endocrinal response, and claimed that if this response occurs, repair
occurs much more rapidly. The idea of any form of osteopathic treatment influencing the endocrine system is not new, however, but Bradbury and Tee were the first to confirm this with laboratory results using
a hormone called sympathin. Many other developments have been
made, but for the most part these cannot be thought of as a complete
school or teaching in themselves, rather a development of the basic
teaching.

Osteopathy is one of the largest unorthodox medical groups in the
world, and is still rapidly expanding. It was originally devised as a
system of treating all forms of disease, but its very success in the field
of acute musculo-skeletal injuries has led to the belief that this is its sole
scope. This is tragic because, like so many other of the fringe sciences,
it is capable of assisting the body to recover naturally from its own sicknesses without the aid of potentially dangerous drugs.

Stephen Pirie

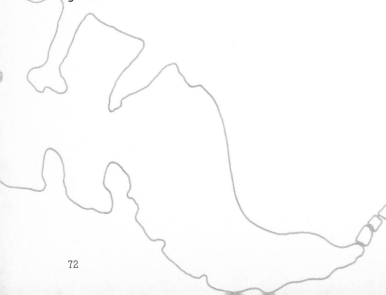

Chiropractic

The word 'chiropractic' is an adaptation from the Greek meaning 'manual medicine' or 'manual practice'. The original Greek expression must certainly be as old as Hippocrates himself since much in the Hippocratic writings is concerned with this subject. Although the founder of modern-day chiropractic, a magnetic healer called Daniel David Palmer, launched the profession in the United States as recently as 1895, the term which he chose is a clear reference to the Hippocratic tradition and the principles of the revived 'kheir praktikos' were not unlike those of the original.

There was perhaps one important difference, for between Hippocrates and Palmer came Plato and Aristotle, who admitted the 'soul' into philosophy, including that of healing. The work and influence of Galen and Vesalius added the last essential ingredient; anatomical knowledge. Palmer provided a synthesis by putting forward the proposition that: (1) we should look well to the spine for the cause of disease (a Hippocratic admonition) because: (2) it contains and protects the spinal cord (as shown by the anatomists), through which *vital forces* flow and are mediated to all parts of the body through the spinal nerves. Palmer then postulated a system of health care based on the hypothesis that misaligned spinal segments interfere, by way of impingement on nerves coming from the spine, with the passage of vital forces which are now known to be nerve impulses. Manual adjustments of the involved parts of the spine were thought to promote the health of the tissues supplied by the appropriate nerves.

The method and its theory attracted students, and colleges were established to train them. But the pooling of different attitudes soon caused conjecture, and as a result, differing emphases were taught in the various colleges. Nevertheless, the American public's interest had been aroused, and the treatment came into demand. Seen against the medicine of the times, chiropractic probably came out rather well, and it rapidly grew. Today it is the largest drugless healing profession in the world (see chart).

The reader might be forgiven for assuming from the foregoing that there is a chiropractic alternative to any other form of health care. This is not the case. Recent surveys of practice in Australia, Canada, and the United Kingdom, suggest that about half of the patients who consult chiropractors seek help for low back pain. About a quarter attend for neck and arm pain and only about ten percent are likely to seek help for anything other than 'rheumatic' complaints.

The reason for this probably lies in the fact that over the years, chiropractors have become increasingly acquainted with the complexities of the musculo-skeletal system. At the same time, the incidence of these complaints has risen and while the public generally has high expectations of orthodox medicine in many other health areas, there is disillusionment with this particular one.

Notwithstanding the contribution of general practice and hospital rehabilitation, the cost in cash and suffering of the conditions that chiropractors treat is great. Many painful episodes eventually remit with rest alone, but the time taken can be considerable. Moreover, prolonged rest does not leave the spine in good condition to sustain what might seem to be modest use, and recurrences are exceedingly common in patients who have been left to their own devices.

Apart from physical suffering, the time factor is often of major concern to patients. In cash terms, their incapacity is reflected in lost wages, lost production and sickness benefits. Such potential losses may account for the widespread use of chiropractors by the self-employed who value the short waiting time for an appointment. Employers sometimes send their employees to chiropractors in the hope of early rehabilitation and prophylaxis; but this does not imply that

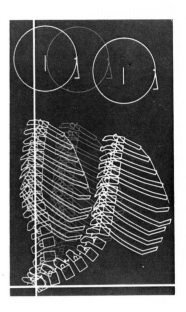

The effect of a 50 kph car crash on the human trunk as shown by drawings derived from a computer. On the left is a normal spine; the centre and right views show the trunk's position 20 and 40 minutes, respectively, after impact.

Chiropractic

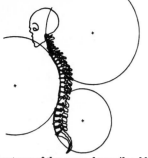

Centres of the arcs described by the three primary spinal curves.

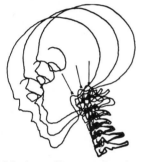

Multi-phase diagram showing relative displacements of neck vertebrae during nodding.

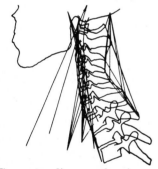

Computer diagram showing forces exerted on neck vertebrae by spinal muscles.

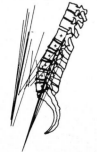

Side view of the lumbar spine illustrated with computer spatial displacement analysis lines.

chiropractors claim, or even expect to achieve, instantaneous cures. What scientific evidence exists to date, however, strongly suggests that chiropractors enjoy success in their major treatment areas.

Palmer realized, despite his lack of formal training, that the therapy he had founded was not a panacea; but he could not have foreseen the dramatic drop in infectious disease which was to follow. Nor did he anticipate the relative rise of malignancy and heart disease in this century. Yet there is another area, of great interest to chiropractors, where their intervention often seems to have a profound effect. Problems such as persistant amenorrhoea, infertility, asthma, migraine, seizures and nerve deafness succumb with a frequency too great to be dismissed as coincidental. There is general agreement that this has to do with nerve supply, but the mechanism seems to be exceedingly complex.

Chiropractic Theory

Chiropractors started with the belief that joints; especially spinal joints, cause the least trouble when they are correctly positioned. This came to be referred to as the study of locomotor statics. Later, largely influenced by European chiropractors, the profession learned to deal with disorders of movement, or dynamics. Because they were involved with painful conditions, much attention was given to the results of research into the way in which pain is generated, transmitted and appreciated. They soon came to realize that many combinations were possible, and began to recognize and predict the courses of common syndromes.

In examining the spine, the chiropractor is likely to assess its movement as a whole, either by measurement or visual assessment. The appreciation of individual joint position and movement by palpation, or 'feel', follows and is probably the most frequently used procedure. This is an art which takes some years to learn and many to perfect. Also of importance is posture, gait, symmetry, weight-bearing, occupational factors, patient attitudes and evidence of underlying disease. X-Ray has always been an important aid to diagnosis because abnormalities of both position and movement can be visualized and the mechanical effects of treatment seen (see illustrations). Common pathologies such as osteoarthrosis can be evaluated and other abnormalities assessed and identified. Occasionally, systemic or other disease is discovered on X-rays and chiropractors use the conventional sequence of case history and physical examination to help to detect this. Such patients are normally referred to orthodox medicine.

To find a concise theory of chiropractic today is difficult, and little evidence exists of rigid adherence to any preconceived idea of health and disease. The definition held by the European Chiropractors' Union reads: ''Chiropractic is a discipline of the scientific healing art concerned with the pathogenesis, diagnostics, therapeutics and prophylaxis of functional disturbances, pain syndromes and other neurophysiological effects relating to static and dynamic disorders of the locomotor system, particularly the spine and pelvis. Its therapy consists of specific manual treatment and supportive measures''. This definition suggests that much attention is paid to joints, and the term 'subluxation' was adapted as a general label to describe a functional abnormality of the joints within their anatomical range of movement. Subluxation has been wrongly alleged to denote a fictitious lesion upon the removal of which all health depends.

The relationship of the findings to the circumstances of the complaint usually suggests the treatment, which varies in complexity. The term 'adjustment' is preferred to 'manipulation', because it seems more suggestive of the discriminatory approach which is thought desirable. The procedures are fairly numerous and are applied in different ways. The commonest method is a rapid manual thrust aimed at inducing a sudden force across an individual joint causing the release of a 'fixed', or immobile joint. But chiropractors employ techniques other than those used to influence joint position and movement; various reflex techniques are used, as well as exercises, advice, nutritional guidance, shoe, seat, bed or work position changes. These measures may be used to help to ensure that treatment benefits are sustained and recurrent problems are avoided. The whole approach is reasonably uniform throughout the chiropractic world because of the constant interchange of updated information from the colleges and other research sources.

Relationship with Osteopathy

Some comment might usefully be made on the conceptual relationship between chiropractic and osteopathy. The professions both started in the USA and had a parallel evolution, although osteopathy originated a number of years earlier.

The difference between the professions is easily explained on the basis of original principles and theories. Andrew Taylor Still, the founder of osteopathy, postulated that blood supply was the essential factor in healthy tissue, whereas Palmer emphasized the nerve supply; but this can no longer be considered informative. Certainly, the two practices treat the same complaints, use mostly manual methods and are both concerned with the functional integrity of the musculoskeletal system. Osteopaths tend to associate the use of high velocity manipulative thrust techniques with chiropractors, while they associate rhythmic movements and massage with osteopaths. Both,

Chiropractic

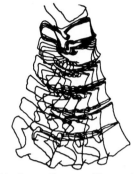

Multi-phase diagram illustrating the forward and backward bending of the lumbar spine.

Front-view X-rays of the low back of a patient before and after corrective treatment for low back pain. The spine is straighter after treatment when the patient is free from pain. This patient had been suffering from back pain for one year.

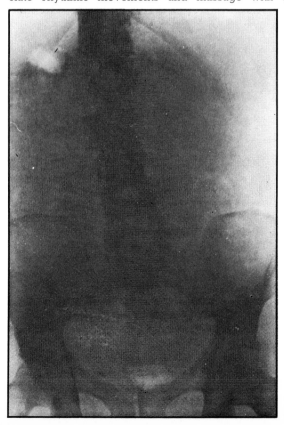

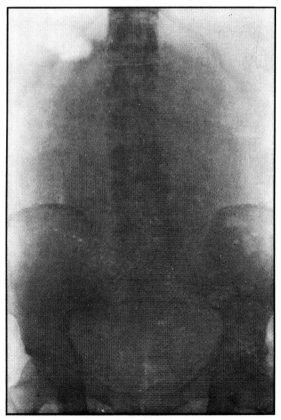

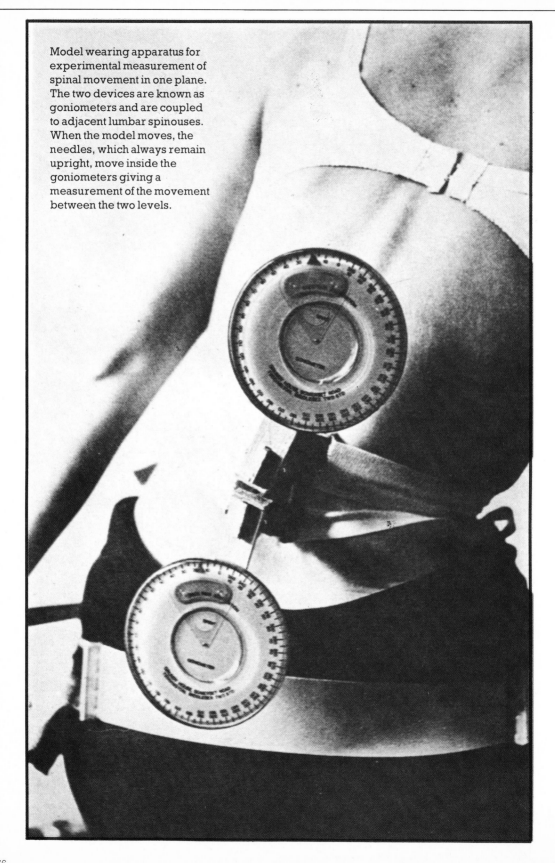

Model wearing apparatus for experimental measurement of spinal movement in one plane. The two devices are known as goniometers and are coupled to adjacent lumbar spinouses. When the model moves, the needles, which always remain upright, move inside the goniometers giving a measurement of the movement between the two levels.

Chiropractic

however, select techniques for the needs of individual patients, and the difference may be small. But we can easily imagine from history how group cohesion kept them apart. Not surprisingly, differences in nomenclature, especially as regards treatment methods, are at the focus of the division, and the situation is complicated by the heterogeneity of osteopathic organizations. The only certain difference is that chiropractors are more likely to make use of diagnostic X-rays than are osteopaths.

Evolution of Chiropractic

In general, the chiropractic discipline has become more scientifically orientated with the passage of time. Its colleges require over 4,000 hours of full-time training before a qualification is granted and by and large, its research reflects the Cartesian attitude of critical doubt. Increasingly it is becoming state-licensed and included in health insurance schemes. Yet it remains distinctly unorthodox. The reasons are complex; it has almost traditionally been at odds with orthodox medicine, particularly in the United States, and the loss of identity of osteopaths after their recognition there has had a profound effect. But there are perhaps other reasons. The efficiency of the service is served, to a large extent, by its remaining uninstitutionalized; furthermore, it tends to give at least as much attention to what is relevant in health care as to what is statistically significant. In this way, chiropractic patients are perhaps more often encouraged to take a critical interest in their own conditions than those under orthodox care. R. L. Kane and co-workers researching the practice in Utah, associated the high level of patient satisfaction with a more egalitarian practitioner-patient relationship than in conventional medicine. Chiropractic may have dispensed with a certain amount of Aesculapian authority in favour of the freedom to implicitly oppose what Ivan Illich has termed "social iatrogenesis", the self-imposed ill health of a society which is dominated by industrial technology, drug over-use and at times a pathetic dependence on monopolistic medical care.

Conclusion

Like many forms of unorthodox practice, the future for chiropractic seems exciting. For while chiropractors are striving for greater knowledge, there is evidence that their point of view is being taken more seriously, and sympathetically by the establishment. A meeting of minds seems inevitable and this has already begun with dialogue initiated by the United States Department of Health Education and Welfare through the National Institute for Neurological Diseases and Stroke (NINDS). In Britain, the Society for Back Pain Research numbers both chiropractors and non-medical osteopaths among its members, so that all who are prepared to do scientific research and submit their results to criticism may participate. Barriers to progress, however, remain substantial. Chiropractors tend to mistrust the therapeutic nihilism which orthodoxy seems prone to adopt in approaching the treatment of common locomotor complaints. Orthodox workers, on the other hand, have only scant access as yet to modern chiropractic theory and tend to be more familiar with its original form which was, and remains, scientifically untenable. Moreover, all groups have their own terminology.

It is humbling to recall Hippocrates' warning "You can discover no weight, no form nor calculation to which to refer your judgement of health and sickness. In the medical arts there exists no certainty except in the physician's senses". But if unorthodox medicine is to give its best, humility will be an essential ingredient.

Alan C. Breen

Doctors of Chiropractic per head of population (1976)

USA	1: 13,060
Canada	1: 20,277
New Zealand	1: 44,700
Denmark	1: 46,875
Australia	1: 56,000
Switzerland	1: 74,324
Norway	1: 81,395
Belgium	1:125,000
Sweden	1:336,957
France	1:516,670
United Kingdom	1:635,542

From Wight, J.G. et al. 'Contact', 1976

Some of the material in this article appeared originally in Mims *magazine (Vol. 2, 1 March 1978) and is reproduced by kind permission of the Publishers.*

Impact Therapy

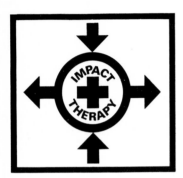

The symbol of Impact Therapy shows the basic principles of mechanics which the method uses. Any force meeting resistance causes pressure (+) which expresses itself laterally – at right angles to the opposing forces. An example is the soft rubber which when pressed between finger and thumb expands from the centre.

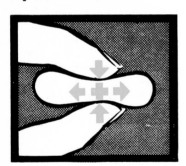

Impact Therapy is a safe and painless pressure wave treatment for the mobilization of joints, for the relief of pain, stiffness, tenderness and congestion in and around joints, in tendon sheaths and in muscles. Both osteoarthrosis and rheumatoid arthritis have responded to this treatment and in addition, many vague residual symptoms in complicated joints that resist every other form of treatment have been relieved by a progressive analytical form of impact therapy.

When a piece of rubber is pressed between finger and thumb, it spreads out from the centre of a compressed area and returns to its original shape, due to elasticity, on release of the pressure. In the same way, when the soft tissues of a limb including a joint are compressed between sand bags, and this pressure is emphasized by an impact wave, they likewise spread out from the centre, causing minimal but appreciable distraction at the joint. Such pressure waves have a cumulative effect due to the tendency of all living structures to return to the normal anatomical alignment. This is the extrinsic effect of Impact Therapy: mobilization by realignment.

Injury or arthritis may cause irregularities in the lining of a joint which may be built up by one other phase movement, causing locking or clicking. Distraction at the moment of locking or clicking will allow the irregularity to flatten and so restore or increase the range of the movement, as in the action of Mobile Impact Therapy. This is the intrinsic effect of impact therapy.

Impact Therapy also has vascular effects. Even pressure over the damaged part of a limb, including normal tissues, will encourage the drainage of fluid products of injury from the damaged area into the normal circulation of the surrounding tissues. Repeated pressure waves cause a pumping action and promote drainage, thereby reducing swelling and tension.

The method of Impact Therapy is simple enough to make it possible for every doctor to practise it in his surgery. On a firm base is placed a soft sand bag. The disabled part is embedded into this, so that it closely fits and evenly supports the whole of the underside. A second soft sand bag is placed on top to complete the protection and buffering above and on either side. A third half-filled heavy sand bag is raised and lowered on top of the second sand bag with a tamping action. On impact this causes a pressure wave which gives the name to the method. The disabled part, fully and firmly supported, and painless under heavy hand pressure, is now ready for treatment.

There are three basic forms of Impact Therapy: Static, Mobile and Spinal. In Static therapy the joint is kept motionless during treatment. The impact bag is gripped firmly by the ears, placed on top of the buffer bag and raised and lowered rhythmically at 100–120 beats a minute, until it progressively reaches a rise and fall with a clearance of from nothing to 3–6 inches. The force of the falling sand bag is converted on impact into a pressure wave which passes through the joint and into its surroundings. A succession of, say, 20–30 such waves effects a reduction of pain and swelling and a mechanical readjustment of displaced parts, which shows itself as a mobilization of the joint.

Mobile Impact Therapy is similarly performed but requires the use of loosely-filled millet-seed bags to allow the joint to be moved during therapy. Each movement of the joint is taken by the patient through a pain-free phase to the point where pain is just experienced and then back again repeatedly, (say, six times) until the tolerance limit on reassessment is found to be considerably increased.

Spinal Impact Therapy requires especially heavy buffering and soft impact force to be both safe and effective. Lighter, sharper rise and fall in pressure waves would give rise to headaches and should not be used. With experience, the greatest demonstrable effect is seen in the

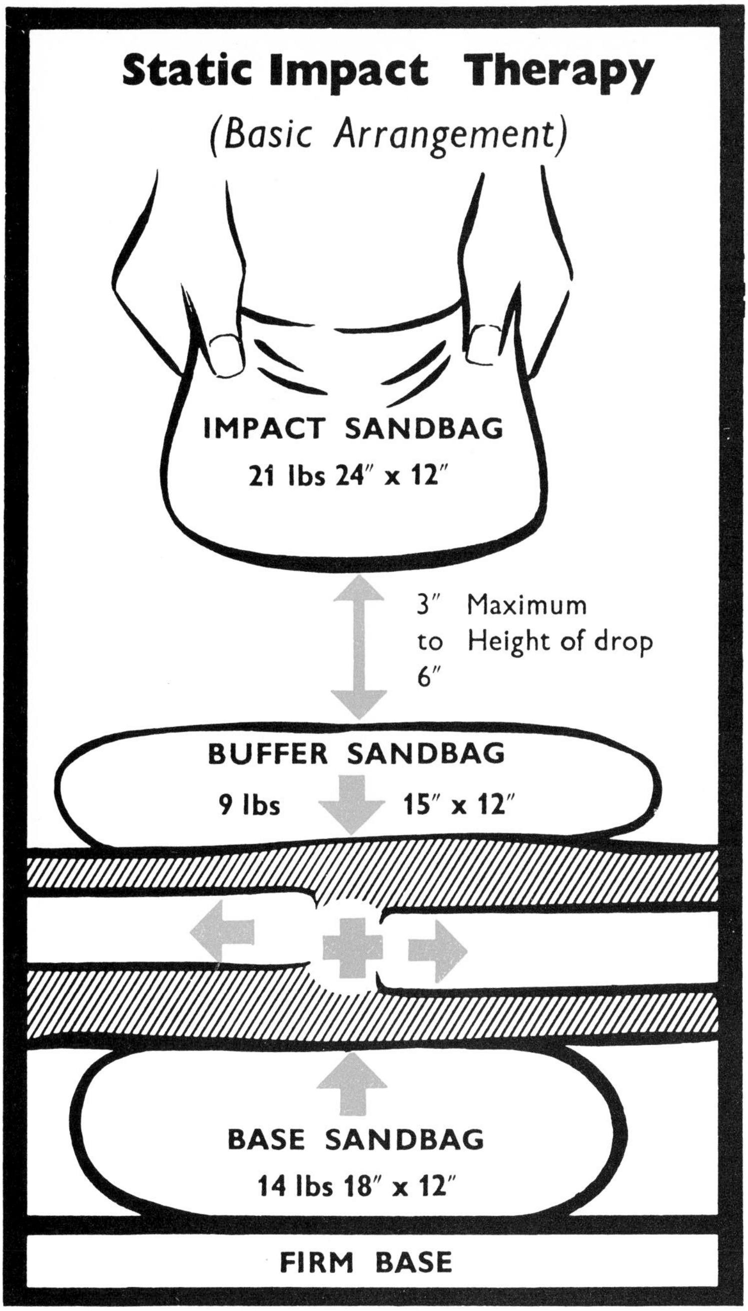

Impact Therapy

Static Impact Therapy
(Basic Arrangement)

IMPACT SANDBAG
21 lbs 24″ x 12″

3″ Maximum
to Height of drop
6″

BUFFER SANDBAG
9 lbs   15″ x 12″

BASE SANDBAG
14 lbs 18″ x 12″

FIRM BASE

The basic method of Impact Therapy showing the weights and sizes of the various sand bags. The forces of the buffer and base sand bag tend to press the enclosed limb outwards from the centre. This action is built up, in Impact Therapy, by a painless pressure wave from the soft impact of a third sand bag falling from a height increasing from zero to 3–6 inches over the centre of the joint. This causes a powerful momentary axial distraction, which, in a disordered joint allows the natural tendency of displaced parts always to return into anatomical alignment, to take place. The cumulative effect of a succession of such distractions at 100–120 beats per minute corrects the displacement, and restores painless mobility.

mobile cervical region, where the relief of 'stiff neck', cervical disc lesions and brachial neuritis can be painless and most dramatic, together with the cure of occipital headache and vertigo arising from cervical tension.

In summary, Impact Therapy is a contribution to physical medicine which has been designed to retain a simplicity which makes it applicable in the home, in the surgery, and in the wards and physiotherapy departments of hospitals. It is painless, safe, and immediately effective, and offers the advantages of economy of time and expense in the rehabilitation of a wide range of physical disabilities.

J. B. Tracey

Some of the material in this article appeared originally in The Practitioner *and is reproduced by kind permission of the Publishers.*

Rolfing

This schematic outline, which is of a child with whom Ida Rolf worked, has become the symbol of rolfing. The segments of the child's body are enclosed in blocks and indicate the relation of these segments to each other in the field of gravity before and after her work with the child.

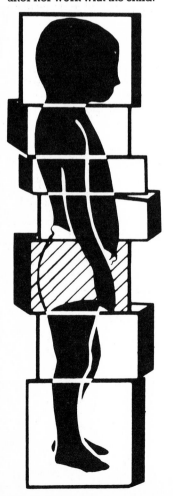

Rolfing was developed by Ida Rolf in the 1930s in the United States, but much of its fame was only achieved in the 1960s with the rise of the humanistic growth movement centred around the Esalen Institute, Big Sur, California. Sometimes known as structural processing, structural integration, postural release or structural dynamics, it is a method of very deep massage, in which the rolfer manipulates the body in order to return it to a normal structural or postural position. The method draws principally upon the work of Wilhelm Reich and Moshe Feldenkrais and consequently rolfing is not simply a physical massage, but an increasingly deepening technique of freeing the body and also the mind and emotions, from their conditioning. Emotional and psychological ways of relating to the world and other people are reflected physically in the body; the body, and particularly muscular imbalance, can be a shield or armouring, protecting a person both from the emotional discomforts of life as well as from conscious experience of the deep, inner hurts that have accumulated throughout life. These armourings or regions of tension by their pull on the body cause distortion, a limitation of movement and rigidity. Thus the body's attitudes reflect mental and emotional attitudes, and the relation between our bodies and our minds is represented as one problem, not two. We are a unity in response to all that has happened to us, not two separate entities responding separately to various influences.

This realization is at the core of all the body/mind therapies currently in use in the West, including rolfing, but it is a realization long familiar in the East.

A further concept important in rolfing is that of the influence of gravity, for the distortions of the body that occur throughout life are accentuated by gravity. Therapy, then, must ensure that ultimately a patient's posture is correctly aligned with the earth's gravity field. "Gravity not only upholds a man, it feeds him . . . thus in an erect man it should be possible to draw a straight line through the ears (bisecting the external meatus), the shoulder (head of the humorus), hip-bone (head of the femur), knee and ankle (external malleolus)." (Ida Rolf). Modern sub-atomic physical research has shown that all 'materializations', including man of course, are impermanent actualizations of forces, here one second and gone the next and then re-appearing. We are simply the result of spiral forces acting upon us. The apparent separation of mind from body and emotion is only, for us with our limited vision, a necessary convenience for descriptive purposes. We are indeed an inseparable whole. The physical work of rolfing by acting on the body at a deep level necessarily prompts reactions in the mind. Energies locked up in armour and defence mechanisms are freed for living and with this freedom there comes concurrent insight into all the fears and inhibitions which have so narrowed down our responses.

Rolfing helps an individual to be balanced and thus free amongst the forces of gravity acting upon him. He is supported by them rather than bent under them. He becomes a living force again; his potential is naturally increased and he is no longer bound by hate, fear, jealousy and similar negative emotions.

The practice of rolfing involves both the loosening and lengthening of specific muscles and fascia. This latter is the thin envelope of connective tissue which houses the structures of the body, including muscles and tendons, lymph nodes, ligaments, nerves and so on. Fascia is the unifying organ of the body and any distortion of it, such as by shortening or thickening, also distorts the whole body. Loosening of the fascia and muscle leads to a repositioning of the muscle fibres and a migration back to their natural position. As a result, by manipulation of the fascia, the whole body can be radically altered. Granted a

Rolfing

freedom of response, the body will naturally revert to its optimum function. Bony malalignments which may have been distorted by previous accidents or illness, by the pressure of fear and other conditioning, will, when the soft tissues, muscles and fascia have been freed also resume as far as possible their normal relationships. Rolfing can perhaps be likened to rebuilding a sagging or bulging wall, rather than trying to prop it up by artificial means.

A course of rolfing usually entails ten sessions over five to ten weeks. The first seven sessions attempt to remove ingrained stress patterns, postures and old ways of bodily relating to the world. More particularly, the first three sessions are concentrated primarily on freeing fascia, while subsequent sessions are more concerned with freeing specific muscles and fascia.

The first session is aimed at opening up breathing throughout the chest areas, unlocking the hips, loosening the outer fascial layers of the body and freeing the muscles in the area of the rib cage to improve the breathing, with a little additional work on the legs in preparation for the second and subsequent sessions. The second session concentrates on the feet and ankles. The importance of the feet psychologically, is to ground the patient, to get him in touch with reality and gravity. Successful foot-work can make a tremendous difference, both literally and metaphorically, to how a person stands in the world.

The goal of the last three sessions of rolfing is to integrate the newly loosened and flowing body into new patterns of movement, by manipulating the layers of fascia in the appropriate directions. ''The unique aim of rolfing is to serve the inner dynamics of the flesh that tend toward the fullness of bodily function in relation to the earth's field. The goal is not 'openness', but freedom of choice''. (Don Johnson). Ida Rolf has said that if the first seven sessions are largely a matter of technique, then the last three can be considered as art.

From the beginning, it is necessary for the therapist to be aware of the attitudes of mind and emotion which the set of the patient's body reveals. As the work proceeds deeper and deeper, so will tensions and resistances become more apparent and it becomes increasingly important for the patient to realize the inherent nature of these 'blocks'. The therapist will point them out and try to dissolve them with his hands. It is however, the patient with his increasing self-awareness who will truly experience the various conflicts within him of which he was previously ignorant. Forces of consciousness which were bound up and fixed in the attitudes held by the patient as childhood defences against pain, fear and disappointments, will virtually unprompted, other than by this freeing of the body's energies, find welcome expression and thus permanent release. Through this therapy a man can move from stereotypy through autonomy to spontaneity.

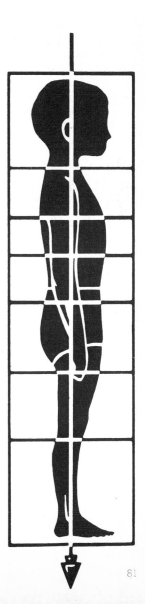

© 1958 Ida P. Rolf.

Manipulative Therapy

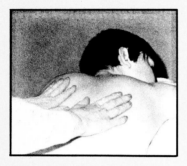

A therapist employing *effleurage* (palmar stroking) technique over the entire back in order to improve circulation and induce relaxation in major muscle areas; at the same time the trained fingers of the therapist carefully palpate for sensitive areas in the muscle tissue.

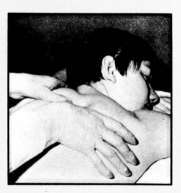

Deep thumb frictions alongside the vertebral column ease the stress on muscular and ligament attachments to the spine and further help to induce a general relaxation of the patient. Tender areas are noted for special attention later in the treatment.

Massage may well lay claim to be the oldest form of medicine known to man. Even the derivation of the word 'massage' is lost in obscurity. Some consider it to be derived from the French word *masser*, meaning 'to shampoo', whilst others consider that it owes its origin to the Greek *massein* meaning 'to knead', or to the Arabic *mas'h* which means 'to press softly'. Perhaps we should settle for the Greek source, and assume that the English and French words have the same derivation.

Notwithstanding the fact that in the ancient works of Kung Fu there are references to the Chinese system of massage about 3,000 BC, we have evidence of the emergence of massage as a therapy in the Western world from the early records of the Greeks. Hippocrates preached the benefits of massage in his teachings: "hard rubbing binds, much rubbing causes parts to waste and moderate rubbing makes them grow". He also tells us that "rubbing can bind a joint that is too loose and loosen a joint that is too rigid" – a reference to the therapeutic benefits of massage.

Homer wrote in *The Odyssey* about the beautiful Greek women who rubbed and anointed the returning war heroes to rest and refresh them. The Greek physician, Asclepiades, employed massage combined with active exercises during his treatments. Gymnasia were prominent therapeutic and cultural centres throughout the cities of Greece and, of course, the Greek Games were frequent and popular events which called for the anointing of the body with oils and powders.

The Romans too, left plenty of evidence of their uses of massage. Julius Caeser used to be pinched daily as a means of treating neuralgia. The Roman physician Celsus wrote that, "chronic pains in the head are relieved by rubbing the head itself" and "a paralysed limb is strengthened by rubbing". The Emperor Hadrian saw an old soldier rubbing himself against a wall at the Baths and promptly gave him two slaves to do the rubbing for him. When others tried the same approach the following day, Hadrian wasn't inclined to give more slaves away, and instead directed that the old men rub one another!

The name of Galen stands far superior to those of his Roman contemporaries, for no one did more to establish a scientific application of massage. He urged its use in treatment of injuries and in the preparation of gladiators for combat in the arena.

As very little is known of progress in any field of medicine between the period of the decline of the Roman Empire and the early Middle Ages in Europe, it is some centuries later that we find evidence of further research into the therapeutic benefits of massage. The Frenchman, Ambroise Pare, described friction massage and praised the healing properties of massage in stiff and injured joints. Early in the nineteenth century, a Swedish professor, Peter Henry Ling, established his school at Stockholm for the teaching of massage and remedial gymnastics, and to this day the term 'Swedish Massage' is used in tribute to Ling to denote the therapeutic application of massage as opposed to the vigorous body pummelling employed at the Turkish baths, etc. At the same time as Ling was establishing massage in Sweden, his contemporary Metzger was doing similar work and research in Holland.

Massage had now become a remedial science. It was introduced to the United States in 1877 by Dr S. W. Mitchell. In 1894, in Britain, a group of women formed the first professional organization, the Society of Trained Masseuses. By 1920, several other groups of masseurs and masseuses were in existence and several excellent textbooks on massage were published around that time. Also, by 1920, schools for massage were to be found in the major cities throughout Britain. The Northern Institute of Massage, established in 1924, survived the changing trends of the past half-century, and still exists today with a busy intake of students for training in therapeutic massage.

With the introduction of electrical treatments, the application of massage began to diminish in the orthodox medical hospitals and to disappear gradually from the teachings of the physiotherapy schools. Physiotherapy in the orthodox hospital service today has consequently now developed along such widely differing paths from its cradling in massage that it virtually represents a different profession altogether, with the emphasis on electrotherapy and group exercise therapy. It has been left to the hard core of masseurs in the unorthodox spheres of medicine to further the proven remedial and therapeutic effects of the laying on of hands, and to such practitioners who consider electro-therapy as a supplement rather than an alternative to massage. The trend appears to be for such therapists to leave the designation 'phy-siotherapist' to the 'new' profession, and to classify themselves more as 'physical therapists', 'remedial masseurs', or 'manipulative thera-pists'.

Manipulative therapy is so akin to the original concept of remedial massage as to be almost inseparable. The development of soft-tissue manipulative techniques invariably leads at an advanced level to the manipulation of the joints of the body, and to a skilled and sensitive touch of the trained therapist.

Whilst manipulative therapy embraces both the techniques of osteopathy and chiropractic, the manipulative therapist does not necessarily subscribe to their theories or philosophies – 'the rule of the artery' or 'the interference to nerve supply'. Like these more recent therapies, manipulative therapy has developed from the 'bone-setters' of yesteryear, but the manipulative therapist regards his work predominantly as physical, not organic, medicine, with the emphasis on the treatment of the joints of the body for physical improvement. Consequently, trained manipulative therapists have earned a great deal of respect from the orthodox medical practitioner over the years, and are not quite so unconventional in their beliefs as their osteopath or chiropractor colleagues. The manipulative therapist regards mani-pulation as being an adjunct to massage, the major part of his therapy being one of remedial massage and resorting to manipulation only when absolutely necessary in the treatment. He sees little point in manipulation without massage itself being the prime therapy. Manipu-lative therapists therefore practise in the sphere of massage, manipu-lation and electrotherapy, rather than specifically manipulation.

K. Woodward

Manipulative Therapy

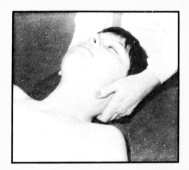

Gentle manual traction (stretching) of the neck muscles helps to ease the tension and remove the postural stress factor from this area of the body; the therapist's sensitive fingers again friction around the muscular attachments of the neck and head.

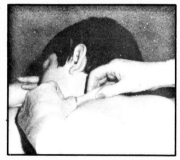

Skin rolling followed by other *pétrissage* ('picking-up') techniques such as wringing and kneading, gently manipulate the soft tissues of

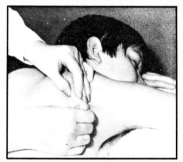

the upper back, shoulder and neck muscles, improving arterial nourishment and assisting lymphatic and venous drainage.

Touch for Health

The concept of Touch for Health is preventive medicine at work in the truest sense. As a course, has been devised specifically for lay people interested in preventive health care, by a group of chiropractic doctors in the United States.

Based on the now widely used principles of applied kinesiology, it brings the simple system of muscle testing used by professional therapists to the home environment. It provides a very effective way of reaching out to other human beings in a spirit of service, to help them feel fitter and bring relief from distressing symptoms.

Touch for Health is a means of diagnosing and relieving not specific illnesses, but imbalances of any kind in the body energy systems. Ancient Oriental understanding of vital life forces can be illustrated dramatically using muscle tests. Anyone can learn to check each of the twelve major body systems, stomach, lungs, pancreas, etc, by testing the related muscles, which if found to be weak, will respond to appropriate therapy on one or more reflex points – become strengthened – sending a surge of life-giving energy where it is most needed. The testing procedure eliminates guesswork, as the body reveals its own weaknesses.

For instance, if a muscle related to the stomach meridian is tested and found to be weak, it could indicate a nutritional deficiency. Astonishingly, if some food, or a dietary supplement containing the nutrient the body needs, is placed in the mouth whilst the muscle is retested, it will immediately be stronger. If the weakness is due to some other energy imbalance, the food substance would have no effect. On the other hand, if the muscle tested strong in the first instance, and a substance harmful to the body, such as white sugar or instant coffee, is placed on the tongue, the strong muscle instantly becomes weakened. Through Touch for Health and applied kinesiology, we can ask the body individually whether it welcomes any given substance or not.

When someone has backache, tests may reveal a weakness in the abdominal muscles, or in those of the pelvis. After application of one or more of the Touch for Health balancing techniques is completed, the previously weak muscles will test strong, and the pain invariably subsides. Another real benefit is the control of the debilitating effects of emotional stress. In many cases, having tested the related muscles, a

Muscle test of the *upper trapezius*, which is related to the function of eyes and ears and is governed by the kidney meridian.

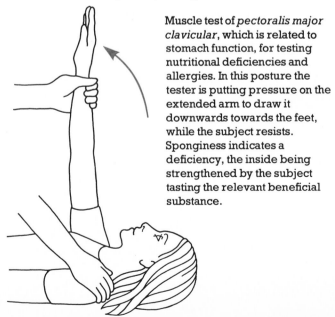

Muscle test of *pectoralis major clavicular*, which is related to stomach function, for testing nutritional deficiencies and allergies. In this posture the tester is putting pressure on the extended arm to draw it downwards towards the feet, while the subject resists. Sponginess indicates a deficiency, the inside being strengthened by the subject tasting the relevant beneficial substance.

Touch for Health

gentle application of the fingertips on the neurovascular points on the forehead whilst the person concentrates on the trauma for a few minutes will give great relief, and upon retesting, the muscle will be strong even though the trauma is being re-lived. This strengthens the individual's ability to cope with the situation in a calmer and more balanced frame of mind, and drastically reduces the need for tranquillizers.

Many people today studying aromatherapy, nutrition, reflexology, shiatsu, yoga, massage and other related therapies will find that Touch for Health provides a fascinating diagnostic means of evaluating the effectiveness of those treatments.

The best way to gain proficiency is to take a short instructional course, since the material only really comes alive in the light of practical experience under the guidance of a qualified instructor. Whilst the basic course does not qualify one to be a therapist, it does provide a sound foundation for the completely safe use of these techniques on family and friends. The use of applied kinesiological techniques associated with Touch for Health does not suggest in any way a cure for pathological conditions, but their regular use will act to stimulate the innate healing resources of the body towards radiant health.

Brian H. Butler

Skin Brushing

When we look at another person, what we see is literally dead tissue, for the surface of the skin is entirely dessicated – dead tissue in the process of flaking away. As the cells in the lower epidermal layers are renewed and push outwards, so the uppermost layers of skin die; the only exception is the sclera covering the eye-ball which is kept constantly moist through the action of blinking.

It is not generally realized, however, that the skin is the largest functioning organ we possess; it is an organ of elimination and is no less important than the other organs of elimination – lungs, kidneys, colon and so on. The skin is constantly disposing of poisonous wastes through the pores, irrespective of whether or not the body is sweating.

Primitive man, in his daily activities of exploring and food gathering was continually having his skin brushed by shrubs, branches and long grasses – even the wind would have ensured that the dead cells were constantly removed from the surface of his skin. Clearly, with the multiple layers of clothing that modern man wears, as well as the oils and powders with which he clogs the pores of his skin, we run the risk of trapping the body's waste products.

While it is helpful not to wear clothing in bed and so allow the skin to function properly for eight hours a day, a more effective solution is to give the skin a good stiff brushing regularly. In Australia and America one can purchase a skin brush with a long detachable handle similar to a bath brush, but with firmer bristles. Such brushes are not available in Britain however, although an adequate substitute is a dog brush from any pet shop.

For the first four or five sessions, brush the skin lightly all over, starting at the face and neck, stroking in a downward direction only; subsequently one can brush more vigorously in all directions. It must be emphasized that for the best results, the skin must be dry – not damp or sweaty. One can actually see the effect of skin brushing by standing at a window in a sunny position, putting one foot up on a chair and brushing the leg lightly in an upward direction. The sunlight will illuminate the thousands of tiny flakes of dead tissue. Scrubbing oneself with a loofah or rough cloth while in the bath is a very poor substitute.

H. W. Williams

The Bates Method of Eyesight Training

Dr W. H. Bates was a successful and distinguished American opthalmologist practising in New York at the beginning of the century. One thing bothered him. Although most of his patients were responding favourably to treatment, many of them continued to complain of headaches and a sense of eyestrain. He was also perturbed by the fact that the majority had to have their prescriptions for glasses regularly strengthened.

One day, sitting in his office relaxing after a series of lengthy consultations, he took off his glasses and wearily leaning his head in his hands, covered his eyes. After ten minutes or so, and feeling refreshed by the silence and the dark, he removed his hands and immediately became aware that the colours and objects in the room seemed brighter and clearer than they were before. At that moment the whole idea behind the Bates Method of Eyesight Training, as it exists today, sprang into being.

The Bates Method was developed simply to teach people to use their eyes in a relaxed and easy manner. Its principal aim is to restore the natural habits of seeing that are lost whenever strain and tension are present. The most important thing to remember about the art of seeing (an art, in the sense that it is half gift and half acquired) is that proper vision cannot be commanded or forced; it must, as it were, just happen. Sight is one of the five senses – vision is pure sensation.

As with other senses – hearing, feeling, tasting and smelling – the brain interprets the data that is presented to it by the organs of sight without the intervention of intellect. What conditions and determines the accuracy or otherwise of that interpretation however, is the quality and intensity of the attention we pay to whatever we are looking at, tasting, smelling or hearing. Attention is the key. It must always flow outward in one direction, embracing its object without distraction, thus allowing the brain to interpret successfully. In the case of vision, it is a matter of being mentally quiet and letting sight come. Except where the eye itself is diseased or has suffered injury, almost all defects of vision (such as near sight and far sight) can be traced to the neglect or disregard of this principal, which the Bates Method is designed to instil and to foster.

Surprisingly perhaps, the most valuable single habit to cultivate is one that almost everyone thinks he already has – the simple act of blinking. Everyone does it of course, but not often enough. This is nature's own way of lubricating the eyes. It counteracts the harmful effect of staring, of keeping the eyes fixed for any length of time focused or unfocused on one particular object, so creating strain. One should purposely blink far more often than seems necessary during the day, until it becomes automatic. A good idea is to practise 'butterfly' blinking which, as the name implies, is a light and rapid fluttering of the eyelids. For obvious reasons, it is wiser to perform this exercise within four walls and preferably at home.

When the eyes are tired, there is nothing more helpful than to palm. This is the name given to the act of 'palming', which is second only to blinking as an aid to relaxed and easy vision. It should be done for short periods and as frequently as possible. It rests the mind as well as the eyes and is therefore doubly beneficial. The method is as follows: cover the closed eyes with the cupped palms of both hands, taking care that no part of the hand should actually touch or press upon the eyeball. The elbows should be resting on a desk or table with the head supported easily on the cushion of the palms. When performing this exercise, it is important that the mind should not be allowed to wander. Think about, but do not concentrate on, some pleasant past or anticipated experience – a holiday in some beautiful place, or an idyllic scene from a book you have read. Alternatively, palm to the

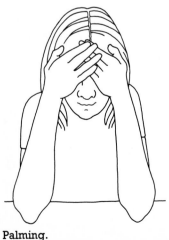

Palming.

The Bates Method of Eyesight Training

sound of music, or to a talk or play on the radio. It is important to palm for as long as possible, and to get real benefit. at least ten minutes should be devoted to the exercise.

Another useful means of relaxing and restoring the eyes is to splash them alternately with warm and cold water. This should be done twice daily using a sequence of twenty splashes for each eye (with closed lids). On rising in the morning, splash them first with fairly hot water and then with cold; last thing at night, reverse the sequence – first with cold and then with hot water. The effect of this is to stimulate the circulation in and around the eyes and to relieve congestion.

A different kind of exercise altogether is needed to strengthen the muscles and to improve the functioning of the eyes. One of the best exercises is, as usual, the simplest. It consists of constantly and deliberately changing focus from near to far, whatever one is doing, throughout the day. Walking, sitting down, working or eating, one should look at and blink at objects alternately close and at a distance; to keep the eye fixed for any length of time in one focus is extremely tiring and a source of strain. When driving, for instance, one should shift one's attention regularly from beyond the windscreen to the inside of the car, focusing mainly on the road of course, but glancing from time to time at the instruments on the dashboard or looking into the driving mirror. For people who spend much of their time in a car, this is an invaluable exercise.

Contrary to common belief, strong sunshine and bright light are generally beneficial to the eyes. The practice of wearing dark glasses in all kinds of weather, indoors and out, can be very harmful, and result in photophobia – a neurotic fear of light – and a gradual weakening of the optic nerves. A 'sunning' drill, favoured by teachers of the Bates Method is as follows: sit facing the sun with the eyes closed, and slowly turn the head from left to right, brushing across the sunlight. Allow the light to seep, as it were, through the closed eyelids. Do not attempt to open the eyes, but feel the pleasant sensation of warmth as the face is turned from side to side. After two minutes, stop and palm until all the different colours that seem to bloom in the darkness fade and disappear. When this happens, quietly take your hands away and open your eyes. You will immediately notice how soothed and relaxed they feel and how much sharper your vision is.

These few techniques are only pointers, a few random suggestions as to how vision may be improved without mechanical aids or recourse to medicine. There is nothing arcane about the Bates Method for it follows the rules of nature itself, and is based on a single premise that can best and perhaps most memorably be expressed in the words of a song from a famous American musical of the 1950s, "Doing what comes naturally".

Michael Ronan

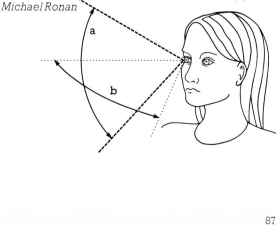

Moving the eyes up and down (a) and from side to side (b).

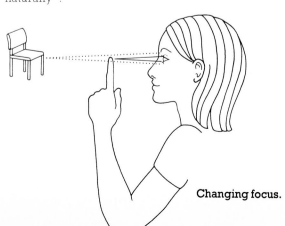

Changing focus.

Heat

Blood both conveys nutrients from the stomach to the tissues, and waste matter from the tissues to the excretory organs. It also serves the purpose of maintaining normal body temperature by carrying surplus heat to the skin surface, where it is dissipated by conduction, radiation and evaporation. Nine-tenths of the heat loss from the body occurs from the skin. One-seventh of this heat loss is due to evaporation; sweating increases the heat loss. The chemical composition of sweat is similar to that of urine, except that sweat is more diluted with water. The skin, therefore, is an important organ for both heat regulation and elimination of waste products from the body.

The thermal effects of dry heat can be used to great advantage in the therapies discussed below. It is important to bear in mind, however, that hyperaemia induced by dry heat must be terminated by a quick cold douche at the end of the treatment so that the natural forces of action and reaction come into play and total circulation is both balanced and stimulated.

Sauna Baths

The sauna bath combines the best features of the moist Russian bath and the early, dry, Roman bath. Like the 'sweat lodge' of the Indian tribes on plains of the western United States, which was a place for both physical and spiritual purification, the sauna has always been a communal meeting place – for physical purification at least.

Saunas are invariably built of wood and consist of a small to medium-sized room with benches set at different heights around the walls; the higher benches are those where the heat is most intense. Heat for the bath is supplied from heated stones or rocks inside the sauna room itself. The ideal temperature for the bath is between 190°F and 200°F; when water is poured onto the stones to create a moist atmosphere, however, temperatures up to 289°F can be withstood by

Sauna room in Karhunpesä, Finland.

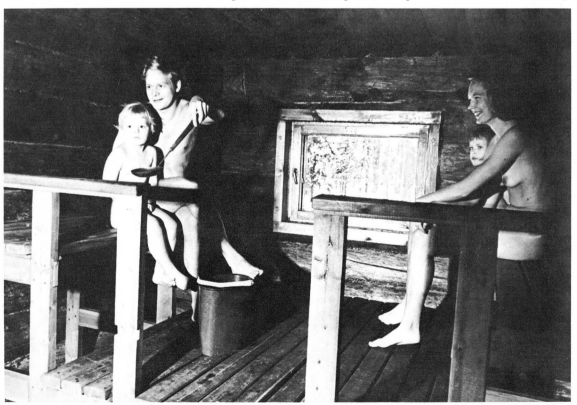

Heat

the body. Ideally, the sauna should be used in three phases: an initial dry heat, which causes a copious perspiration to cleanse the skin, followed by the addition of water to the hot stones to create a hot, moist atmosphere which tones up the whole body, and a final wash or shower in cold water. The moist phase of the sauna is useful for skin diseases, rheumatism and the early stages of catarrh of the nose, throat or respiratory organs. The sauna is not recommended for acute inflammation of the eyes or nose, in angina, or in persons who suffer from high or variable blood pressure. In general, the sauna is useful for obesity, for making the limbs supple and to assist sleep.

The true Finnish sauna also entails 'whisking' of the skin with birch leaves to further tone the skin, followed by a plunge into icy water.

Hot Blanket

This form of therapy is normally supplied by specially made electric blankets. The blanket is usually large enough to completely envelop the body, with increased effects obtained by wrapping the patient in a large plastic sheet before being encased in the blanket. It is a form of dry heat which can be applied with great success in cases of obesity, rheumatic ailments, arthritic conditions and similar conditions. Profuse sweating is possible in hot blankets. By applying cold towels (or iced pads) to the head and neck it is possible to some extent to reduce discomfort, decrease the effect of increased temperature on the brain and heart and lengthen the duration of the treatment.

A less drastic measure is to completely wrap the patient in dry blankets to cause an accumulation of body heat and lessen heat elimination. Hot water bottles can be used to increase the thermal effect and induce perspiration. This is a form of hot blanket pack. Hot, dry sand can be used for the same purpose.

Hot blankets are of great benefit in chronic rheumatism and afflictions of the neuro-muscular system. The hot blanket pack differs from the wet sheet pack in that it is an excitant measure, whereas the wet sheet pack is primarily sedative.

Infra-red

Normal visible light consists of electromagnetic radiation of wavelengths between 4,000 and 7,500 Å (Angström unit). Longer wavelengths, beyond the red end of the visible spectrum, are known as infra-red and are those wavelengths which carry heat.

Every substance emits infra-red rays as soon as its temperature is raised above absolute zero. However, an object can only receive infra-red rays from something hotter than itself. There are two types of infra-red in general use. One is a luminous type with a coiled tungsten filament within a glass tube, which generates invisible infra-red along with a proportion of visible red and yellow radiation, while the other is a porcelain embedded dark emitter generating invisible infra-red rays only. Any hot body, however, emits infra-red radiation and an ordinary electric fire – particularly a bowl-shaped fire – is a good source of infra-red radiation. Infra-red rays produce hyperaemia – vasodilation and a local rise of temperature deeply within the subcutaneous tissues of the irradiated area. By creating local or general hyperaemia, infra-red treatment is a good preparation for ultra-violet irradiation, while both can be used simultaneously to increase the effectiveness of the ultra-violet rays.

With the luminous type of infra-red, it may be necessary, especially in the case of the fair-skinned person to take precautions against overheating of the skin. Application of sunflower or some other oil, or lanolin to the skin, can be used as a precautionary measure. In all cases, if the face is being irradiated, the eyes should be protected.

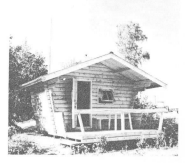

A typical Finnish log-built sauna house.

Heat

General treatment of the whole body surface with infra-red promotes circulation and excretion via the skin. A general infra-red irradiation reduces the red corpuscles of the blood, diminishes the calcium content of the body and increases the output of urea. General treatment by infra-red is invaluable in cases of rheumatism and allied complaints, while local treatment is advocated for lumbago, nephritis, gall-bladder inflammation and in most acute conditions of pain and injury, though not all inflammatory states. Victims of diabetes do not usually tolerate heat well and burn easily.

Locally, infra-red treatment can produce a blood temperature exceeding that of a high fever. Local circulation is increased by dilating the blood vessels and overcoming stasis thereby improving elimination. The distance between the area being treated and the equipment employed varies with personal sensitivity and the type of equipment used. The distance from the lamp should be not less than six inches with the length of treatment varying from fifteen minutes to an hour.

Radiant Heat

Radiant heat is usually given under a tunnel-shaped cabinet placed over a bed. The inner surface of the cabinet is lined with reflective material and three to four rows of electric light bulbs supply the heat. Such cabinets are also built for patients to sit in for exposure to heat and temperature of a very high degree. A dry temperature of around 200°F (93°C) can be endured without discomfort for fifteen minutes. All such submission to great heat must be terminated with a quick, cold bath or shower.

Radiant heat treatment is extremely beneficial for all muscular/skeletal complaints, sciatica and obesity. It would not be recommended for the very young, aged or enfeebled person and would be contraindicated in heart cases and hypertension. Where the thermal effects of infra-red or radiant heat are employed on extensive areas of the body it is always advisable to keep the head and neck cool with the aid of cold towels or ice pads.

Wax Baths

Wax baths are particularly useful in the treatment of all rheumatic aches and pains. It is especially adaptable for the treatment of arthritis in the hands and wrists. Paraffin wax with a melting point of around 115°F (46°C) is placed in a thermostatically controlled tank. The affected part is dipped in the molten wax some ten times until it is well coated. It is then wrapped in wax-proof paper in a plastic bag and draped in a towel for about twenty minutes. The wax is then painlessly removed and the treated part placed under running cold water for half a minute to a minute.

Where local treatment of arthritic hands and wrists is required, wax baths form a valuable medium. Wax is very inflammable and it should, therefore, always be heated in a double saucepan when being used in the home.

Alan Moyle

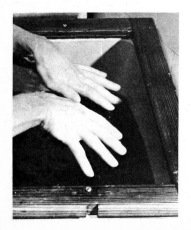

Wax bath treatment of the hands and wrists.

Radiant heat treatment. Note that the bed is positioned so that the patient's head projects from the heated cubicle.

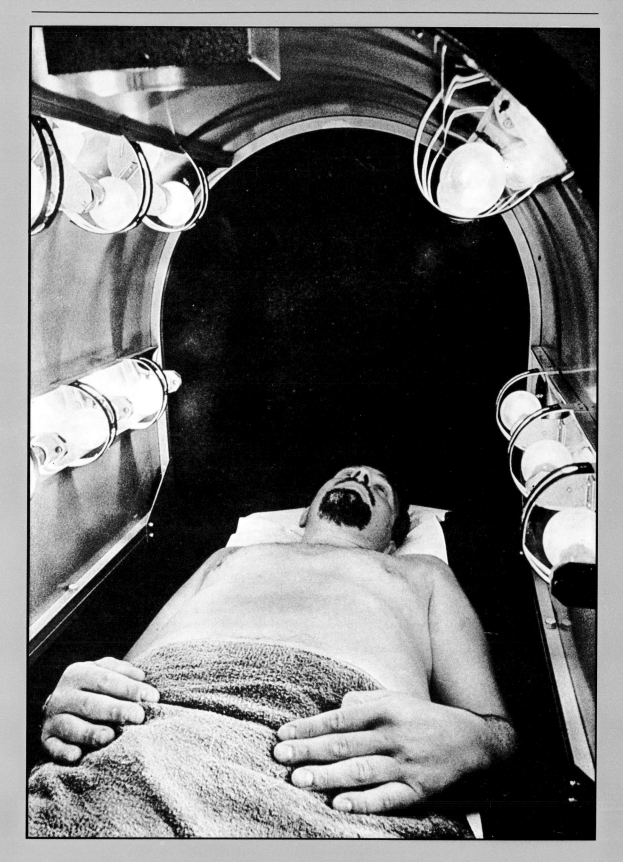

Air and Light

It is axiomatic that air is the most important nutritional factor in life, yet being blessed with a super-abundance of air, we take it for granted. Nevertheless, it is only possible to live for a few minutes without it. What is seldom realized is that most people have lost the ability to breathe properly; they have become shallow breathers, and this unfortunate practice condemns us to a life of oxygen deficiency, lack of vitality and high toxic threshold. The skin also plays a vital role in the respiratory process, and is sometimes referred to as the 'third lung'. The story of the small boy who was painted with gold-leaf at a carnival and thereafter died from respiratory failure is well known; yet most people totally disregard the importance of fresh air and a healthy skin by persistently closing all windows, breathing stale and polluted air, covering their skins with all kinds of chemical preparations and wearing many layers of thick clothing.

All of these factors are detrimental to health and cause people to become vulnerable to changes in temperature. Those who complain most about the cold are usually those who cannot tolerate the heat. In winter they wear thick clothing, yet are still cold; their dwellings are like hot-houses and they themselves frequently suffer from respiratory problems. Healthy people, on the other hand, wear little clothing and allow their bodies to be exposed to the air as much as possible. The air bath, in which the whole body is exposed to the air, is highly beneficial for the skin and for general health, but should be a regular activity and not an annual effort! In modern times it is normal for people to be scantily dressed on the beach and to expose most, if not all, of the body to the air and sunshine. This is good, for it was not so long ago that such activity would have been regarded as immoral – and still is by a small minority. Unfortunately, many people are still unable to avail themselves of this health-giving procedure, while for others it is possible for only a few days a year.

Breathing

Deep breathing is an integral part of healthy living for it charges the body with vitality as well as facilitating favourable oxygen tension in the blood and tissues. Orientals have known since antiquity that special breathing techniques are capable of bringing about the extraction of a certain energy from the air which the Indians term *prana* – yogic breathing is sometimes called *pranayama*. The main intake of prana is through the respiratory tract but it may also be assimilated in other ways. However, the quality of the energy absorbed probably differs, hence the extreme importance of breathing properly. In some areas of the world there is a high concentration of prana, particularly at the seaside, at high altitudes and in an abundance of sunshine. Sanatoria are almost always sited in these locations. Prana is an etheric force which is received, transmuted and transmitted to various parts of the body via the chakras which are centres or vortices of vibrant energy.

In general, deep breathing entails abdominal, thoracic and clavicular movement and all breathing should be nasal except in cases of extreme oxygen debt. In terms of Western physiological knowledge alone, nasal breathing is known to have a much more beneficial effect on lymphatic drainage than mouth breathing.

Opposite: Dr Rollier's Sun School in Switzerland.

The revolving solarium at Aix les Bains, France, designed by Dr Jean Saidman.

Sun Bath

The sun bath should, ideally, be taken early in the morning when the therapeutic effects of the sun's rays are at a maximum and adverse effects are at a minimum. In hotter climates, the patient is advised to begin with 10–15 minutes and work up to a maximum of 45 minutes. In countries where prolonged sunshine is rare, however, a sun-lamp may

Air and Light

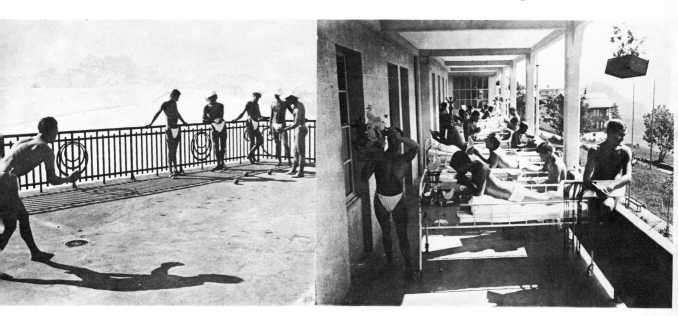

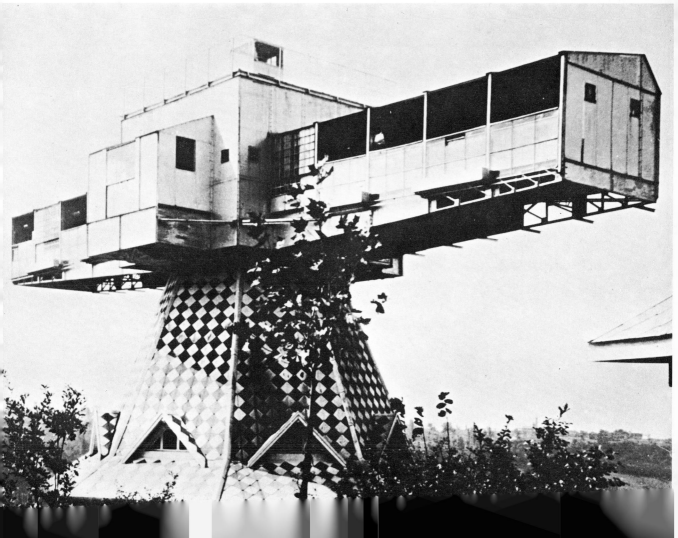

Air and Light

have to be employed, but although they can be used to deliver more accurate doses than with natural sunlight, they are never as good. The benefits of sun treatment are enhanced considerably by the concomitant use of hydrotherapy. A wet cloth is wrung out and placed over the body from neck to knees. The face should be shielded by two pieces of folded wet cloth placed over the eyes and mouth. The sun bath should be followed by a spinal bath.

Many other varieties of sun bath are used and local, diseased parts are often exposed to the sun. Water which has been exposed to direct sunlight is also beneficial and is said to contain etheric vitamins which are associated with negative ions. The air is always charged with both negative and positive ions, which are produced in abundance by cosmic radiation, sunlight, lightning, wind and in any place where water changes its physical state. Sometimes, climatic disturbances are heralded by the presence of excessive positive ions in the air, which can cause respiratory distress, headaches and depression. Negative ions have the opposite effect – increased well-being, easing of respiratory problems such as those of asthma and hay fever and acceleration of healing. It has been found that certain varieties of synthetic fibre increases the negative ions in ambient air and have even been known to benefit asthmatics and arthritics. Negative ion generators are sometimes used to give relief to patients with particular health problems.

Light

Light is the basis of life on this planet, and apart from its unique ability to promote photosynthesis, it also provides the energy for the transfer of electrons from water to other receptive substances. It is difficult to predict the long-term effects of artificial lighting on people, but it is highly probable that it is responsible for the earlier maturation of children that we see today. This is not unexpected, since light is thought to be absorbed through acupuncture points, from which energy is transmitted via the hypothalamus to the endocrine system.

A cubicle in the solarium at Aix les Bains. The beds are adjustable so that the sun's rays fall at right angles to the bed throughout the day. The rays are filtered in order that ultraviolet only reaches the body.

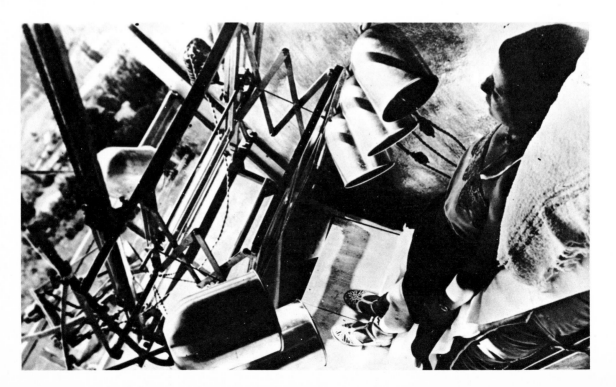

Air and Light

Ultra-violet Radiation

Ultra-violet radiation is that part of the sun's rays between 3,900 Å (the lowest range of visible light) and 136 Å, although the therapeutic portion does not appear to extend much below 2,000 Å. The longer the waves, the more penetrating they are, and those above 3,300 Å penetrate just below the deep epidermis, to be absorbed by the capillary blood. Very short waves are absorbed by the superficial epidermis which protects the underlying tissue from damaging rays of lower wavelengths. Ultra-violet therapy has, for some reason, lost much of its former popularity, but there is no doubt that, properly used, it can be of immense value. Its effects are:

1. Formation of vitamin D from cholesterol.
2. Improved resistance to infection.
3. Development of improved skin and muscle tone.
4. Improved skin functioning and amelioration of many dermatological conditions.
5. Improved calcium and phosphorus metabolism.
6. On blood, bringing about changes in cell-count, increased oxygenation, increased alkali reserve (hence a diminished tendency to thrombosis) and increased bactericidal powers.
7. Analgesia.
8. Respiratory – slowing down respiration and increasing the discharge of carbon dioxide.
9. Normalization of blood pressure.
10. Increase of metabolism. Appetite may be improved and obesity helped.
11. Improved endocrine functioning.
12. Stimulation of mental and nervous activity.

Individuals with very sensitive skins should not be given U.V., and some conditions such as acute dermatitis or eczema may be aggravated by it. In general, it is contraindicated in cases of fever and pulmonary tuberculosis.

Cupping

The earliest form of cupping was probably the love-bite, but there are indications that the ancient Chinese used animal horns which they applied to the skin, sucked from the other end to remove air and then sealed with the finger. Modern cupping is accomplished by using glass or metal cups or even a machine which provides a negative pressure by its pumping action. In traditional acupuncture treatment, cupping is still performed by burning a herb or cotton wool which has been soaked in spirit inside the cup. After it has burnt, the cup is placed upon the skin, taking care that the edge of the cup is not too hot. As it cools down a partial vacuum is created inside the cup drawing the flesh into the cup. It is useful for painful congestion, bronchitis, asthma, pneumonia, pleurisy, boils, swellings, rheumatism and arthritic conditions. Cupping may be done to the spine by placing cups over the spinous processes. This is usually effected by using several cups and changing the position of the uppermost cup from the top to the bottom of the row at regular intervals until the entire spine has been covered. Cups are normally left in position for 5–10 minutes. Cupping to the chest involves placing the cups over the entire area as well as on the solar plexus and others down each side of the abdomen. If desired, the cup may be moved along the muscle after lubricating the surface with a little oil. Cupping can be used to relieve migraine and other types of headaches by first piercing the skin with a special acupuncture needle and then cupping, which draws out a quantity of blood.

M. J. Nightingale

Electro-therapy

Electro-therapy is the treatment of disease and injury by the use of electricity applied directly to the surface of the body or by placing the diseased area in an electrical, electromagnetic or ultrasonic field.

Galvanism

Historically, the first electro-therapy treatment used was a method called Galvanism, or the application of direct current (as opposed to alternating current). Luigi Galvani, from whom the name derives, was a professor of anatomy at the University of Bologna, Italy, who, in 1789 reported the results of a now famous experiment in which he noticed that a freshly dissected frog's leg twitched when it was subjected to an electrical stimulation.

Therapeutically, Galvanism is employed in three distinct ways: medical Galvanism, surgical Galvanism and iontophoresis.

Medical Galvanism involves the use of direct current for (a) its hyperaemia effect, in which the circulation of blood around the body is improved, which in turn speeds up re-absorption of any inflammatory products that may be present, and (b) the nerve irritability effect of direct current may be used in a number of acute and chronic inflammatory conditions such as contusions, sprains, fibrositis and in selected cases of arthritis, neuritis and neuralgia.

The use of Galvanism in these ways however, has declined over the years, even for the treatment of sports injuries for which it was popularly used. The effect of Galvanism in the above treatments is not specific and it is now mostly used when other methods have proved ineffectual.

The caustic or burning effect on a micro scale of direct current has been used for many years in surgical Galvanism, principally for the removal of superfluous hair.

Through the technique of iontophoresis, it is possible to introduce the ions of a number of drugs and medicaments into the skin and mucous membranes by the polarity effect of direct current. Chloride, histamine, magnesium, quinine, iodine and salicylic (aspirin) ions are among the drugs which can be introduced into the body with iontophoresis. Electrodes are placed on the skin and the drug placed under either the positive or negative electrode, depending on whether the drug ions are positive or negative. When the current is turned on, the ions will tend to migrate towards the opposite electrode and hence into the skin. In present-day beauty therapy, iontophoresis is increasingly used for the introduction of enzymes into the body for, say, the dispersal of fat.

Diagram illustrating the principle of iontophoresis. A solution of the drug is placed on a piece of gauze which is then placed between the electrode and the skin. When the current is applied, the drug, in this case magnesium (Mg^+), tends to migrate through the skin towards the opposite electrode. In this way the drug can reach the site of injury or inflammation.

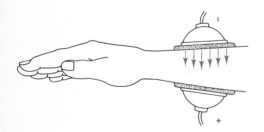

Faradism

In the early part of the nineteenth century, Michael Faraday demonstrated that it was possible to induce an electrical current through the magnetic field set up around a 'primary' current flow of electricity. He gave his name to the Farad, the unit of electrical capacity, and to Faradic currents which are 'pulsating' currents, with varying pulse shapes, frequencies and durations.

It is perhaps in Faradism that the electro-therapist still has today his finest tool. The use of electricity is the only means of testing the degree of degeneration or improvement of nerves and muscles following injury or disease. Also, as an electrical impulse so closely resembles the natural nerve impulse which activates the muscles, it is the only means of stimulating denervated muscle whilst its nerve supply is regenerating. Used in conjunction with Galvanism, (although Galvanism is seldom used in itself for muscle stimulation), Faradism makes it possible, for example, to estimate the degree of reaction of degeneration of the nerve supply to a muscle after injury.

The Faradic current can be employed for the stimulation of both the sensory nerves (although of little practical value), and the motor nerves through the tetanic contraction of the muscles. But it is in the sphere of muscular re-education and rehabilitation that Faradism reigns supreme, and although it has been used in physical therapy now for the best part of this century no subsequent developments in electro-therapy have surpassed that of the Faradic current for its effect on muscular contraction. Although having lost favour in hospital treatments for a while, the 'space age' necessity to exercise the muscles of an astronaut whilst he is confined, perhaps for days on end, in a space capsule saw the reintroduction of Faradism in a more sophisticated form. A further development was the design for the beauty therapy world of multi-output Faradic units, with a varying number of individual circuits which could be used to exercise and tone the muscles of several areas of the body at the same time.

Sinusoidal Current

The sinusoidal current is an evenly alternating low frequency current, similar to that of a 'stepped down' mains supply, and with similar biological effects to Faradic currents in respect of its stimulating effects on both sensory and motor nerves as well as on muscular contraction. Because of its rather irritating effects on the skin during application, however, this type of current is not as comfortable as the Faradic current. Since its effects lie mainly in the area of muscle exercising, which can perhaps be better achieved by active exercising or, in cases of infirmity, with Faradic currents, sinusoidal currents are used far less frequently today.

Interferential Therapy

The low frequency currents involved in Faradism and sinusoidal require a high intensity of current to overcome skin resistance and so reach the tissues beneath. In interferential therapy the benefits and safety of low frequency currents are maintained by applying two separate and slightly varying medium frequency currents to the body through electrodes placed in such positions that the two currents will be superimposed on each other at the required point in the tissues. Where the currents 'interfere' with each other, a very low frequency 'beat' rhythm is produced, equivalent to the difference between the two frequencies employed. For instance, a frequency of 3900–4000 cycles superimposed on a constant one of 4000 cycles would produce a beat rhythm of from 0–100 cycles. Therapeutically a range of effects can be achieved, from analgesia to blood and lymphatic flow improvement as well as benefits derived from the motor stimulation effect of such current.

High Frequency Currents

High frequency currents are generally considered to be those above 100,000 cycles per second, for beyond this frequency there is no tetanic effect. The description 'high frequency apparatus' is often applied to a particular type of equipment in which the current is applied to the skin through an assortment of glass electrodes, although, strictly speaking, the current employed in the modern version of this very old type of treatment is a medium frequency current. A number of exaggerated and rather optimistic claims, for instance stimulation of hair growth, have been made in years gone by for the effects of high frequency currents. Its therapeutic value is limited to its use in raising skin temperature slightly, or to provide a means of cauterization of certain skin conditions.

Electro-therapy

The positioning of the electrodes for the interferential treatment of arthritis in the knee. Low frequency currents require a high intensity of current to overcome skin resistance. By applying two separate and slightly varying medium frequency currents, skin resistance is overcome and where the two currents become superimposed on each other deep within the tissues, a low frequency rhythm is produced equivalent to the difference between the two frequencies employed.

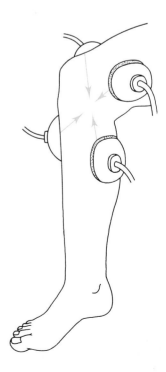

Electro-therapy

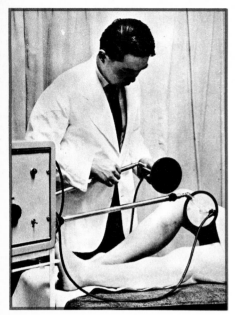

Short wave diathermy treatment of an injured knee.

An ultrasonic generator in use.

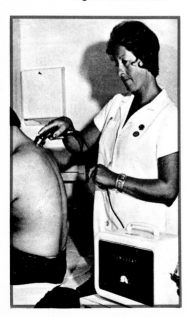

Diathermy and Microwave Therapies

Diathermy is a method of treatment which involves the use of currents at about 27,000,000 cycles per second; currents of such high frequency induce therapeutic thermal effects deep in the body tissues, including muscles and joints. The electrodes between which the current passes, are placed either side of the part of the body or limb being treated, with either air-space or thick separator pads between the electrodes and the skin to prevent surface burning. Particular caution must be exercised to avoid deep diathermy burns within the body, and it is important to ensure that there are no metallic objects such as jewellery, in the path of the current.

Despite the precautions necessary with diathermy therapy, this equipment is an established feature of the hospital physiotherapy department as well as the clinics of alternative medicine practitioners. The popularity of diathermy in sports clubs is now waning with the development of microwave and pulsed high frequency therapies.

Microwave diathermy employs radio waves oscillating at around 3,000,000,000 cycles per second instead of electrical impulses. It utilizes both the electric and electromagnetic fields and has a thermal effect on the body tissues, particularly those containing a high fluid content. However its thermal penetration, although considerably more than infra-red rays, is rather less than that of short wave diathermy. The equipment though, which utilizes only a single electrode in most cases, is easier to apply than short wave diathermy equipment and so perhaps provides a more convenient means of tissue heating, although its benefits are really confined to this effect. In this context, it is probably less effective than correctly applied short wave diathermy. Precautions against skin and tissue burning are also necessary with microwave therapy.

Ultrasonics

Ultrasonic is the treatment of the body with sound pressure waves of such high frequency as to be inaudible to humans. The frequencies used in ultrasonics are too high for mechanical production and are achieved instead by subjecting a quartz crystal to an electric field, whereby the crystal expands and contracts rapidly producing the necessary vibrations. The frequency of the vibrations are determined by the frequency of the electric field applied to the crystal.

Ultrasonics are employed therapeutically for their thermal effects (heat is produced when the waves are absorbed by tissue), for their analgesic effect (partly due to the thermal effect but possibly due to a direct effect on nerves), and for their mechanical effect, which produces a kind of micro-massage in the tissues. Ultrasonic waves will not pass through a vacuum and are reflected by the air, so when being used therapeutically either the limb being treated and the head of the equipment are immersed in water (through which the waves will pass) or the skin is covered with a gel prior to the application of the treatment head. This type of therapy has proved to be very beneficial in the treatment of recent injuries such as sprains and strains, gained on the sporting field.

K. Woodward

Pulsed High Frequency Therapy

In 1934 Dr Abraham Ginsberg of New York developed a theory that the therapeutic benefit of high energy radio waves was derived from their ability to penetrate deep into body tissues and accelerate the body's normal healing process, rather than being related to the thermal effects of such waves. With the help of physicist A. S. Milinowski, Ginsberg devised a method of pulsing electromagnetic energy; the

Electro-therapy

brief period between each pulse of energy thus allowed any heat generated in the tissue to be dissipated. In a typical modern pulse generator, the period of peak power lasts for 65 microseconds followed by a rest interval of 1600 microseconds before the next pulse.

Pulsed high frequency therapy has, over thirty-five years of research and application, been found to be extremely effective in treating a wide variety of complaints from sinusitis, bursitis, rheumatoid arthritis and osteomyelitis, to disorders of muscles, tendons and bones, such as sprains, strains and fractures. Reports on soft tissue injury have shown that the therapy produces definite biological improvement, especially in the reduction of pain and disability. Other reported examples of its use include reduction of tissue swelling following injury, quicker formation of new skin in burns, reduction of excess tissue fluid (oedema) associated with cellular damage and dispersal of normal bruising which follows some types of surgery. Calcification which develops with swollen joints can also be reversed.

The healing of bone and tissue can be accelerated by as much as fifty percent by this therapy, and in fact in any condition where the body is able to heal itself, pulsed high frequency therapy can accelerate that healing by virtue of its ability to reach deep into the treatment area and affect individual cells. When a cell is damaged by traumatic injury or disease, there is a loss of electrical potential in that cell. Where this occurs, the potential difference between the cell and nearby healthy cells sets up a current flow from the uninjured to the injured area, so recharging the damaged cell until its potential is restored and it is once again healthy and functioning. This is the basic healing process that pulsed high frequency therapy accelerates. When the cells are placed under the electrode of the generator, they tend to align themselves with the electromagnetic field during the period of each energy pulse and return to normal during each rest period. The stress induced in the cells by this process increases their receptivity to the natural healing current flow.

Pulsed high frequency therapy is the only electro-therapy that can affect individual cells without damage, and its ability to penetrate deeply into affected tissue has proven itself to be of great therapeutic value, especially in such deep-seated complaints as cystitis and prostatitis. It can treat through clothing, surgical dressings, plaster casts and metal implants. There have been no reports of adverse effects and the only contraindication is if the patient is wearing a cardiac pacemaker. Pulsed high frequency therapy should not be confused with pulsed diathermy which induces heat in tissues and therefore has the same contraindications as diathermy.   *Manning D. Ross*

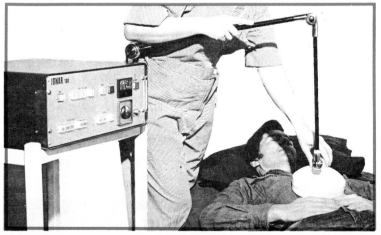

The use of pulsed high frequency therapy to improve generally the blood circulation and so speed up the removal of toxic products from sites of inflammation elsewhere in the body.

Electro-therapy

Endogenous Endocrinotherapy

Many body functions are controlled by hormones produced by the different endocrine glands. In order for health to exist and functions to be harmonized, the endocrine system must be in balance. Many diseases, such as depression, emotional disturbances, lassitude, insomnia, overweight, underweight, some types of heart disease, skin conditions and arthritis are caused by, or associated with, endocrine disturbance.

Orthodox treatment is exogenous, involving the administration of synthetic hormones at a stage when structural changes to the gland have taken place. This encourages further deterioration and may also be dangerous. The naturopathic approach, termed endogenous endocrinotherapy, consists in normalizing the malfunctioning gland.

Numerous methods may be employed to accomplish this, including physiotherapy, acupuncture, homoeopathy, osteopathy, herbs and applied kinesiology. The use of short-wave therapy as elaborated by Dr Jules Samuels is the most dramatic of these and is usually regarded as being synonymous with endogenous endocrinotherapy. The treatment is based upon the knowledge that the reduction time of oxygenated blood in the capillary bed (i.e. the time which elapses between 'pinching off' a fold of skin until the reduction of the oxyhaemoglobin is completed and the bands of methaemoglobin are visible) is normally twenty-five seconds. A remarkable test has been devised in which a spectroscope, an instrument used to examine the chemical structure of different substances, is used to measure the reduction time and, thereby, the normality or otherwise of the endocrine system. Treatment consists of a few minutes irradiation of the offending gland with standard short-wave equipment such as is found in any hospital physiotherapy department. Treatment and progress may be monitored by the spectroscopic test and, of course, by amelioration of symptoms. Treatment usually lasts for about two to three months, but bi-annual checks are recommended. More serious conditions may take longer to treat, but much depends on the patient's way of life.

M. J. Nightingale

Short wave irradiation to correct a malfunctioning pituitary.

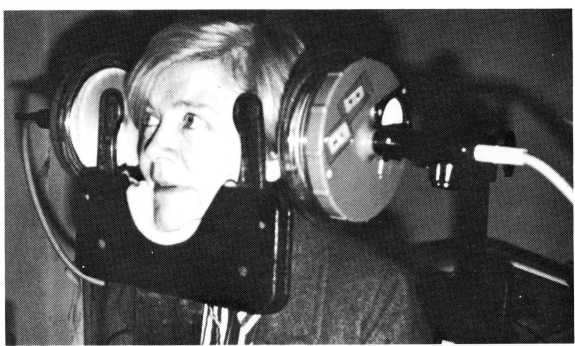

Gems

Throughout history, man has been fascinated by the effect of gems on his body, mind, spirit and soul. He has also related them to health, money, economics, and has accrued a great deal of experience from them.

Gems are essentially related to the spectrum. Colours seen around them are spectroscopic, but not all spectroscopic colours are visible; the visible colours are deflections of each individual person's eye pattern, or retina, and people's individual colour conditioning.

The spectroscope is fundamentally a prism and the white ray, when passing through a prism, breaks down into its seven component aspects: violet, indigo, blue, green, yellow, orange and red. Each colour has its own vibration rate and frequency range. The human body is composed of cells which must also deflect and refract light, and this property results in the phenomenon which clairvoyants and psychic observers call the ura. The colours of the aura also correspond to the spectrum, that is, the seven colours of the rainbow. As contemporary science advances, it has began to recognize the Kirlian method of photography, confirming what ancient, traditional science has known for many centuries. A photograph taken of a human hand in a high frequency field shows that the fingers of the hand radiate all seven colours, as follows:

Thumb	— Mount of Venus	— Indigo
Index finger	— Mount of Jupiter	— Blue
Middle finger	— Mount of Saturn	— Violet
Ring finger	— Mount of the Sun	— Red
Little finger	— Mount of Mercury	— Green
Joint of thumb *and* Index finger, *and* Base of little finger	— Mount of Mars	— Yellow
Outer edge of little finger	— Mount of Moon	— Orange

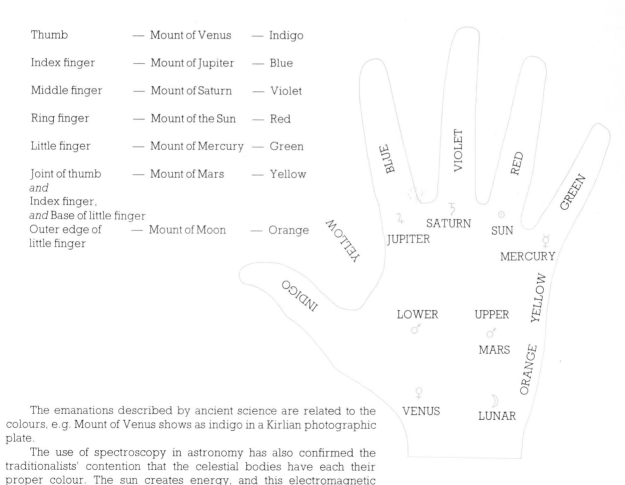

The emanations described by ancient science are related to the colours, e.g. Mount of Venus shows as indigo in a Kirlian photographic plate.

The use of spectroscopy in astronomy has also confirmed the traditionalists' contention that the celestial bodies have each their proper colour. The sun creates energy, and this electromagnetic energy band results in a visible spectrum, as the colours of the rainbow. Gems, stars, the planets and the human body all radiate the colours of the spectrum. We understand and accept that energy is in

Gems

matter and that all living matter has its own energy pattern. Each pattern is connected to the spectrum.

Ancient Yoga related these patterns to the body and divided the physical energies into seven 'chakras' or concentrations. Each chakra represents a colour and controls the energy concentrated in that part of the body, and the seven chakras together correspond to the completed spectrum.

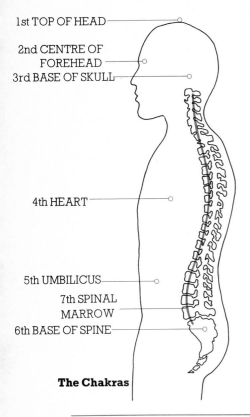

- 1st TOP OF HEAD
- 2nd CENTRE OF FOREHEAD
- 3rd BASE OF SKULL
- 4th HEART
- 5th UMBILICUS
- 7th SPINAL MARROW
- 6th BASE OF SPINE

The Chakras

Chakra	Colour	Number of Chakra
Top of the head	Violet	7
Centre of forehead	Indigo	6
Base of skull	Blue	5
Heart	Green	4
Abdomen	Yellow	3
Base of spine	Orange	2
Spinal marrow	Red	1

The seven chakras also correspond to the major endocrine glands: pineal, pituitary, thyroid, thymus, supra-renal (corticoid and medullar) and ovarian or testicular.

The colours are in turn represented by the astrological symbols we have enumerated above and the ruling planets. Each ruling planet is related through the spectrum to gems.

Gems are also related to numerology, and people are related to gems by their particular number which is determined as follows. To arrive at the number in the simplest way, take your date of birth, say, $4.4.1960 — 4+4+1+9+6+0 = 24$ then $2+4 = 6$. If the number should exceed 9 then you again add the two digits. Say 11 makes $1+1 = 2$. No. 1 represents violet, No. 2 indigo and so on. The eighth and ninth numbers correspond to the Mount of Mars and the Mount of the Moon respectively.

	JADE	TOPAZ	CORAL	DIAMOND	SAPPHIRE	RUBY
Therapeutic values	Chest and heart; whooping cough. Controls psychosomatic conditions, e.g. anxiety causes diarrhoea.	Heart and its autonomic nervous system. Controls tachycardia and bradycardia; depressions of spiritual instrument e.g. 'patient feels he is doomed by the influence of Saturn'.	All face symptoms and head. Diseases of ear, nose, eyes. Psychosis.	Bone and bone systems, including injury to skull.	Sweats, colds, coughs, catarrh. 'Nervous apprehension'. Increases optimism by understanding pessimistic outlooks.	Paralytic fear and paralysis body. Promo better therm balance.
Signs	Virgo	Sagittarius	Taurus	Capricorn	Aries	Leo
Number	5	3	6	8	9 3	1 and Kundalini
Chakra affected	3	5	6	7		4

Gems

Chromotherapy advocates the use of colour as a healing, comforting psychedelic factor, and thus again acknowledges the use of gems, their absorbed lustre colour, their vibratory rate and retinal impressions.

In radiesthesia, two people experimented and established the practice of using gems. Mme Chrapowisky showed the clinical value of the use of gems and colours in an extensive work she published. Mrs Barraclough, using the pendulum in conjunction with the triangle, developed a system of diagnosis based on 'matching' the frequency of a patient's blood sample with a particular gem, and advocated the use of gems for health. Drs Jennings, Jenner and Brown published works on the therapeutic use of gems. The writer has extensively used gems both for prophylactic and curative purposes.

For therapeutic purposes it must be noted that the use of a gem, as in any other therapy, must be determined on the basis of profound knowledge of the patient as a whole, his symptoms, his bodily reactions, his numerological and astrological values.

In the selection of a gem it is primarily important to be aware of the symptom picture associated with it, also its astrological and numerological relationships.

Physicians differ in their choice of the therapeutic uses of gems. While some recommend that a sample of the stone be kept in a prominent place in the domestic or working environment, others require the gem to be worn on the patient's person. According to different views, the gem may be worn in direct contact with the skin, or on the clothing, as a brooch or pendant. The author favours the latter method, advising the patient periodically to remind himself of the gemstone's presence, by fingering or looking at it. A third school believes that the stone should be placed in a vessel of pure water, from which the patient drinks.

C. H. Sharma

ZIRCON	ONYX	EMERALD	HESANITE	CORNELIAN	PEARL
					(most values similar to Moonstone)
Tumours in ear, nose and throat passage. Cataract. Delusions: 'I am God' 'I am damned' 'I am Hitler'.	All diseases which tend to electrolytic imbalance. Water retentive. Cellulitis. Nightmares and enuresis.	Flushes, heats, sweats. Anger. Controls mercurial temperaments. Increases clairvoyance, clairaudience.	Strong vibratory and vitality stone. Use as small a stone as possible. Prevents bone disease, especially of the bone marrow. Useful in cases of meningitis and after-effects of measles, vaccines and immunizations.	Digestive disorders where wind prevails. Eructations, flatulence. Illnesses producing bile and fast pulse; fast bowel action, fast breathing. Restlessness, racing thoughts.	Irritations of solid organs, e.g. pancreas, spleen, brain tumours. Inhibitions caused by mental, physical or psychic pressures. Used in cases of compulsive tidiness.
Libra	Pisces	Gemini	Aquarius	Scorpio	Cancer
6	4	5	8	9	2
6	7	1 and 2	3	5	3 through parathyroid

Copper

The folklore of many countries includes the prescription of copper bracelets, rings and necklaces to alleviate the pain associated with rheumatoid arthritis. According to this same folklore, the usefulness of copper in such conditions extends to animals as well as humans. Lieutenant-Colonel A. Forbes of Cheltenham, England, has supplied copper bracelets and bangles for many years to sufferers of rheumatic conditions, with considerable success. Both dogs and horses have also benefited from specially adapted copper straps made by Colonel Forbes.

Like many folk remedies, the apparent efficacy of copper has been greeted, for the most part, with considerable scepticism by the scientific establishment, and in particular the medical profession. Evidence has been accumulating over the past few years, however, which suggests that beliefs in copper therapy may be well founded.

In 1974 a report appeared in the journal *Medical News* describing the anti-inflammatory properties of a chemical in which both copper and aspirin (acetylsalicylic acid) or salicylic acid are linked (it is inflammation which causes the pain in rheumatoid arthritis sufferers). The possibility now arose that copper from a bracelet or ring could combine with a chemical in sweat, possibly an amino acid, and thereby penetrate both the skin and the venous system, to reach the site of the inflammation.

Professor W. R. Walker at the University of Newcastle in New South Wales, quickly took up the challenge and in a first study of rheumatoid arthritis sufferers who wear copper bracelets, found that the weight of the bracelets decreased by about 40 mg a month. This weight loss could not be accounted for by natural abrasion of the bracelets. Subsequent experiments by Professor Walker showed that copper may in fact dissolve in human sweat. Further, he showed that a chemical in which copper and the natural amino acid glycine are linked, can penetrate the skin of a cat. While this has not yet been verified in humans it would appear that copper therapy no longer belongs to the realm of folklore.

Section of skin containing perfused copper.

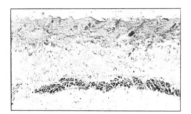

Bracelets worn by sufferers from rheumatism.

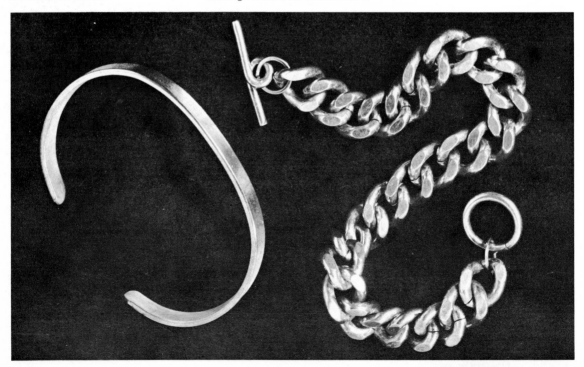

Clay and Mud

Earth has been used for healing purposes for thousands of years and it is recorded that Hippocrates, Dioscorides, Avicenna and Galen all worked miracles with clay treatment. The great healing powers of clay however, can only be partly explained by its chemical composition. The negative ions of clay are able to attract and absorb positively ionized toxins, and even radioactivity can be absorbed by clay. It is capable of detoxifying and even dechlorinating contaminated or chlorinated water. Clay has both antiseptic and antibiotic properties and promotes wound healing – even festering wounds can be successfully treated with it. Intestinal catarrh, excessive stomach acidity, ulcers, sores and dysentery all successfully respond to clay treatment.

Clay treatment should be accompanied by a vegetarian diet and usually preceded by a fast or special eliminative diet thus ensuring that the clay exerts its optimum effect; clay also works best if not combined with any other medication. Only virgin clay – clay that has not been previously employed – should be used.

An ointment can be made from clay by soaking it in cold water for a few hours, pouring off the fluid together with any foreign substances and making a paste by adding lemon juice or an aqueous extract of horsetail or St John's wort. The ointment may be applied to ulcers, sores and so on. A suitable eye ointment may be made by using an extract of eyebright in place of the lemon juice. A clay pack may be made by mixing clay with warm water, making it into a paste and spreading this on a cloth or sheet. This is placed on the area to be treated and covered with a blanket or towels.

Mud baths are also therapeutic and may be used for many conditions, particularly skin troubles. Some muds have special value for treating specific conditions.

M. J. Nightingale

Japanese women taking advantage of the medicinal sands on the shores of Beppu in the south of Japan.

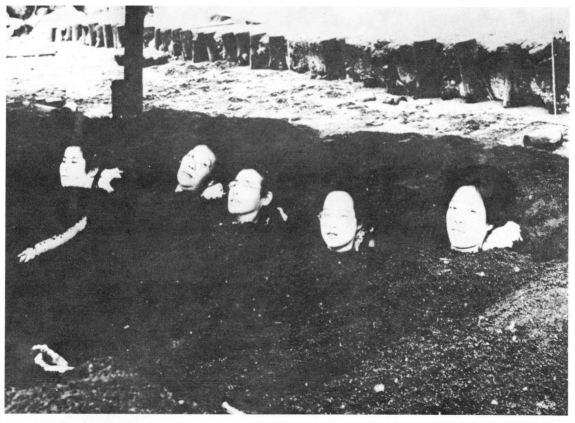

Hydrotherapy

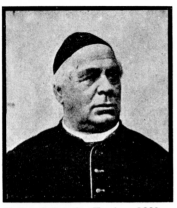

Father Sebastian Kneipp, 1821–1897. A Roman Catholic priest, Kneipp originated the 'Kneipp cure' based on water, fresh air, sunshine and regular activity including walking barefoot through snow.

Water has long been recognized as possessing therapeutic and even miraculous properties, from the early Roman and Turkish baths to the healing waters of Lourdes; even the word hydro (water) became applied to places of healing. It is appropriate that water should be a valuable therapeutic medium for all life depends on its presence. Our body tissues are two-thirds water and while we can live without food for considerable periods of time, water is essential to prevent the tissues from dehydrating and dying. On a biochemical level, the body's water is vital for maintaining normal salt concentrations, making osmosis possible, assisting in the chemical changes of the digestive system and as an aid to peristalsis, the wave-like rhythmic contraction which conveys food from the rear of the mouth to the stomach. Particularly important from the point of view of hydrotherapy is the fact that water provides the medium of transport for removing the body's waste products. Every day, the sweat glands of the body excrete about 30 ounces (850 ml) of water containing about one-twentieth of this weight of nitrogenous waste matter. One of the benefits of hydrotherapy is to increase the efficiency of the sweat glands.

A great proponent of hydrotherapy was Father Sebastian Kneipp (1821–97), a parish priest from Worishofen in Bavaria, whose water cures became internationally famous. Kneipp maintained that the purpose of hydrotherapy was "to dissolve, remove and strengthen. These . . . are the three principle attributes of water, and we maintain water to be capable of curing every curable disease, as its various applications, properly applied, directly attack the root of the evil, and have the result:

1. Of dissolving the germs of diseased matter contained in the blood. 2. Of withdrawing the diseased matter from the system. 3. Of restoring the purified blood to its proper state of circulation. 4. Of bracing the weakened constitution and rendering it fit for renewed exertion."

Water is certainly an adaptable medium to work with in therapy. It possesses buoyancy and, being fluid, is capable of a range of movement and pressures. Water can be used as a jet or in a variety of sprays allowing control of pressure. Since water has thermal properties it can be applied over a wide range of temperatures. Therapeutically, it can be used both internally and externally.

One of the basic laws of hydrotherapy is that of action and reaction. The application of any form of heat to the skin draws the blood to the surface – though this is not a lasting effect, the blood ultimately returning to the deeper blood vessels. The application of cold water has the initial effect of driving blood away from the surface. The secondary, and lasting effect, is that of warmth, since by the law of action and reaction the blood must circulate back to the vessels and tissues from which it was expelled. This law can best be seen at work in the three basic baths of hydrotherapy – cold, hot and alternate hot and cold.

Cold Baths

Short applications of cold water have a tonic and invigorating effect upon the part treated. Initially, a cold application induces pallor and coldness of the skin due to the contraction of the small blood vessels. If the cold is not prolonged, this is rapidly replaced by redness caused by dilation of the small arteries of the skin. This secondary effect is lasting and is the most important hydrotherapeutically. Generally, one of the most effective cold bathing methods is to run water, at a temperature not usually less than 60°F (16°C), into a bath to a depth of about ten inches. The hips are then lowered into the bath and water splashed over the chest. The patient then stands and runs in the water for a few seconds. Total subjection should be from thirty seconds to two minutes.

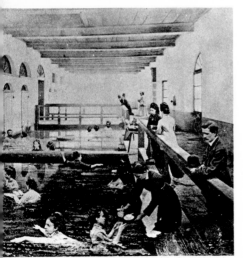

The baths at Loeche.

A simple guide to the use of cold water is that it should be applied to any part of the body suffering from hyperaemia and that it is necessary to equate the severity of the cold application to the vital energy and recuperative powers of the person concerned.

In general, prolonged cold applications should be avoided in children under seven, in very enfeebled and anaemic conditions, heart disease, Bright's disease, old age and in those suffering from nerve tension and hysteria.

Hot Baths

Hot baths are mainly enervating and increase the efficiency of the sweat glands. When heat is applied to the skin, the nearby arteries dilate, the blood slows while at the same time more blood is pushed into the charged arteries causing redness and congestion. If the heat is not removed the blood becomes locked and perspiration occurs. Hot baths commence at 100°F (38°C). Various medicinal and herbal preparations can be added to hot baths, the opened pores of the skin more easily absorbing the active constituents of the preparations.

Seaweed, peat, salt, sea salt, epsom salt, soda and sulphur can be added to the baths for complaints ranging from arthritis, rheumatism, paralysis and poor circulation to general pain and muscle fatigue. Herbal mixtures can also be added; specific herbs have different effects, for instance lime blossom, valerian, chamomile, rosemary and horsetail are all recommended for nervous complaints.

Alternate Hot and Cold Baths

Alternate hot and cold baths make full use of the law of action and reaction, acting like an artificial pump to stimulate blood flow and venous and lymphatic drainage. When applied to congested areas they bring about a rapid reduction of inflammation. They are also used where there is a need to increase local circulation. This bath can take the form of a sitz, arm or foot bath or as hot and cold sprays. The general rule is 2–3 minutes in hot water followed by half a minute in cold water, repeated three times and concluding with the cold application.

The Rising and Falling Bath

This bath doubles the effect of alternate hot and cold baths and has the advantage that it can be tolerated by less vigorous people. The bath commences with tepid water and the temperature raised by the addition of hot water and then reduced to cold by quickly running out some water and adding cold water.

Neutral Baths

Neutral baths, with a temperature of 90–95°F (36.7–37.2°C), can and should last longer than hot baths. The effect of such baths is to produce relaxation and reduce tension. Adding relaxing herbs to the bath makes them ideal in all cases of insomnia, tension, irritability. Some skin conditions can be treated with this bath, while the addition of salt allows these baths to be used for the treatment of burns. Seaweed, pine, oats, bran, salt, soda and herb mixtures of elderflower, peppermint and horsetail all enhance the effect of neutral baths.

Baths Using Movement of Water

Underwater massage

This form of bath combines the thermal and relaxing effect of water with a powerful form of massage. Water is sucked up from the bath and returned as a jet, with the pressure varied to suit individual cases. The jet can be directed to any part of the body and is a very stimulating and powerful form of massage. It is important to rest after such baths.

Hydrotherapy

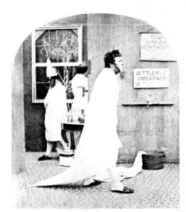

Taking the cold water cure at an English spa in 1860.

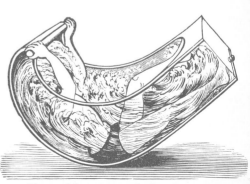

The rocking or wave bath illustrated in F. E. Bilz's *Natural Method of Healing*.

Hydrotherapy

Whirlpool baths

The whirlpool bath uses small electric agitators to produce an effect similar to underwater massage, though much less strenuous. It was used extensively during World War I, in America, for treating arm and leg wounds, fractures and for paralysis. Used at neutral temperatures, whirlpool baths can be used for the treatment of insomnia and tension; at higher temperatures they can be employed where connective tissues, nerves and joints have been damaged.

Aerated baths

In these baths compressed air is forced through small holes in wood or metal to create a mass of bubbles in the water. This is a less powerful but highly effective form of under-water massage which has wide applications for treating fractures and sprains and as a general tonic. Such baths are found naturally in certain spas.

Sitz Baths

The sitz bath is used in two sections. The first is a large bath in which one sits so that the lower abdomen is covered by water with the legs dangling over the side and the knees in a raised position. The second is a small bath for the feet, and has the advantage that it can be kept at a different temperature from the large bath. Sitz baths are particularly useful for illnesses of the lower abdomen – intestinal, genital and urinary disorders, and for disorders of the female reproductive system.

The sitz bath can be adapted as a safe sweating treatment for aged and infirm people by covering the bath with a blanket. In the position adopted in the bath, blood is drawn to the abdomen, and the heart and head are not subject to the higher temperatures involved in other forms of sweating. Some modern sitz baths have anal and spinal douches attached.

Hot sitz bath

In the hot sitz bath, with temperatures ranging from 108–110°F (44°C), all the abdominal blood vessels and tissues become expanded as more blood is attracted to the abdomen. The bath should last for ten minutes with the heat being maintained, while the feet are kept in a bowl of cold water. After the required period the position is reversed, the patient sits in a cold sitz bath and the feet are placed in a bowl of hot water. The cold sitz bath should last for one to two minutes.

The sudden cold bath contracts the abdominal blood vessels and tissues and the blood is forced to other parts of the body. By the law of action and reaction, and particularly because of the large volume of blood involved, the effect is that of increased total blood circulation all over the body. Warm extremities and the relaxation of pressure in the body are the immediate effects of the bath.

Alternate hot and cold sitz bath

While all abdominal complaints will benefit from sitz baths, many conditions, including constipation, haemorrhoids, prostate and anal fissures, etc will derive more benefit from the alternate variety. As the name implies, the patient sits in the hot bath for three minutes, in the cold bath for 30 to 60 seconds with the process repeated three times, concluding with the cold bath. As before, the feet are in cold water when sitting in the hot bath, and vice versa.

The cold sitz bath

The cold sitz bath should last for 30 to 60 seconds according to the temperature of the tap water and the room. It is recommended for its tonic effect and is invaluable in cases of impotence and prostate trouble.

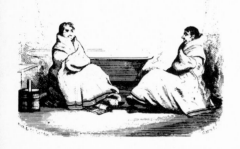

The sitz bath, old and new. Hidden under the towels in this 1855 cartoon are smaller versions of the modern sitz bath which is designed so that the hips and feet can be immersed at different temperatures.

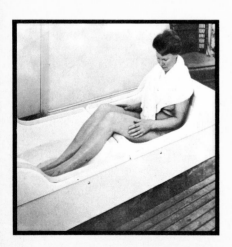

Hydrotherapy

Sweating Baths

The Russian and Turkish baths

The Russian bath, which has a long tradition of use, is similar to the Finnish sauna, except that the steam is generated externally and piped into the steam room or cubicle. In the simplest Russian bath, which is still in use in parts of the Soviet Union, steam is generated by pouring hot water on the uppermost benches of the room, and cooler water (109–134°F) on the lower benches. After fifteen minutes, during which copious sweating is induced, the bather cools himself with a cold water dip, or by plunging naked into the snow.

The Turkish bath is a rather different affair and is ably described by F. E. Bilz in his book *The Natural Method of Healing:*

"We first enter the undressing room. Here the bather takes off his clothes, wraps one cloth around his loins, and another, dipped in water, around his head, to prevent a rush of blood to that part, and enters the second room. The temperature here varies from 100° to 112°F. The heat, however, in this and the further rooms does not arise from steam, but from hot air. The bather remains in this room for 10–15 minutes, till the skin begins to get damp. Then he goes into a third room, with a temperature of 134°–150°F. Here the perspiration flows off in streams, and the bather at the same time experiences a sensation of great mental and bodily ease and lightness. From a quarter to three-quarters of an hour are usually spent in this room. At the end of this time the whole body is massaged by the bath-attendant, and the skin thoroughly rubbed and brushed, a process which removes all dirt and impurities".

Cabinet baths

The cabinet, or steam-box bath, is an individual sweating bath which caters more for specific requirements of a patient than the Russian or Turkish baths. Cabinet baths have the additional advantage that the head is kept cool, the patient breathes pure air and has an attendant at his side to remedy any unpleasant effects such as giddiness and palpitations of the heart.

Douches

A douche is a strong stream, jet or spray of water which is directed either locally or generally onto the body – the simplest form of douche is the ordinary shower. The therapeutic effects of the douche depend upon:

A. Water temperature.
B. Pressure of water jet.
C. Duration of treatment.
D. Type of douche.

Douches can be applied at temperatures higher than normal hot baths but otherwise the law of action and reaction is observed and the full range of water temperatures employed. Pressures employed can range from 10–60 lb/sq in.

The therapeutic benefits derived from douches are similar to those from normal baths with the added advantage of the mechanical effects of the jet or spray.

Bilz's book had this to say about douches:

"The douche . . . is the pearl of all forms of water treatment, and indispensable where the object is to cure most of the chronic diseases. What will it not do, when combined with the horizontal shower-bath, in abdominal complaints, colic, catarrhs of the stomach, throat, and bowels; in neuralgia, sciatica, rheumatic affections, discharges, swelling of the liver and spleen?''

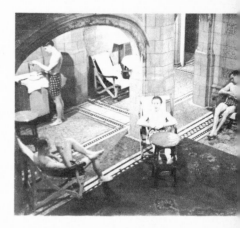

An English Turkish bath in the 1950s. The various rooms of the bath retain the names used in the ancient Roman baths. The bather first rests in the Frigidarium, then moves to the Tepidarium (shown here), where he begins to sweat, before going into the intense dry heat of the Caldarium.

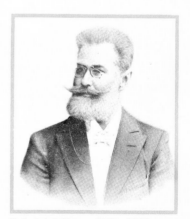

Friedrich Eduard Bilz, 1842–1922. Author of the classic *The Natural Method of Healing*, and founder of the Bilz Sanatorium at Oberlossnitz near Dresden.

Hydrotherapy

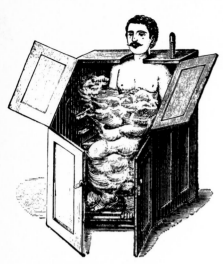

19th century cabinet baths. The steam, generated outside the cabinet, was piped through a rubber hose and entered the cabinet under the seat.

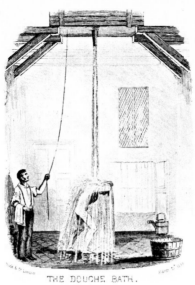

THE DOUCHE BATH.

The douche bath, 1855.

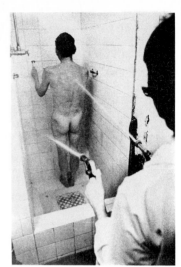

Scotch douche being used on a patient at Tyringham Naturopathic Clinic, Buckinghamshire, England.

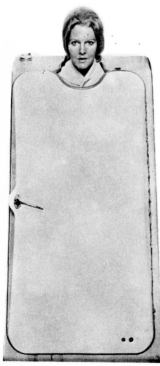

A modern cabinet steam bath.

Douches are contraindicated in the cases of the very young, old and enfeebled and those suffering from nervous irritability.

Scotch douche

This consists of the application of hot water for 1–5 minutes, followed by a cold application lasting for 5–30 seconds. The temperature can be varied to suit the individual.

The alternative douche

This douche consists of subjecting the person to applications of alternate hot and cold water of equal duration, of about 15 seconds each, but concluded with the cold.

The neutral douche

This neutral douche lasts about five minutes with the temperature of the water around 99°F (37°C).

Douches can be applied to any part of the body: spine, buttocks, chest, feet, etc but not on varicose veins or any condition where pressure effects may damage tissue.

Steaming

When water is applied to hot stones, as in saunas, a fine vapour is produced. A similar effect is obtained with a steam kettle in a cabinet bath.

A more direct effect can be obtained by employing a steam kettle to play steam upon the face or chest directly. This form of water treatment is advocated in all cases of colds, influenza, sinusitis and all respiratory ailments. It is also excellent for acne and 'spotty' skins. Pine, peppermint, eucalyptus, Friar's Balsam and a herb mixture of chamomile, lime flower, lady's mantle and yarrow can be used with these baths.

Packs, Compresses and Fomentations

Packs are lengths of linen or towelling, usually used wet, which are wrapped around that part of the body to be treated.

Packs can vary from a full pack which extends from the armpits to the feet, to three-quarter packs which extend to the knees only. Abdominal packs are applied around the abdomen and lower spine while T-packs are wrapped with the horizontal bar around the abdomen and the vertical bar drawn through the legs to connect with the back of the horizontal bar. In addition to these, local packs can be applied to the chest, throat, arms, knees or feet. Throat packs should never be applied alone because they draw blood to this restricted area, and it is necessary to apply an abdominal pack at the same time.

The cold pack is somewhat of a misnomer, since the end result of the pack is neutral and calming. The cold, wet sheet pack is an extremely safe and simple manner of producing a decongesting, strengthening and calming effect upon the body. It can be used where manipulation would be contraindicated, to reduce swelling and stiffness in the joints and muscles. With the addition of sufficient hot water bottles, packs can be used for sweating, but the predominant result of the cold pack is that of moist heat.

The wet sheet pack makes good use of the law of action and reaction. The initial effect is to drive blood away from the treatment area, but the secondary and lasting effect is that of moist warmth, enhanced by body heat (and the addition of hot water bottles where necessary) and the dry covering or bedclothes. Elimination of waste matter via the skin is increased by the pack and it is particularly indicated in painful swellings and inflammation of the joints.

The method of application is simple. The requirements, in the case of body packs, are a piece of rubber or plastic sheeting to protect the undersheet, a piece of linen or cotton sheeting large enough to cover the required area, and a similar (or slightly larger) piece of blanketing. The sheeting is dipped into very cold water and well wrung out. This is placed on the blanketing which has been spread over the protective sheeting. The patient lies on the wet sheet which is then quickly pulled over him and, followed by the dry blanketing; the whole is secured with safety-pins. The top bedclothing is then pulled over and at least one hot water bottle (more if it is desirable for the patient to sweat) is installed. The patient can sleep in the pack in the normal manner. The pack should be kept on for six to eight hours. The same rules applies to all packs with the exception of those on one limb only. These can be for a shorter period, and repeated after a few hours.

Compresses and fomentations

Cold compresses or local packs are applied to any part where excess blood has been attracted, i.e. sprains, swellings, bruises. The cold reduces hyperaemia and pain and relieves congestion. Hot compresses or fomentations are applied where pain without swelling is the predominant factor and where it is necessary to attract more blood to the part treated. Witch-hazel, arnica and extract of chestnut can be used with compresses for bruises, swellings and sprains.

Ice packs

These come under the same category as cold compresses but with a quicker and more direct effect. Unlike packs, compresses and hot fomentations must be renewed every ten to fifteen minutes.

Alan Moyle

Hydrotherapy

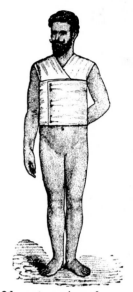

A 19th century view of a shoulder pack and chest compress . . .

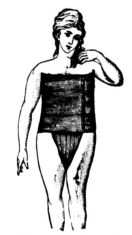

. . . and a T-pack and trunk pack.

Hydrotherapy

Colonic Irrigation

A standard part of the therapeutic regime at many health spas and naturopathic clinics is colonic irrigation. Based on the same hygienic principles as the enema it is, however, a more elaborate piece of equipment and cleanses a greater area of the lower bowel (colon). The whole procedure may take thirty to forty-five minutes during which water, at body temperature, is injected into the rectum and then flows out again through a two way tube.

The irrigation reaches above the normal defaecation area into the descending and transverse colon and so its action is more effective than that of an enema. Furthermore, the repeated washing in and out of the water helps to loosen adherent faecal matter.

Colonic irrigations are only suitable for patients who have been fasting for several days in whom the normal faecal matter and digestive residues have passed through the colon. They are of value for patients who suffer from constipation and other chronic conditions in which healthy bowel elimination may be of vital importance, such as chronic catarrh, gastric troubles and skin disorders. In such disorders the irrigation would be used as part of a broader therapeutic regime, involving dietary control and other physical treatments.

There are distinct contraindications to the use of colonic irrigations, such as diverticulitis, certain types of colitis, malignant growths and cases of greatly reduced vitality.

A further disadvantage of the colonic irrigation is that the vital *Lactobacillus communis*, which play such an important part in the digestion of cellulose, tend to be washed out. They can be quickly re-established by return to a diet high in natural fibre, consisting of whole grains, fresh fruits and vegetables and goats' milk yoghourt.

Enemas

Man's preoccupation with his internal as well as external cleanliness has lead to a variety of devices to achieve that idyllic state. Perhaps the most bizarre practice is that of some eastern mystics who swallow a length of material, passing it right through the gastro-intestinal tract to absorb and scour impurities. Advanced disciples of yoga are reputed to be able to draw water into the rectum and lower bowel by the action of their abdominal muscles and give what is, in effect, an enema. The man-made enema, a device for injecting water, food or medicinal substances into the lower intestine, is probably a more recent, if rather mechanical device based on the ancient hygienic principle. The subsequent evacuation of the water cleanses the lower bowel of unexpelled faeces.

Enemas are used in hospital practice to cleanse the bowel prior to some abdominal operations, or for x-ray investigations of the large intestine when a radio-opaque substance, barium, is injected. As a form of hydrotherapy however, they have long been popular with practitioners of various types of natural hygiene. In conjunction with fasting and controlled dietary programmes, enemas are a valuable part of the eliminative regime. They are said to remove waste which may otherwise lodge in folds of the rectum and be bypassed by normal faecal flow.

Apart from the cleansing function of enemas, the gradual injection of cold water can be of assistance in reducing fevers. Small amounts are injected, starting at body temperature, and reducing to 60°F.

It is unwise to rely on enemas as a treatment for constipation because an artificial aid of this nature tends to reduce the normal function of the bowels. Repeated enemas also disturb normal mucus secretion and bacterial function in the colon. Enemas should normally only be used when undergoing a short fast or controlled light diet.

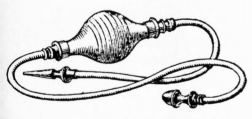

An enema of the bulb type which was in general use in the early part of this century.
The catheter was inserted in the rectum with the aid of soap or other lubricant and the opposite end in the container of water at body temperature. The pumping action of the bulbous portion helped to inject the water into the rectum.
In modern practice a gravity feed type of container is used.

Hydrotherapy

Inhalation

The first physician to recommend 'a change of air' for his patients could be regarded as the true originator of inhalation therapy. In fact the practice of applying substances in a vaporized form, primarily for respiratory diseases, is a very old one which has embraced some unusual modalities. Among the more empirical recommendations of early days was the breathing of the vapours, in newly ploughed fields for whooping cough. The air in caves was once considered beneficial for sufferers from pulmonary tuberculosis. Asthma sufferers in Russia were sometimes sent to the salt mines of Siberia following the observation that the miners there seldom suffer from the complaint.

The respiratory membranes are an active and receptive surface which is well illustrated by the use of smelling salts (spirits of ammonia) as a stimulant for people who faint. Inhalation is also used, however, to support the respiration as well as to remove obstruction to the airways, whether in the form of catarrh or broncho-spasm (spasm of the bronchial tubes, as in asthma).

Catarrh of the sinuses and throat is often effectively mobilized by inhalations of steam. Various herbal extracts or aromatic oils can be added to the water. The most famous is Friars Balsam, a resinoid from the plant. Extract of Lupulinum allays irritability of the respiratory organs whilst the inhalation of the fumes from burning Strammonium will relax spasm of involuntary muscles of the bronchial tubes. Herbal chest balsams which can be rubbed on the skin achieve some of their benefits through inhalation.

Although a somewhat elaborate and time-consuming procedure, inhalation therapy is effective and economical when correctly selected herbal vapours are used. The modern use of aerosols in conventional medicine does not diminish the value of this traditional measure.

"Improvised steam inhalation tent" of the type recommended by F. E. Bilz in the 1890s.

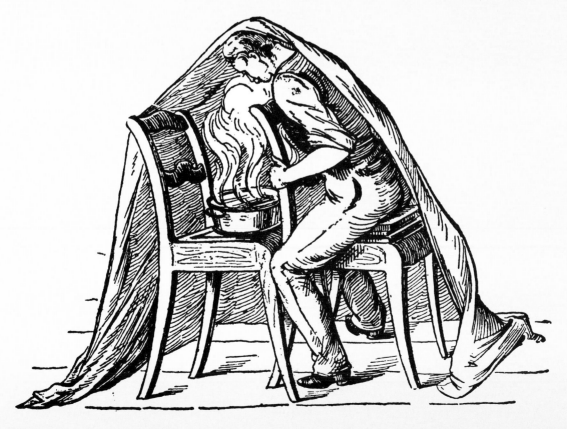

Hydrotherapy

Mineral Water Therapy

There can be few therapeutic modalities which have been so much a part of a fashionable life style, as well as contributing phrases to our language, as mineral water therapy. The practice of drinking and bathing in natural spring waters where these are believed to have special therapeutic benefits has given rise to such terms as 'taking the cure'. In the eighteenth and nineteenth centuries, a few weeks spent taking the waters in a spa where these natural springs are to be found, became an important part of the social calendar for the wealthy classes.

The term 'spa' was adopted for such centres after the name of the Belgian town of Spa, whose mineral springs had been known for their therapeutic benefits since Roman times. But it was not until the late eighteenth century that Spa became a fashionable and famous resort, as did many other European sources, such as Leamington, Baden Baden, and Bath. They were regularly patronized by members of high society and even royalty. Peter the Great and the Emperor Joseph II were regular visitors to Spa.

The therapeutic properties reputedly lie in the mineral content of these waters. Because of the geological structure of the rocks in certain areas, there has been imparted to the water a particular concentration of minerals. However, the common feature of these waters is that the amount of solid mineral constituents is small and that of the gaseous constituents is large. The waters are therefore considered to be of low mineralization in which the natural mineral constituents are present in the form of free ions, and in this ionized form they are more potent in their action than the mineral salts. The ability of the body to utilize minerals in their ionized form is known to be greater.

As the age of leisure and elegance faded, the fashion for mineral water treatment also declined. Furthermore the advent of more immediate forms of symptomatic relief for chronic ailments made the spas less popular. From being an accepted and widely recommended form of orthodox treatment, the mineral water therapy has become one of the more remote forms of unconventional medicine in which the therapeutic claims are regarded with some scepticism in many scientific circles. Even in its heyday, mineral water therapy had its opponents. Bilz, the nineteenth-century German natural therapeutic doctor, strongly criticized the "senseless drinking of enormous quantities of water" which he maintained overstimulated the heart and nervous system.

Was mineral water therapy a fashionable fad, or is there in fact any scientific basis for its application? The equilibrium of many bodily functions depends on the correct composition of the minerals in the blood and serum. The minerals in the body fluids are known as the serum electrolytes and their balance is maintained by the process of osmosis and transport across cell membranes. Minerals perform a number of essential functions in the body. For example, they are required for the metabolism of all cells; they form the greater part of the hard structures, such as bones and teeth; they regulate the permeability of the cell membranes and capillaries; they regulate the excitability of muscles and nervous tissue. Minerals play an important role in the maintenance of the acid-base balance of the body; they are constituents of glandular secretions and play an essential role in the regulation of the osmotic pressure of the cells. Any deficiency, or disturbance in the availability of essential minerals to the body, may contribute to a decline in general vitality or a deterioration of the natural immunity as well as to more serious disease processes.

Mineral water therapy is believed to exert its benefits by restoring the equilibrium of the electrolytes in the body fluids through the provision of mineral substances in an easily assimilable form. Many of

---

Analysis of the Saline Waters at Leamington Spa (calculated in parts* per 100,000)

Electro-Positive Ions

Sodium	(Na^+)	345.12
Potassium	(K^+)	1.56
Magnesium	(Mg^+)	24.56
Calcium	(Ca^+)	68.01
Iron	(Fe^+)	0.105

Electro-Negative Ions

Chloride	(Cl^-)	580.00
Bicarbonate	(HCO_3^-)	7.08
Silicate	(SiO_3^-)	0.24
Sulphate	(SO_4^-)	181.90

In their respective characters, the Leamington Waters closely resemble those of the Continental Spas – Hamburg, Wiesbaden and Kissengen.

*provided by Warwick District Council Information Bureau.

the spa waters contain a high content of ionized calcium, a mineral which plays an important part in many aspects of body metabolism. Others are rich in nitrogen or sulphur, both of which are considered to be of benefit for chronic ailments, particularly in the rheumatic sphere. The waters of many European spas are considered beneficial for rheumatic disorders. Those of places such as Baden Baden are known to be valuable for respiratory problems and gynaecological disorders. Vichy, the famous French resort, has mineral springs the waters of which are beneficial to the digestive system, as also is Marianske Lazne (Marienbad) in Czechoslovakia, a favourite resort of King Edward VII.

Today the mineral waters of many famous resorts are bottled at source and sold throughout the world. They are valuable adjuncts to other forms of dietary and naturopathic treatment. Because of their purity (strict regulations control the bottling of mineral waters at source to prevent possible contamination with impurities or artificial additives), these waters are excellent for use during fasting treatments.

Whatever their therapeutic properties, the refreshing taste and freedom from chemicals, such as chlorine, found in normal drinking water, make the spa waters excellent table water for use with fruit juices, or by themselves.

Roger Newman Turner

Hydrotherapy

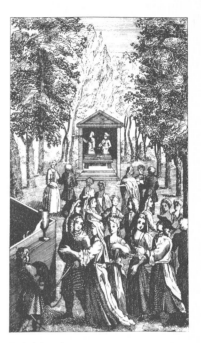

Drinking the waters at Tunbridge Wells in 1664.

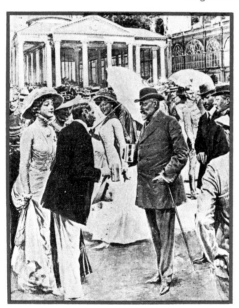

King Edward VII taking the waters at Marienbad.

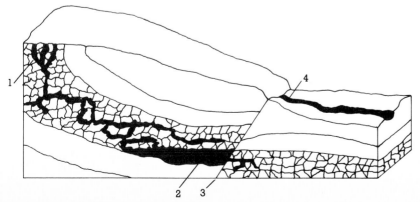

FORMATION OF MINERAL SPRINGS

Surface water, carrying carbon dioxide from the atmosphere, seeps into underground channels (1). It accumulates in large underground basins formed by the geological strata (2) where in the course of time it absorbs mineral substances from the surrounding rocks.

Geological faults (3) may later develop, compressing the underground reservoirs and forcing mineral rich water to the surface where it emerges in natural springs (4).

Herbal Medicine

Herbal medicine may be defined as the art and science of restoring a sufferer to health by the use of plant remedies. These remedies, often referred to as 'herbs', may actually be derived from trees, ferns, seaweeds or lichens. In this context 'herb' is used differently from its usual botanical and gardening connotation. One important feature of herbal medicine is that the remedies used comprise the whole biogenetically produced complex in the plant and not isolated or synthesized chemicals extracted from a plant or elaborated in a laboratory. The purpose of herbal medicine is to assist the recuperative processes in the body, sometimes named homoeostasis, as they re-establish the physiological balance of health. This balance is restored by the use of remedies elaborated in the context of a living cell and given as a biodynamic whole. Clinical observation has shown that the whole plant remedy, consisting of active principles together with complex proteins, enzymes, trace elements (such as iron, fluorine, copper) and other primary metabolites, is readily assimilable and free from the toxic side-effects of drug therapy.

Origins

The origins of herbal medicine are lost in antiquity. All animals are dependent upon plants for their supply of food and for the oxygen they require for life. What is more natural than the discovery and use of plants in prehistoric times as a means of correction in ill health? Virgil's wild goat knew the value of the herb dittany (*Origanum dictamnum*) as an antiseptic and vulnerary when wounded by the hunter's arrow. (*Aeneid* XII 412). Recently, a bitch belonging to a colleague developed mammary cancer and suddenly revealed an insatiable craving for violet leaves. This instinct, widespread in animals, as any farmer will testify, has become almost extinguished in the city dweller of our technological civilization. While traditional herbal medicine is believed to date back several millennia BC in India, China and Egypt, the earliest written records have been discovered in Egypt (Ebers Papyrus *c*. 1500 BC) and Assyria (650 BC). Scores of the herbs named in these documents, and by the Greeks, have been identified as remedies in therapeutic use today. The action of plants in medicine was used by Dioscorides and by Galen as a basis for classification, a practice followed by English herbalists such as John Parkinson, whose *Theatrum Botanicum* (1640) contains descriptions of 3,800 plants arranged according to their medicinal properties. Modern herbals by Otto Gessner (1974) and Schauenberg and Paris (1977) follow this method of grouping remedies under their main constituents and pharmacological actions.

What are herbal remedies?

In herbal medicine, the various organs of a plant may be used, such as root, rhizome, stem, leaf, flower, fruit or seed; or tissues such as bark and wood; or gums and resins which are collected as exudates from incisions in the plant. Many small annual herbs are used whole. In medicine, the fresh herb may be utilized, often taken in an infusion, like making a cup of tea, or the herb may be dried, cut and powdered. Woody remedies are boiled in a little water for twenty minutes to produce a decoction. Preparations from herbs are widely used, especially in dispensing the prescriptions of the herbal practitioner. They include tinctures, often one part of the herb in five parts of diluted alcohol, or liquid extracts which contain one part by weight of the herb in one part by volume of the extract. Tablets, pills, lotions, suppositories and inhalants are also dispensed from herbal remedies. Every continent yields its quota of valuable herbs for use in medicine, and it is common practice to include a cosmopolitan choice of herbal

Herbal Medicine

preparations in the dispensary. Indigenous herbs may be gathered, taking care to avoid proximity to roads and other sources of chemical contamination, not to mention herbicide and insecticide sprays. Harvesting is usually best carried out during the flowering period of the plant for sub-aerial parts, or in the autumn for roots and storage organs. Collection should take place in dry weather conditions, before noon, and the herbs dried rapidly in warm air. They should be stored in airtight containers and protected from light to avoid deterioration. Most herbs will keep well for a year if thoroughly dried and stored carefully.

How herbal remedies act

It is of great importance to ensure the correct identification of a medicinal herb. In the case of a freshly growing herb, complete with flower, the botanical identity may be rapidly confirmed by the use of a botanical *flora*. The dried and powdered remedy presents certain problems which are the concern of the science of pharmacognosy. This consists of an accurate diagnostic description of the herb in various degrees of comminution. Microscope data are given for identification and standards are set for the permitted maximum of foreign plants e.g. grass, of ash after incineration and after treatment with acid. The last establishes a standard for freedom from soil and sand. Many herbal remedies are standardized according to their content of volatile oil, a characteristic of the labiates, including the mints. These requirements for a herb of acceptable quality for use in medicine are set out in the British Herbal Pharmacopoeia, the US Dispensatory and other pharmacopoeias. The monographs on each remedy often include chromatographic and other standards to ensure that the herb is not only correctly identified but that after harvesting and storing, it contains the actual ingredient needed for a successful therapeutic use. In addition to the volatile oils already mentioned, herbs may depend for their medicinal action upon the presence of nitrogen compounds called alkaloids, upon a wide range of substances compounded with various sugars and called glycosides, upon astringent tannins, upon resins, oils and fats, upon carbohydrates and mucilages, and upon complex proteins and enzymes. Vitamins occur widely in plants, and trace chemicals needed for health are supplied by herbs e.g. zinc from the coltsfoot *(Tussilago farfara)*. By the application of the science of pharmacology, which deals with the mode of action of substances upon the organs of the body, we now understand a great deal about the pathways of the herbal constituents from the digestive tract into the blood stream and how the remedial actions are brought about. Such knowledge enables specific treatment to be prescribed for any person, while at the same time building up the general health by the combined action of the other constituents in the natural herb.

Diseases Treated

So wide is the range of constituents present in plants and so enormous is the number of botanical species that it is no surprise to find records of herbal treatment for practically all known diseases of man. Many of these records are based upon clinical observation or on the pharmacological studies of various constituents and sometimes of the whole plant preparation. These diseases include those of the digestive system, liver and pancreas, the pulmonary system, the heart and blood vessels; the nervous, endocrine, reproductive and urinary systems; immune disease, blood dyscrasias, neoplastic disease and skin conditions. No more complete system of medical treatment could be imagined.

Herbal Medicine

COMMON CONDITIONS AND THEIR HERBAL TREATMENT

For the convenience of readers a selection of the herbs used in the treatment of various conditions follows. These herbs are arranged in order of decreasing activity (potency), the most useful is given first. The selection has been made on the basis of clinical experience and traditional usage supported in most cases by the demonstrable properties of constituents present in the plant. Strong remedies, suitable only for prescription by a herbal practitioner, have been omitted. Conditions not listed such as high blood pressure, heart disease, kidney and bladder complaints etc. are not appropriate for self-treatment. If you think you may have a complaint not in the chart, or if you are not making good progress with your selection of remedies, you are advised to consult a herbal or other practitioner for an accurate diagnosis and professional advice.

Note: The same common name may be used of entirely different plants in various localities. To avoid the confusion and serious mistakes which this may cause, the botanical name and authority is also given.

Anxiety, excitability
Hops, *Humulus lupulus* L.; scullcap, *Scutellaria lateriflora* L.; lime flowers, *Tilta platyphyllos* Scop.; *Tilia cordata* Mill.; damiana, *Turnera diffusa* var. *aphrodisiaca* Urb.; pulsatilla, *Anemone pulsatilla* L.; American valerian, *Cypripedium pubescens* Willd.

Appetite – to improve appetite, increase salivation and aid digestion
Centaury, *Centaurium erythraea* Rafn.; gentian, *Gentiana lutea* L.; burdock, *Arctium lappa* L.; chamomile, *Chamaemelum nobile* L.; dandelion, *Taraxacum offinale* L.

Asthma
Senega, *Polygala senega* L.; gum plant, *Grindelia camporum* Greene, Euphorbia pilulifera, *Euphorbia hirta* L.; squill, *Urginea maritima* Baker; sundew, *Drosera rotundifolia* L.

Bedwetting – nocturnal urinary incontinence
Ma huang, *Ephedra sinica* Stapf.; horsetail, *Equisetum arvense* L.

Boils and carbuncles
Burdock, *Arctium lappa* L.; black sampson, *Echinacea angustifolia* (D.C.) Heller, *Echinacea pallida* (Nutt.) Britt.; wild indigo, *Baptisia tinctoria* R.Br. A compress or poultice of marshmallow root, *Althaea officinalis* L.; linseed, *Linum usitatissimum* L.; slippery elm, *Ulmus fulva* Mich., and thyme, *Thymus vulgaris* L. may be applied.

Bronchitis and cough
Gum plant, *Grindelia camporum* Greene; coltsfoot, *Tussilago farfara* L.; white horsehound, *Marrubium vulgare* L.; squill, *Urginea maritima* Baker; licorice, *Glycyrrhiza glabra* L.; comfrey, *Symphytum officinale* L.; boneset, *Eupatorium perfoliatum* L.

Catarrh – nasal
Black sampson, *Echinacea angustifolia* (D.C.) Heller; garlic, *Allium sativum* L.; cayenne, *Capsicum minimum* Roxb.; red eyebright, *Euphrasia officinalis* L.; rosemary, *Rosmarinus officinalis* L.; hyssop, *Hyssopus officinalis* L.; low cudweed, *Gnaphalium uliginosum* L.

Circulation – poor
Prickly ash, *Zanthoxylum americanum* Mill.; cayenne, *Capsicum minimum* Roxb.; hawthorn, *Crataegus oxyacanthoides* Thuill.; galangal, *Alpinia galanga* Willd.

Colds and influenza
Yarrow, *Achillea millefolium* L.; elder, *Sambucus nigra* L.; cayenne, *Capsicum minimum* Roxb.; peppermint, *Mentha piperita* L.; boneset, *Eupatorium perfoliatum* L.; ginger, *Zingiber officinale* Rosc.; catnip, *Nepeta cataria* L.; coltsfoot, *Tussilago farfara* L.

Constipation
Cascara, *Rhamnus purshiana* D.C.; senna, *Cassia angustifolia* Vahl., *Cassia acutifolia* Del.; buckthorn, *Rhamnus cathartica* L.; licorice, *Glycyrrhiza glabra* L.; barberry bark, *Berberis vulgaris* L.; dandelion, *Taraxacum officinale* L.

Contusions and bruises
Apply only to unbroken skin – St John's wort, *Hypericum perforatum* L.; witch hazel, *Hamamelis virginiana* L.; comfrey, *Symphytum officinale* L.; fenugreek, *Trigonella foenum-graecum.*

Corns – *see Warts*

Cramps
Cramp bark, *Viburnum opulus* L.; prickly ash, *Zanthoxylum americanum* Mill.; wild yam, *Dioscorea villosa* L.; cayenne, *Capsicum minimum* Roxb.; rosemary, *Rosmarinus officinalis* L.

Depression
Oats, *Avena sativa* L.; damiana, *Turnera aphrodisiaca* Urb.; ginseng, *Panax shinseng*, *Panax quinquefolium* L.; kola nuts, *Cola nitida* A.Chev., *Cola acuminata* Schott & Endl.; vervain, *Verbena officinalis* L.

Diarrhoea
Oak bark, *Quercus robur* L.; tormentil, *Potentilla tormentilla* Neck.; spotted cranebill, *Geranium maculatum* L.; agrimony, *Agrimonia eupatoria* L.; herb bennet, *Geum urbanum* L.

Dyspepsia – flatulent indigestion
Chamomile, *Chamaemelum nobile* L.; lemon balm, *Melissa officinalis* L.; meadowsweet, *Filipendula ulmaria* L.; hops, *Humulus lupulus* L.; peppermint, *Mentha piperita* L.; marshmallow, *Althaea officinalis* L.; dandelion, *Taraxacum officinale* L.; caraway, *Carum carvi* L.

Eczema and skin affections
Internal use – burdock root, *Arctium lappa* L., *Arctium minus* Bernh.; cleavers, *Galium aparine* L.; fumitory, *Fumaria officinalis* L.; yellow dock root, *Rumex crispus* L.; figwort, *Scrophularia nodosa* L.; nettle, *Urtica dioica* L.; red clover, *Trifolium pratense* L. External application – chickweed, *Stellaria media* (L) Vill.; marshmallow, *Althaea officinalis* L.; chamomile, *Chamaemelum nobile* L.; thyme, *Thymus vulgaris* L.

Gall-bladder complaints – *see Liverishness*

Gout
Goutwort, *Aegopodium podagraria* L.; guaiac, *Guaiacum officinale* L.; celery seed, *Apium graveolens* L.; meadowsweet, *Filipendula ulmaria* L.; bean pod, *Phaseolus vulgaris* L.; queen of the meadow, *Eupatorium purpureum* L.

Haemorrhoids
Plantain, *Plantago major* L.; pilewort, *Ranunculus ficaria* L.; marigold, *Calendula officinalis* L.; witch hazel, *Hamamelis virginiana* L.; herb bennet, *Geum urbanum* L.; ground ivy, *Nepeta hederacea* (L.) Trev.

Headache – *see also Migraine*
Passion flower, *Passiflora incarnata* L.; Jamaica dogwood, *Piscidia erythrina* L.; hops, *Humulus lupulus* L.; wood betony, *Betonica officinalis* L.; St John's wort, *Hypericum perforatum* L.

Incontinence, urinary – *see Bedwetting*

Indigestion – *see Dyspepsia*

Influenza – *see Colds*

Insomnia
Hops, *Humulus lupulus* L.; valerian, *Valeriana officinalis* L.; passion flower, *Passiflora incarnata* L.; American valerian, *Cypripedium pubescens* Willd.; pulsatilla, *Anemone pulsatilla* L.; lime flowers, *Tilia species*.

Liverishness – liver and gall-bladder complaints
Barberry bark, *Berberis vulgaris* L.; fringe tree bark, *Chionanthus virginicus* L.; wahoo, *Euonymus atropurpureus* Jacq.; dandelion root, *Taraxacum officinale* L.; yellow dock root, *Rumex crispus* L.

Lumbago – *see Rheumatism*

Menstruation – excessive
Beth root, *Trillium erectum* L.; American cranesbill, *Geranium maculatum* L.; bistort, *Polygonum bistorta* L.; St John's wort, *Hypericum perforatum* L.; black haw, *Viburnum prunifolium* L.; witch hazel, *Hamamelis virginiana* L.; periwinkle, *Vinca major* L.

Menstruation – painful
Pulsatilla, *Anemone pulsatilla* L.; black haw, *Viburnum prunifolium* L.; passion flower, *Passiflora incarnata* L.; Jamaica dogwood, *Piscidia erythrina* L.; blue cohosh, *Caulophyllum thalictroides* Mich.; wild lettuce, *Lactuca virosa* L.; false unicorn root, *Chamaelirium luteum* (L.) A. Gray; marigold, *Calendula officinalis* L.

Menopausal – depression
St John's wort, *Hypericum perforatum* L.; oats, *Avena sativa* L.; rosemary, *Rosmarinus officinalis* L.

Menopausal – flushes
Life root, *Senecio aureus* L.; goldenseal, *Hydrastis canadensis* L.

Migraine – *see also Headache*
Valerian, *Valeriana officinalis* L.; meadowsweet, *Filipendula ulmaria* L.; mistletoe herb, *Viscum album* L.; vervain, *Verbena officinalis* L.

Nausea and vomiting
Black horehound, *Ballota nigra* L.; chamomile, *Chamaemelum nobile* L.; lemon balm, *Melissa officinalis* L.; peppermint, *Mentha piperita* L.; galangal, *Alpinia officinarum* Hance.

Neuralgia
Hops, *Humulus lupulus* L.; passion flower, *Passiflora incarnata* L.; Jamaica dogwood, *Piscidia erythrina* L.; pulsatilla, *Anemone pulsatilla* L.; scullcap, *Scutellaria lateriflora* L.

Rheumatism
Black cohosh, *Cimicifuga racemosa* Nutt.; bog bean, *Menyanthes trifoliata* L.; celery seed, *Apium graveolens* L.; guaiac, *Guaiacum officinale* L.; meadowsweet, *Filpendula ulmaria* L.; juniper, *Juniperus communis* L.; parsley, *Carum petroselinum* Benth. & Hook.

For external application – wintergreen oil, *Gaultheria procumbens* L.; ragwort, *Senecio jacobaea* L.

Sciatica – *see Neuralgia*

Throat affections
Wild indigo, *Baptisia tinctoria* R.Br.; myrrh, *Commiphora molmol* Eng.; poke root, *Phytolacca americana* L.; black sampson, *Echinacea angustifolia* (D.C.) Heller, *Echinacea pallida* (Nutt.) Britt.; cayenne, *Capsicum minimum* Roxb.; red sage, *Salvia officinalis* L.; raspberry, *Rubus idaeus* L.; thyme, *Thymus vulgaris* L.

Ulceration – mouth ulcers
Paint with myrrh, *Commiphora molmol* Eng.; ipecacuanha, *Cephaelis ipecacuanha* (Brot.) A. Rich; red sage, *Salvia officinalis* L.; oak bark, *Quercus robor* L.

Ulceration – leg ulcers
Apply as compress, lotion or ointment, comfrey, *Symphytum officinale* L.; marshmallow, *Althaea officinalis* L.; marigold, *Calendula officinalis* L.; American cranesbill, *Geranium maculatum* L.; chickweed, *Stellaria media* (L.) Vill.

Ulceration – of stomach or duodenum
Chamomile, *Chamaemelum nobile* L.; hops, *Humulus lupulus* L.; comfrey, *Symphytum officinale* L.; lemon balm, *Melissa officinalis* L.; bur-marigold, *Bidens tripartita* L.; meadowsweet, *Filipendula ulmaria* L.; peppermint, *Mentha piperita* L.

Vomiting – *see Nausea*

Warts and corns
External application – greater celandine, *Chelidonium majus* L.; spurge latex, *Euphorbia peplus* L., *Euphorbia species*; arbor-vitae, *Thuja occidentalis* L.; garlic, *Allium sativum* L.

Wounds – to aid healing
Comfrey, *Symphytum officinale* L.; marigold, *Calendula officinalis* L.; American cranesbill, *Geranium maculatum* L.; plantain, *Plantago major* L.; slippery elm, *Ulmus fulva* Mich.; black sampson, *Echinacea species*.

Herbal Medicine

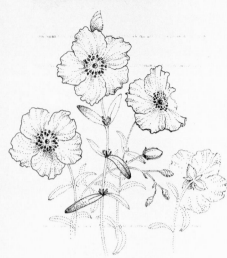

Rock rose

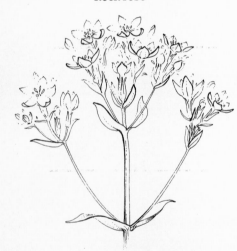

Centaury

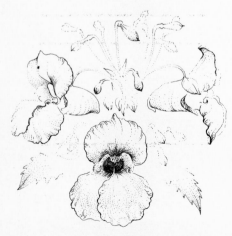

Impatiens

The Herbal Practitioner

It should be evident from a perusal of all of these disease conditions that most of these are much too serious to be suitable for self-diagnosis and medication. Should there be no marked improvement or alleviation of symptoms after taking a herbal tea for say 'indigestion' or 'headache', it would be wise to seek the advice of a herbal practitioner who is qualified after a lengthy course of training in accurate diagnosis and in the herbal materia medica. The National Institute of Medical Herbalists of Great Britain was founded in 1864 and maintains a Tutorial School of Herbal Medicine which prepares applicants for the written and practical examination for membership of the Institute. Members are engaged in herbal practice, not in the retail supply of remedies, although many have their own dispensaries. The practice of herbal medicine, protected in Britain under a law of Henry VIII, has recently been given statutory recognition in sections 12 and 56 of the Medicines Act (1968). The appointment of a herbal practitioner to two sub-committees under the Medicines Commission and to the Committee on the Review of Medicines is important and indicates a growing awareness of the valuable contribution of herbal therapy to medicine.

Herbalism in North America and Europe

While medical herbalists in Britain last century were uniting to form the National Institute, the effectiveness of herbal remedies used by the indigenous races was being rediscovered in North America. Pioneering practitioners such as Samuel Thomson (1769–1843) in New Hampshire, publicized the valuable herbs growing in the United States, including such remedies as *Lobelia inflata*, *Dioscorea villosa* (Wild Yam), *Zanthoxylum* (Prickly Ash), *Cypripedium pubescens* (American Valerian), and so on. The principle of therapy called *physiomedicalism* was established in which the sick person is regarded as suffering from a disturbance of the normal equilibrium which we know as health. The function of the physician is to aid the natural restorative processes with non-poisonous herbal medicines and the adoption of a health-maintaining dietary regimen. The theory that disease was due to micro-organisms was discounted. Emetic and colonic lavage were used to 'cleanse the system from effete matter'.

Such was the therapeutic success of physiomedicalism that hospitals and medical colleges were founded in many States and were recognized by the legislature until well into this century. This movement in North America influenced the development of herbal medicine in Britain and there was a reciprocal interchange of practitioners across the Atlantic. Dr A. I. Coffin brought physiomedicalism to Lancashire and to London in 1838. He found that a similar growth in herbal philosophy and practice had arisen independently from the work of Samuel Tilke, born in Devon (1794). The American and British systems were amalgamated in the work of John Skelton (1853) and succeeding practitioners. As a result, many valuable herbs in use today by British herbalists are imported from America as they have been for a century.

There appears to be no diminution in the interest in herbal remedies – judging by the numerous enquiries from citizens of the US for information on herbs or for courses of training in their therapeutic application. American Schools of Pharmacology have launched ambitious programmes to examine large numbers of plants in an attempt to discover constituents useful in medicine. In the process, hundreds of folk medicine reports have been recorded and much valuable information adduced. It is still possible for the public to obtain medicinal herbs through retail outlets, but the practice of medicine, and that includes herbal medicine, is restricted to the registered physician in the US and Canada, as in many other countries today.

Herbal Medicine

A large number of herbs prescribed and used in Britain are derived from mainland Europe whence the knowledge of their health-restoring activity first came. Such well-known remedies as the chamomile and lime flowers are among herbs imported to Britain from Europe. In most countries of Europe, the position is similar to that which exists in America as far as availability of herbs is concerned. The general practitioner of Western Germany includes the use of herbs, both in material and in homoeopathic dosage, in his therapy. He is licensed to practise according to the regulations in force in various regions and he is served by manufacturing firms as Madaus of Cologne, where extensive research on herbal remedies is carried out.

Advancing Knowledge

There is today a resurgence of interest in herbal medicine. Millions of people take plant remedies, and there is a significant change of climate towards natural treatment evident in Europe, Scandinavia, Russia, China, India, Australasia and some parts of Africa. The screening of many thousands of species for antitumour and antiviral activity by Professor Farnsworth and the search for alkaloids in plants by Dr Smolenski and his workers, both investigations centred in the United States, have discovered a number of valuable remedies in hitherto unknown herbs. It is estimated that there are 250,000 species of flowering plants and only a tiny proportion of these has been examined for therapeutic activity. More advances have been made in this field during recent decades than in any other. It is arguable that malignant disease might well have been under control if the effort put into chemotherapy had been expended in the study of plant antitumour remedies. History records the rise and fall of many fashions in medical treatment, but herbal medicine has a future as secure as its venerable past.

F. Fletcher Hyde

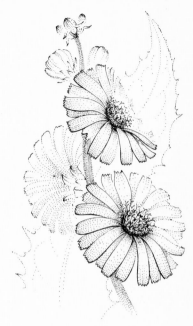

Chicory

Vita Florum

Elizabeth Bellhouse has been working with alternative forms of therapy since 1938 and with flower potencies since 1945. A selection of flowers, some common, some rare, some growing locally and others from all over the world, are held in water in sunlight until their power passes into it. The method is exacting and tedious since the flowers are not cut or bruised in any way. The choice of flowers is not random, for Mrs Bellhouse is led to them by Divine guidance. She says that the potentized water contains the radiations of the Creator for which the flowers are the vehicle.

While Exultation of Flowers acts on the psyche, Vita Florum heals the body because it is a harmonizing agent that opens the way for psychological and spiritual growth. Vita Florum differs from the Bach Flower Remedies in that the flowers are not cut, and from homoeopathic potencies because the principle is not one of like curing like. Mrs Bellhouse has coined the word 'Homoeovitic' for this "principle new to science" (Dr Alec Forbes), stating that Vita Florum has the same base as vitality or life.

Quoting Andrew Weil *(The Natural Mind)* she says: " 'Man has an innate normal desire to alter consciousness.' By capturing and limiting our awareness, illness and pain chain or imprison us, restricting our consciousness drastically, for, if we functioned as we should do, we would spend every bit as much time in other states of being and consciousness as we do in awareness of the physical world and of our physical bodies."

Vita Florum gives three kinds of help:

(i) "help in positively directing our other inner-consciousness into calm, unitive, constructive states of being and awareness, so that

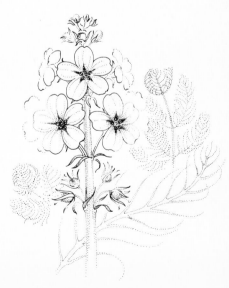

Water violet

Vita Florum

our other-consciousness can contribute peace and harmony to our physical selves:

(ii) "immediate help to get over pain and illness so that we can live fully, not only in this mortal physical life, but also in the other states of being and consciousness that we should inhabit:

(iii) "courage, strength, and understanding so that we do not repeat the same sort of mistakes and so that our other-consciousness can contribute to our physical and our general well-being at all times."

Vita Florum works on everybody and every living thing as a general tonic, and, in more frequent doses, as a therapeutic agent. A great many people have vouched for the efficacy of the preparations, which are currently also used by many orthodox doctors. It comes in a water base for internal use; in a lotion, an ointment, a massage oil and a talcum powder for external application; as water and salve for animals; as a foliar spray and as a soil conditioner.

Prepared from information supplied by Elizabeth Bellhouse

Exultation of Flowers

Exultation of Flowers was first offered to the public by Alick McInnes in 1956. This preparation consists of the potencies of many flowers. For each flower there is an ideal time when the transference may be effected, usually when the flowers are at their peak, sometimes around the time of the full moon. Potencies from the rose, for example, are taken in midsummer. When the flower radiations are transferred to the water, they remain indefinitely, with no preservative added.

Since the death of Alick McInnes in 1975, Kay McInnes has continued to market this preparation. She uses eighty-four different species growing in her garden and in the fields around her house, holding the blossoms close to the water, but not immersing them. She says that the action of butterfles, bees and other insects intensifies the radiations.

In 1961, following a trial under the Trades Description Act, the Court ordered that all bottles of Exultation of Flowers be labelled as containing one hundred percent water, since the radiations cannot be identified by chemical analysis.

Exultation of Flowers is not a specific treatment for any particular disease. It operates on the radiations flowing through the human body and in so doing raises the general vitality. An average dose is five or six drops. Animals also benefit and, in a garden spray, it can be used on flowers and fruit.

Prepared from the introductory booklet on the Exultation of Flowers by Alick McInnes

Bach Flower Remedies

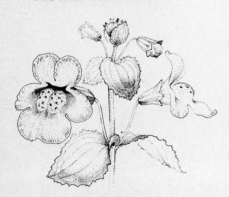

Mimulus

Dr Edward Bach MB, BS, MRCS, LRCP, trained and qualified at University College, London and gained the Diploma of Public Health (DHP) at Cambridge in 1913. He died in 1936.

During his medical training, he began to see that his interest lay not so much in treating physical symptoms, but in the patients themselves, their personalities and their emotional states. He realized that the body is the mirror of the mental condition, for if the patient is without hope, fearful, worried or depressed he makes slow progress, whereas the hopeful, cheerful man, determined to recover, does so far more rapidly. The sufferer therefore requires help to overcome his negative thinking, the basic cause of his ill health. A new and practical treatment was needed, for it was of little use just to say to a worried man: "Don't worry, be happy".

When he had qualified, Dr Bach determined to test for himself other methods of conventional medicine and, after practising as an orthodox consultant for some years, he turned to bacteriology, gaining a considerable reputation for his researches into that branch of medicine. The work did not satisfy him, however, for he was still

Bach Flower Remedies

treating bodies, not people. He then came into contact with homoeopathy and was delighted to discover that Hahnemann, the founder of homoeopathy had said: ''The patient is the most important factor in his healing''. Dr Bach became a homoeopath, working for several years in the laboratories of the Royal London Homoeopathic Hospital. There he successfully prepared seven nosodes for chronic diseases, given by mouth. A significant discovery was to follow. It became clear that all the patients with the same emotional problems needed the same nosode, irrespective of their varying physical ailments. From that moment onwards, he based his prescriptions entirely upon the nature of the patient's temperament. The results were excellent.

Bach was now convinced that physical disease was not of physical origin, but the 'consolidation of a mental attitude'. But homoeopathy was a lifetime's study; a simple, harmless treatment must quickly be arrived at which would restore peace of mind and hope to the sick. He believed that he would find such remedies amongst the trees and plants of Nature, for all our needs are provided for in Nature by our Creator. Bach already knew that the basic principle of his new method would be ''treat the patient and not his disease''. In 1930 he abandoned all his professional work in London and departed, without a backward thought, to live in the country.

Throughout his years of medical practice, he had been seeking for scientific proofs, using his intellect. A change now came about. He became extremely sensitive to his intuitive faculty, for he found that by holding his hand over a flowering plant he would experience in himself the properties of that plant. When seeking a particular flower for a negative state of mind, he himself would also suffer in an acute form that distressing condition, but upon finding the right flower his serenity and peace of mind were immediately restored.

During the next seven years, he isolated thirty-eight benign wild flowers to cover the negative states of mind from which mankind can suffer. He used only the flowers that grow above ground in air and sunlight, holding in their hearts the seeds, the continuous life of the plant. These flowers he prepared in the field where they grew, placing the flower heads upon the surface of water in a plain glass bowl, in full sunlight, for three hours. Nature then took over without further human interference. The heat of the sun drew the life-force of the flowers into the water, which became sparkling and full of tiny bubbles – living water. The flowers were then gently lifted out of the bowl and the water bottled and preserved. For early-blooming flowers, mostly the tree flowers, he used a different method. These he placed in a sterile saucepan, brought them quickly to the house, covered them with water and gently boiled them for half an hour. The flowers removed, the water was filtered, bottled and preserved by adding a small amount of brandy. The Bach Remedies are always prepared in this way.

These remedies are not homoeopathic, nor do they have different potencies, for the power set free from the flowers is the unalterable life-force itself. They are not prescribed for any particular physical complaint, but for the basic cause, the patient's apprehension, depression, jealousy, worry, lack of confidence.

Dr Bach divided the thirty-eight remedies into seven groups to treat fear, uncertainty, insufficient interest in present circumstances, loneliness, over-sensitivity to influences and ideas, despondency and over anxiousness for the welfare of others. One of the most popular products is the *Rescue* remedy which combines five remedies to form this emergency first aid. It can be used in all cases and concepts of shock, terror, panic, sorrow, sudden bad news, great or small accidents.

Nora Weeks

THE THIRTY-EIGHT REMEDIES
(grouped under sub-headings)

FEAR
Rock Rose, Mimulus, Cherry Plum, Aspen, Red Chestnut

UNCERTAINTY
Cerato, Scleranthus, Gentian, Gorse, Hornbeam, Wild Oat

INSUFFICIENT INTEREST IN PRESENT CIRCUMSTANCES
Clematis, Honeysuckle, Wild Rose, Olive, White Chestnut, Mustard, Chestnut Bud

LONELINESS
Water Violet, Impatiens, Heather

OVER-SENSITIVITY TO INFLUENCES AND IDEAS
Agrimony, Centaury, Walnut, Holly

DESPONDENCY OR DESPAIR
Larch, Pine, Elm, Sweet Chestnut, Star of Bethlehem, Willow, Oak, Crab Apple

OVER-CARE FOR WELFARE OF OTHERS
Chicory, Vervain, Vine, Beech, Rock Water

(It is necessary to obtain *The Twelve Healers* booklet on prescribing to ascertain which remedy is appropriate to individual states of mind)

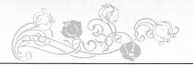

Aromatherapy

Although its roots can be traced back to the early Egyptian empire some 5000 years ago, therapy with essential oils is relatively new as a healing discipline in its own right. The term 'aromatherapy' was coined about fifty years ago by René Maurice Gattefossé, a French cosmetic chemist. His interest was aroused when preliminary research showed that essential oils in general have a profound effect on the skin. Further investigations revealed that these essences could be successfully used not only as cosmetic agents, but also to treat medical skin conditions, such as dermatitis. Gattefossé wrote of ''a sphere of research opening enormous vistas to those who have started exploring it''.

Gattefossé realized the tremendous value of essential oils as antibacterial agents and their potential for treating all kinds of infections. Although interest in this area was considerably dampened with the advent of antibiotics, it is very possible that plant essences present a viable alternative which is also natural. It is true that essences are not always as effective as antibiotics, but at the same time they do not have the drawbacks of antibiotics. Recent research in the USSR has revealed that a type of eucalyptus oil is effective against a common influenza virus. Antiviral agents are rare indeed and virtually unknown in the realm of nature.

A colleague of Gattefossé's, Godissart, set up his own aromatherapy clinic in the United States, where he developed a treatment for skin cancers based on lavender oil. His successes with essential oils also included the treatment of gangrene, osteomalacia and facial ulcers, all of which were healed in record time.

Following the earlier work of Gattefossé and other pioneers in Europe, two important figures, Marguerite Maury and Dr Jean Valnet, emerged in the late 1950s, both of whom made considerable contributions to the development of aromatherapy.

Marguerite Maury, who died some ten years ago, has become something of a legend. Her book *The Secret of Life and Youth* is perceptive and thought-provoking. Dr Jean Valnet, a French doctor and ex-army surgeon, is the author of another classic book *Aromatherapie*. Their individual approaches to aromatherapy were, however, very different. While Madame Maury attempted to treat the whole person – mind, body and psyche – and used the oils externally for massage. Dr Valnet was more orthodox in his approach and prescribed them to be taken by mouth as would an orthodox doctor or a herbalist.

Some see aromatherapy as a branch of herbal medicine, and in fact many herbs owe their properties to the essential oil they contain – clove, eucalyptus, peppermint and so on. However in practice essences are very rarely used by herbalists; there is a basic difference between the healing effect of herb and essence. Many essences can be prescribed in the same way as herbs, i.e. a carminative such as coriander oil, is prescribed for indigestion; an antispasmodic, like marjoram oil, is given for asthma. The difference is due in fact to the ethereal nature of the oils (they are highly volatile) which gives them a profound effect on the mental/emotional level, an effect comparable to the Bach Flower Remedies. The effect of essences on the mind can sometimes be even more powerful than their action on the body and so aromatherapy lends itself to a wholistic, mind/body approach which goes beyond normal herbal practice. An important factor in 'psychological aromatherapy' is the actual perception of fragrance by the patient, and this seems to come nearer to the literal meaning of aromatherapy than any other approach.

Dr Paolo Rovesti, at Milan University, has been studying the effects of essential oils on the mind. Sometimes he gives the oils on sugar, which is then allowed to slowly dissolve in the mouth. Because the perception of the fragrance is so important they are often simply

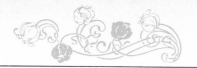

Aromatherapy

sprayed around the patient from an aerosol can. Rovesti has successfully used essences which are basically nerve stimulants or sedatives to treat the opposing states of depression and anxiety. The effect of odours on the emotions has been known for centuries, but it is only in the last thirty years or so that we have begun to realize the healing potential of this deep, inherent response to fragrance. From my own experience with aromatherapy, essences can be found for the whole spectrum of emotional dis-ease; from anger (chamomile), to grief (hyssop), to jealousy (rose).

In use, essential oils are extremely versatile. They are ideally suited to massage since they dissolve in vegetable oil (they are too strong to use neat) and are readily absorbed by the skin. This absorption and subsequent dispersal of essential oil through the tissues of the body, formed the basis of Madame Maury's therapy. In this way the oils can be used not only to stimulate or relax, but also to treat most types of internal problem. It is interesting to note that essences in general and in particular bergamot, chamomile and lavender, have been found to possess the property of stimulating the production of white blood cells, but that this effect only takes place when the essence is either rubbed on the skin or inhaled. Thus these oils can stimulate the body's natural defences against any infection and can be used either to treat infection or simply to maintain a high level of resistance.

The other principal method of application is to give the oils orally- usually about three drops on a little sugar. In this way they can be prescribed like herbs or drugs, to treat all types of complaints, mental and physical.

Essential oils lend themselves admirably for use in therapeutic baths; they can also be easily incorporated into creams, gels, ointments, lotions, capsules, syrups and aerosols.

The use of essences and products made with them, is now very popular in beauty therapy, for these oils not only permeate the skin with great ease but many of them have a particular action on the skin. For example, lavender oil is for oily skin, sandalwood for dry skin and chamomile for inflamed or sensitive skin. Chamomile oil contains the chemical azulene, which is now known to be an effective anti-inflammatory agent. Azulene is increasingly used in both cosmetic and medicinal creams and lotions.

Azulene, as the name suggests, is a deep blue colour; blue is also the colour used in colour therapy to reduce inflammation. This leads on to an entirely different approach to aromatherapy which, to my knowledge, is little used. We can see essences, not as chemical mixtures but as 'liquid vibrations', each one having a certain resonance which corresponds with a particular colour and sound. Cinnamon oil, for instance, corresponds with the colour orange, which is associated with the sun, traditionally the ruling planet of cinnamon. The sun comes under the element of fire, and in oriental terms cinnamon is a yang essence. This picture corresponds well with the fact that cinnamon is basically warming, stimulating the heart and circulation and causing a slight rise in temperature. A similar correspondence can be seen with each essence, and in this way they can be used rather like colours, to treat on a level which relates to the subtle body of the patient.

This approach enables one to treat physical and emotional disease in a very precise manner, each remedy being tailor-made for the patient. Such accuracy of prescription is a fine art requiring much experience and, eventually, an intuitive grasp of aromatherapy.

Robert Tisserand

The Rules of Eating

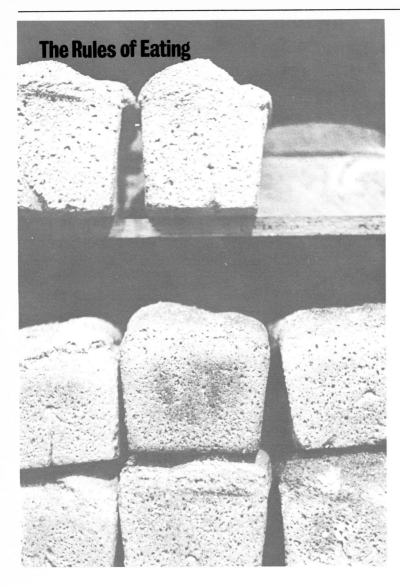

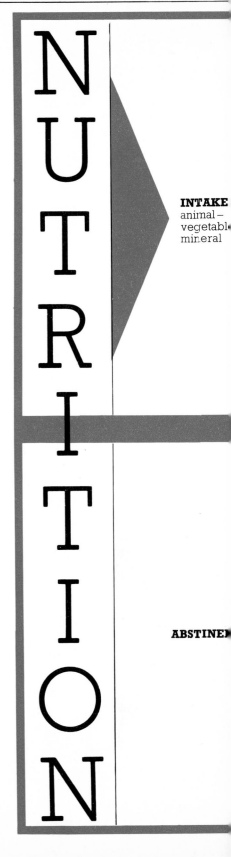

INTAKE
animal –
vegetable
mineral

ABSTINE

Sensible eating is only one of the factors essential to the securement and maintenance of good health. Without fresh air and sunlight, ample movement, adequate rest and sleep, pure water and joyful emotions there cannot be lasting health.

If NUTRITION is taken to mean the provision of life-maintaining nourishment to any tissue or cell of the body – without which that tissue or cell would ail and die – it is implicit that:

1. there must be an intake of foodstuffs biologically suitable for the person concerned;

2. the organs of mastication, digestion, absorption and assimilation must be efficient;

3. there must be unimpeded disposal of the non-food elements ingested as well as of the waste products of metabolism;

4. the mental and emotional climate must be such as to avoid interference with nervous and hormonal activity which is the controlling and co-ordinating mechanism of all nutritive processes.

A NUTRIENT is that which provides nutrition and is a constituent of food.

FOOD (becomes a healthy part of the living being)	MACRONUTRIENT	PROTEIN / CARBOHYDRATE / FAT	BUILDING / REPAIRING
	MICRONUTRIENT	MINERAL SALTS / TRACE ELEMENTS / VITAMINS / ENZYMES	ORGANICALLY PROTECTIVE / CATALYTIC
NON-FOOD (the body strives to dispose of dilute or render harmless)	ESSENTIAL	PRESERVATIVES non-toxic / PURIFYING AGENTS / ROUGHAGE	ELIMINATIVE / CHEMICALLY PROTECTIVE
	NON-ESSENTIAL	CHEMICALS additives, pesticides, fertilizers / DRUGS medical, habitual / POISONS	DESTRUCTIVE / PSEUDO-PLEASURABLE

FASTING	PHYSIOLOGY abstinence between meals	
	RELIGION	
	POLITICS protest	
	SELF-DISCIPLINE	
	HYGIENE	physiological rest / physiological compensation
	PATHOLOGY stenosis, anorexia	
	INJURY	
	CAPTIVITY	

STARVATION	ACCIDENT or DESIGN
	ISOLATION in foodless environment
	PATHOLOGY stenosis, anorexia
	FAMINE

The Rules of Eating

FOOD comprises all those materials which by their nature can contribute to the energy supply of an organism or provide the components necessary for the growth and repair of its tissues. No substance in a foodstuff can be considered as food if it is not a source of potential energy which can be converted into heat and nervous or muscular work (carbohydrate, fat, protein); or a means of conserving the material of the body (protein); or a catalyst or a protective element (vitamin, mineral, trace element, enzyme). Food, by this definition, is that which becomes one with the living body and *assists in its continued survival.*

NON-FOODS may include some possibly desirable elements, such as those that enhance flavour or appearance, prevent decomposition, especially of animal products, or provide roughage. Most non-food components are potential hazards to the living body which will try to dispose of them or render them harmless. If the stomach is irritated, for example, there may be vomiting. If the hazard passes through the stomach into the small intestine, there may be increased peristalsis and eventual diarrhoea of the contents of the lower bowel. Should the toxic substances remain within the alimentary canal, there is likely to be an increase of secretions in an effort to dilute or wash them away. Immovable irritants may be encysted. If the normal eliminative efforts are insufficient to prevent absorption of the toxic material into general circulation, other systems may be called to the body's defence. Kidneys and bladder, lungs, skin may all show so-called symptoms. Bile secretion may be retched up, urine become thickened, the skin erupt or heat up with fever; there may be excessive catarrhal mucus, swollen lymph glands, coughing, sneezing or discharging from any orifice or wound. All are indicative of the extent to which the overloading has involved other organs and systems.

A satisfactory FOODSTUFF therefore must, when eaten, be free from deleterious substances that could:

1. harm the body, such as chemical poisons;

2. prevent other components of the foodstuff from fulfilling their function;

3. cumulatively force the body to mobilize its defence mechanisms in order to survive.

Sources of Food

1. Primarily, green plants. The healthier the soil, the more nourishing its produce.

2. Animals or plants which depend for their own metabolism on green plants, e.g. cattle, mushrooms.

3. Bacteria which live in human intestines and synthesize, for example, certain vitamins; hence one of the dangers of liquid paraffin or antibiotics which ultimately are detrimental to intestinal flora.

Quality

People reflect the quality of the produce they eat even into future generations. The quality and dietetic value of food hinge on factors such as the following:

a. maturity or 'ripeness';

b. foods in season and indigenous;

c. the relative proportions of a foodstuff's different components – ratios of sodium to potassium and calcium to phosphorus, for example, are all-important;

d. fertility of the soil;

e. freshness (minimal storage, processing and cooking);

f. not least, the requirements of the ingesting organism.

The Rules of Eating

Requirements of the Ingesting Organism

Individual needs must be assessed according to:

1. Age. Older people need less food; growing children have special requirements; it may be easier for young people to change their habits than for those set in their aged ways.

2. Health. Certain diseases will either preclude or demand certain foods (see *Supplementary*, *Restricted*). In some degenerative conditions, such as of the heart or kidneys, the total withholding of food would be contra-indicated (see *Fasting*).

3. Likes and dislikes. The nature of the individual often dictates food peculiarities, ranging from the obsessional to the imitative: "that's the way I am"; "that's what I eat".

4. The role of food. Some eat merely in order to stay alive. There are others for whom eating is the sole pleasure. Food may also be linked with social or business activities. For many, eating is a compensation for lack of affection or for any of a number of psychologically associated experiences; guilt, punishment or spite, for instance.

5. Convention, religion, compassion, economics. (See *Fasting*, *Vegetarianism*, *Veganism*).

6. Availability. There are three types of availability: of the food to the eater (soil, market, finance); of the food component to the eater's body, (quality, food combinations, wholeness); of the digested nutrients to the tissues (general health, supporting systems providing oxygen, waste elimination, nerve and hormone control).

Principles of Food Selection

1. Avoid fanaticism. Fear of 'wrong' foods is as counter-productive as fear of germs.

2. A healthy soil is the one indispensable requisite for healthy produce and therefore a healthy chain of consumers – bacteria, plants, animals, people. This implies a minimum of artificial chemicalization, respect for the cycles of fertility and climate, organic composting and judicious crop rotation.

3. Consume foodstuffs that are as close to their original state as is possible, i.e. unrefined, unprocessed, fresh, raw (if so edible) and uncontaminated by non-food elements (see *Wholefood*, *Raw Food*).

4. Keep meals simple; three or four items at a meal are unlikely to strain the digestive organs or to create the problems attendant upon unwise food combining (see *Hay*, *Bircher-Benner* and *Natural Hygiene*).

5. Except on social occasions, drink only when thirsty. Only water is capable of activating the thirst-regulating mechanism in the brain. Sweet drinks, or tea and coffee tend, like alcohol, to be taken for reasons other than thirst and as such are usually taken to physiological excess. While fruit and vegetable juices are extremely useful, it is inadvisable to drink more than one would eat if the sources were in their original state. A glass of juice expressed from ten oranges, say, will flood the system out of all proportion to the potential benefits of oranges. (See *Supplementary Diets*).

6. Eat no more than is necessary. Overeating, whether of good, bad or indifferent food is the prime dietetic error.

Health improves with sensible nutrition. There will be better blood supply, clearer complexion, improved glandular function and the return of youthful vigour, with a heightened sense of taste and smell. This will eventually ensure a re-establishment of the nutritional instincts missing from the average individual. Animals in the wild and certain societies before they were spoiled by the short-cuts of civilization are and were healthy because they knew how to eat, what to eat and when to eat. *Joseph Goodman*

Wholefood

Wholefood in the simplest sense is food which exists in the natural, living state and comprises fruit, vegetables, grains and edible seeds. In the context of this book there is a further qualification. It should be 'organically' grown, which is to say without the aid of most chemical fertilizers and free from pesticides and weedkillers.

Fifty years ago, the concept of wholefood was new. What has compelled wide attention to it more recently is the impact of factory farming and food technology in industrialized countries and in particular the use of chemical sprays, fertilizers and food additives, either to stimulate growth or to preserve, colour and flavour food. It is known that many of the chemicals used are lethal to plants and to human life. The theory that only infinitesimal doses are absorbed by the consumer is in conflict with the known cumulative effects of such toxic materials. The fact that a certain chemical spray or additive is ultimately banned because of its toxic effect is again neutralized by the constant additions made to the list.

Apart from wholefoods which are consumed raw, such as fruit, vegetables and nuts, there is a second category which must be processed, such as wheat and sugar.

When wheat is grown naturally and then stone ground, the result is a flour which retains the vital wheat germ, but removes sufficient of the fibrous matter (bran) to make it palatable and digestible. The extraction rate is then around 80–85 percent, which means that 85 pounds of flour are produced from 100 pounds of wheat.

Sugar is a natural food present in most fruits and many vegetables. However, to extract sufficient sugar from those foods would entail consuming masses of fibrous matter – an impossible task for human economy and for most normal digestive processes. When cane sugar was first used, it was as much for its medicinal purposes as a luxury item of diet. Extraction was limited and the sugar was dark and contained many of the vitamins, amino acids and mineral salts possessed by the plant in its original state. Efficiency in refining methods increased productivity and eroded nutritional quality. Gradually, white sugar arrived at its present 99 percent sucrose content, but all essential nutrients are removed in the process, leading to unbalanced and deficient food.

The introduction of the steel roller mill to produce flour, the volatile growth of sugar refining from both cane and beet pose a menace to health by altering natural food articles from nutritious substances to near 'dead' foods containing little or nothing of the natural elements essential to health. This process, furthermore, creates a dangerous concentration of calorific matter which disturbs the body's balance. The danger was not serious when white bread and white sugar were luxury items. But as refined wheat and sugar extended their hold on the market, those who recognized the dangers began to talk about wholefoods. Two wars provided vital evidence that when the consumption of white flour and white sugar products were curtailed and more extensive use was made of wholegrains, public health increased.

Feeding the world's population requires industrialized processes for mass production. The problem is to maintain nutritional levels. The increasing number of healthfood shops in city centres points to a growing awareness of the importance of wholefoods by an enlightened minority. The critical question is how to make wholefoods available to the public worldwide through education and technological advances.

Alan Moyle

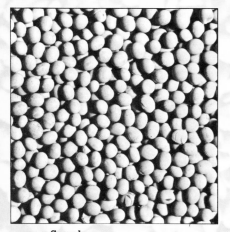

Soya beans

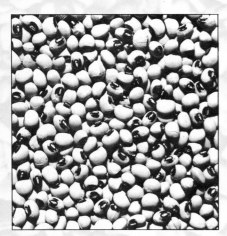

Blackeye beans

Vegetarianism

Vegetarianism is often thought of as being a relatively modern attitude to nutrition, but in fact it is as old as civilization itself. In many parts of the world, the exclusion of meat from the diet has been part of the religious and philosophical way of life for thousands of years. Traditionally, neither Buddhist nor Hindus are meat eaters and Taoist writings state that a meatless diet is essential for spiritual development. The priestly classes of the Aztecs and particularly the Incas were vegetarian. In Europe, the Pythagorean School of the 5th century BC laid down strict rules of conduct for the three hundred young men who formed its select society. Blood sacrifices were unknown and cakes and fruits were the only ceremonial offerings allowed. Pythagoras enjoined abstinence from the flesh of living beings because, he said, it conduces to peace. Seneca wrote an attack on butchery and later Francis Bacon wrote on compassion for dumb animals. Subsequent literary references are legion.

It is a curious irony that modern developed countries regard the ability to afford beef as a mark of material success, while the Third World is less fortunate. In fact, the incidence of coronary diseases and rheumatic disability is markedly less prevalent in the under-developed countries than is the case in the comfortable West. A further irony is that while in the East it was the élite, the educated or priestly class that chose to be vegetarian, the lower orders of society were often meat eaters.

The modern case for vegetarianism is based on moral, economic and therapeutic grounds. The ethical case has been reinforced in recent years by the methods of modern factory farming. It is generally accepted that however many safeguards are built into the rearing and slaughtering of animals for food, cruelty cannot be divorced from the process. The production of veal is a particularly unnatural and cruel procedure.

On economic grounds, there is an equally good case for vegetarianism. In terms of nutrition, meat is expensive and inefficient. The amount of food and space taken up by cows and pigs in the course of their existence is unrelated to the eventual value of the animal when slaughtered. Far more protein, calories, vitamins and fats are available from non-animal sources for considerably less time and space. It is estimated that the conversion rate of domestic animals (including dairy cows) into actual food is never much higher than 4:10 and probably considerably less. Some quote a ratio of 1:10. But whatever the precise figure, there is no doubt that in terms of the food they consume, the return is low. Half the total grain consumption of the world is fed to domestic animals. When this is added to the pasture land that could be used for tillage it is obvious that meat is nutritionally uneconomic.

On health grounds, the case is equally firm. While fruit and vegetables are alkaline in reaction, meat is highly acid (especially pork and offal). Vegetarians usually have an alkaline urine, while that of meat eaters is invariably acid. Excesses of meat are known to be partially responsible for cases of rheumatism, chronic arthritis, gout and other diseases of the musculo-skeletal system. Meat is a high cholesterol food which damages the arteries and is toxic to the bloodstream. The toxic factor is increased by the chemicals in animal feeding stuffs and those drugs and vaccines with which the animal is treated. Meat is also a highly stimulating food, whereas fruit and vegetables tend to have a calming influence.

Early vegetarians had little idea of correct nutrition. In their concern to avoid flesh foods they tended to eat too much starch (even white bread and refined cereals) and to make up the protein deficiency with nuts, eggs cheese and pulses. Modern vegetarians, how-

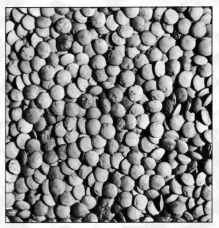

Lentils

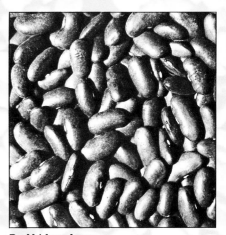

Red kidney beans

Vegetarianism

ever, have a clearer concept of balanced nutrition and lay more emphasis on wholefoods. One raw salad meal and one raw fruit a day is advocated, and they stress the importance of wholewheat bread, unrefined cereals, fruit, vegetables, sprouting shoots and seed oils.

There is no doubt that complete vegetarianism would not suit every individual. Much has been made of vitamin B12 deficiency in vegetarians. This is only true in some cases, and the same deficiency also occurs in meat eaters. Some vegetarians compromise by eating fish, but this is not the complete answer. It is also possible that long-standing vegetarians, especially those born of vegetarian parents have adapted the alimentary tract to the extent that they can exist quite normally on the small amount of B12 contained in their diet.

Alan Moyle

Veganism

The Vegan Society was formed in 1944 as a more fundamental form of vegetarianism. Followers of vegetarianism are lacto-ovo vegetarians which means that they will eat dairy and poultry products, whereas Vegans live exclusively on the produce of the plant kingdom. For Vegans, the concern with man's exploitation of the animal kingdom and the environment is therefore more far reaching, though both movements have many common concerns.

The Vegan diet is limited to wholegrain cereals, nuts, pulse foods, fruit, vegetables, seed and vegetable oils and 'milk' made from non-animal sources, such as the soya bean. Herbs, wild plants and seaweed are also adopted in the diet. Emphasis is placed on wholefoods and a great deal of raw food (cereals, fruit, nuts, and vegetables) are consumed. Of necessity, more of the protein-containing pulse foods are recommended in this diet, and soya flour plays a large part in Vegan recipes. The 'cheese' used by Vegans has a soya base.

Wholefoods are undoubtedly a factor in preventing deficiencies in the Vegan diet. Limited variety, however, may possible create a shortage of amino-acids in the body. This problem also applies to some vegetarians and the answer must largely lie in the quantity and range of protein food consumed.

The fact that there are thousands of healthy Vegans proves that normally accepted principles of nutrition are not necessarily correct. Health can be maintained – and improved – when flesh foods are totally removed from the diet, but such regimes might not be suitable for every individual. In both vegetarianism and Veganism, ethical and health considerations are major factors. The economics speak for themselves.

Alan Moyle

Macrobiotics

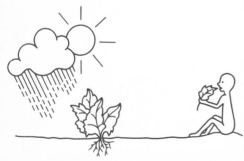

Man and the environment.

The use of the term macrobiotics was first applied to this diet by the Japanese philosopher George Ohsawa. He felt that the term reflected the spirit of what a healthy person should feel: *macro*, meaning large or great, and *bios*, meaning life. In other words, with proper diet we can experience a great life, full of adventure, freedom and creativity. Ohsawa spent the better part of his life spreading macrobiotic philosophy and dietary reform throughout the world. Since his death in the mid-1960s, several of his friends and students have carried on his work, primarily Michio Kushi in America.

The macrobiotic approach is one which takes into account the evolution of humanity, our relationship to the environment and our individual needs. The diet is not only a preventive one, aiming to maintain good health and to decrease the incidence of sickness; it is also used therapeutically, for those who are already ill and wish to use natural means of healing.

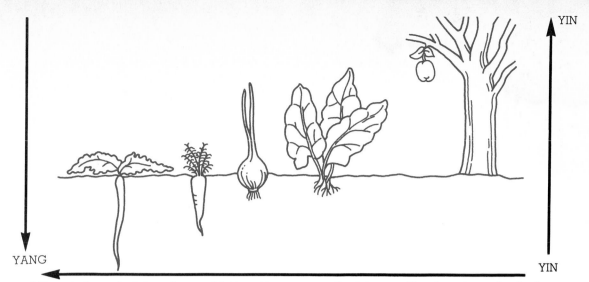

YANG

YIN

YIN

YIN

The yin and yang foods of our planet.

Although the principles of macrobiotic eating are practised in many traditional cultures, the philosophical basis of macrobiotics is the study of yin and yang, the basis of all Oriental medicine. (For an explanation of yin and yang *see* the section on Oriental medicine.)

Macrobiotics is a dietary approach rather than a specifically defined diet. Since we are all different, live in differing environments, have diverse needs and do different work, individual diets will vary.

Diet and Health

The importance of proper diet for good health has been largely lost in modern times. Among more primitive societies this basic fact was well recognized and used as the basis of medicine. Food is our source of being. Through the vegetal kingdom, all the basic forces of life are combined in a form that can be used by the human organism. Sunlight, soil, water and air are taken in through the medium of the vegetal kingdom. To eat is to take in the whole environment.

The classification of foods into categories of yin and yang is essential for the development of a balanced diet. Different factors in the growth and structure of the foods can indicate whether the food is predominantly yin or yang.

Classification

YIN	YANG
Growing in a hot climate	Growing in a cold climate
Containing more water	More dry
Fruits and leaves	Stems, roots and seeds
Growing high above the ground	Growing below ground
Causing an acid reaction in the body	Causing alkaline reaction in the body
Hot, aromatic foods	Salty, sour foods

To classify foods we must see the factors which dominate, since all foods have both yin and yang qualities.

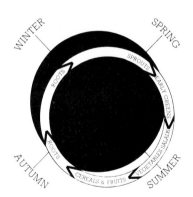

Diagram of changes in the seasonal cycle.

Yin and Yang and Growth Cycles

One of the most accurate methods of classification is by seeing the cycle of growth in food plants. During the winter, the climate is cold and damp (yin); during this time of year the vegetal energy descends into the root system. Leaves wither and die as the sap descends to the roots and the vitality of the plant becomes more yang. Plants which are used for food and grow in the late autumn and winter are more dry and have more vitality. They can be kept a long time without spoiling. Examples of these plants are roots such as carrots, parsnips, turnips, cabbages etc. During the spring and early summer, the vegetal energy ascends and new greens appear as the weather be-

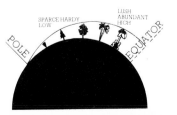

Growth patterns of yin and yang foods.

Macrobiotics

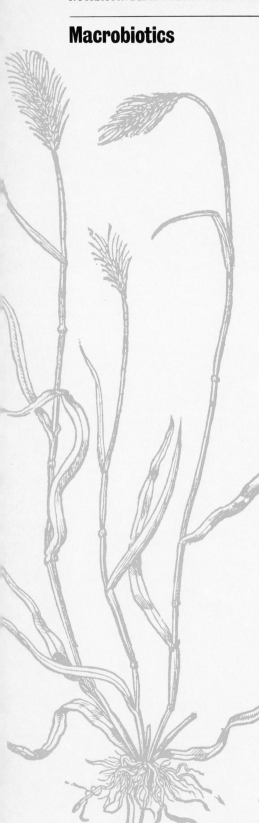

comes more hot and dry (yang). These plants are more yin in nature. Summer vegetables are more watery and perish quickly. They provide a cooling effect which is needed in warm months. In late summer, the vegetal energy has reached its zenith and the fruits become ripe. They are very watery and sweet and develop higher above the ground.

This yearly cycle shows the alternation between the dominance of yin and yang as the seasons turn.

This same cycle can be applied to the part of the world in which a food originates. Foods which find their origin in hot tropical climates where the vegetation is lush and abundant are more yin, while those foods which come from more northern climates are more yang.

Among different foods which grow at the same time of year we can classify by seeing the general growth pattern. The root system is governed by yang energy, the tendency to descend. The stem and leaves are governed by yin energy. This is expressed in the dominant direction of growth.

The Importance of the Cereal Grains

For centuries, humanity has looked to the cereal grains as the primary food. This is especially true of the great civilizations of the world. The importance of the cereal grains in the evolution of humanity cannot be overlooked. Recently the consumption of whole grains has sharply fallen and has been replaced by animal quality foods, such as dairy foods, meat and refined carbohydrates such as sugar and refined flour. It is now widely recognized that this shift in diet has resulted in many of the major sicknesses that our technological civilization is prone to.

The cereal grains are unique among our foods; they are both the beginning and end of the vegetal cycle, combining seed and fruit.

SEED .... ROOTS .... STEM .... LEAVES .... FLOWER .... FRUIT
GRAINS

It is for these reasons as well as the great ability of cereals to combine well with other vegetables to provide a wholesome diet that cereals form the most important single food in the macrobiotic regime.

Preparation

Macrobiotic cooking is a high art. The ingredients are simple and cooking is the key to producing meals which are both nutritious, tasty and attractive. The cook has the ability to change the quality of the food. More cooking, the use of pressure, salt, high heat make the food more yang. Quick cooking and little salt preserves the yin qualities of the food. A good cook controls the health of those she cooks for.

Chewing is an important aspect of the macrobiotic diet. It can also be thought of as a form of preparation. A meal should be eaten calmly with gratitude. One of the best ways of expressing this gratitude is by chewing well so that the food we eat can be used by the body more efficiently and digested well.

The Macrobiotic Way

Macrobiotics is really a commonsense approach to eating. In light of the incidence of degenerative illness and general poor health which plagues the world, the macrobiotic approach is a sensible alternative to our overprocessed and devitalized foods. Recent studies by the World Health Organization and the American government have stated that diet is the single most important factor in the rise of degenerative illness. The return to a diet more in keeping with that of our ancestors is in order if humanity is to regain its health and vitality.

William Tara

Macrobiotics

WHOLE CEREAL GRAINS. These foods would comprise 50–60 percent of daily consumption, including: brown rice, whole wheat, millet, barley, oats, buckwheat, maize and rye – either as whole grains or used in the form of flour for making bread or noodles.

FRESH VEGETABLES. Vegetables would comprise 20–30 percent of the total volume of food. The majority of them would be cooked, using a variety of methods, and the rest used raw in salads. The raw vegetables would be more appropriate in summer or in hot climate, whereas cooking would be more common in the winter or in a cold climate. Vegetables should be used in season of growth and compost-grown where possible. The nightshades such as potato, tomato and aubergine are usually avoided because of their extreme yin effect.

BEANS. Beans, cooked in soups, stews or on their own comprise 10–15 percent of the normal diet. The most commonly used are the aduki bean, lentils and other small varieties.

SEA VEGETABLES. These foods are used as an important supplement, taken in small quantities comprising about 5 percent. Such local varieties as dulse and Irish moss are used as well as dried imported varieties such as kombu, wakame, mekabu and nori. These provide an abundance of trace minerals.

FERMENTED SOYA BEAN PRODUCTS. The soya bean has been used in the Orient for centuries as a valuable vegetable source of protein. The beans are used in the form of *miso*, a thick paste with a savoury flavour, or tamari soya sauce. These condiments are an important addition to the macrobiotic cuisine used as a base for soups or sauces or used as a cooking condiment.

FRUITS AND NUTS. These foods are eaten as occasional desserts or snacks, but are considered pleasure foods for the most part. Tropical fruits are not used in northern or temperate climates, and all fruits are used in season.

SEEDS. Sunflower seeds, sesame seeds and pumpkin seeds are often used as a garnish or snack, usually slightly roasted and salted.

FISH. Macrobiotics is not a vegetarian approach to eating, although many macrobiotic people prefer to avoid all animal foods. Some people may include fish in one or two meals a week depending on the climate. Fish is usually used in more cold conditions and in the winter.

MILK, CHEESE, BUTTER, EGGS. These products are usually avoided but are sometimes used on special occasions but then only in small quantities. They are not considered as necessary foods.

POULTRY AND MAMMAL MEAT. These meats are almost always avoided for health reasons. If used at all, the white meat of poultry is preferable.

REFINED FLOUR AND SIMPLE SUGAR. These two foods are avoided, and considered to have especially harmful effects. For sweeteners, if used at all, fruit concentrate, barley malt or dried fruits are used in cooking. Honey is seldom used.

PROCESSED, RECONSTITUTED AND CHEMICALIZED FOODS. These have no place in the diet at all.

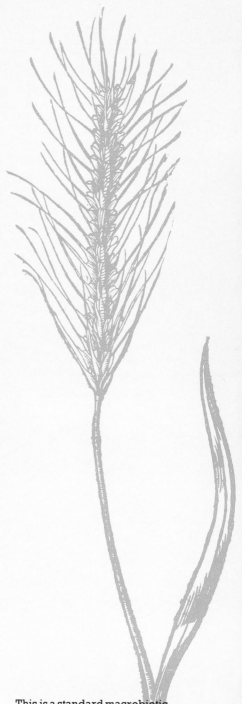

This is a standard macrobiotic diet, now in use. The diet would be changed depending on the individual's condition, environment and activity. All percentages relate to the volume of food eaten daily.

The Bircher-Benner System

Dr Bircher-Benner founded his now-famous Zurich clinic in 1902. The dietary system named after him represents an attitude to nutrition based upon a belief in the importance of raw plant foods and is thus related to other raw food regimes and to the Food Reform movement.

There are six basic principles involved, which are as follows:

1. Half the daily intake should be fresh, uncontaminated raw plant food, grown in healthy soil. (Heating destroys enzymes and vitamins and alters the physical and chemical properties of plants.)

2. Begin each meal with raw food, i.e. start with raw and proceed to cooked food.

3. There should not be a day without green leaves (chlorophyll).

4. If protein is required, eat lacto-vegetarian proteins, e.g. eggs, cheese, etc., not meat.

5. For flavouring, use aromatic herbs, biochemic salt, yeast products like Marmite, barbados sugar or honey. Avoid all condiments that blunt the palate, e.g. ordinary cooking salt, vinegar, pepper.

6. Cereal food should be whole-grain and include the germ.

The chart below shows how constructively the Bircher-Benner system works in practice.

Joseph Goodman

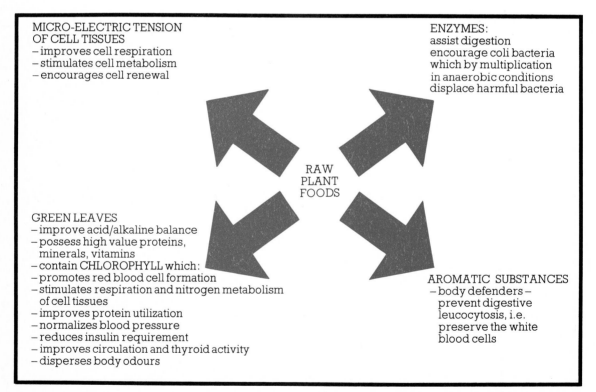

MICRO-ELECTRIC TENSION OF CELL TISSUES
– improves cell respiration
– stimulates cell metabolism
– encourages cell renewal

ENZYMES:
assist digestion
encourage coli bacteria
which by multiplication
in anaerobic conditions
displace harmful bacteria

RAW PLANT FOODS

GREEN LEAVES
– improve acid/alkaline balance
– possess high value proteins, minerals, vitamins
– contain CHLOROPHYLL which:
– promotes red blood cell formation
– stimulates respiration and nitrogen metabolism of cell tissues
– improves protein utilization
– normalizes blood pressure
– reduces insulin requirement
– improves circulation and thyroid activity
– disperses body odours

AROMATIC SUBSTANCES
– body defenders –
prevent digestive
leucocytosis, i.e.
preserve the white
blood cells

Raw Food

Raw food includes all those fruit and vegetables, cereals, nuts, seeds and herbs which can be consumed without any form of preparation apart from the necessary cleaning and, where applicable, peeling. It can, in the wider sense, include cheese. Salads of raw vegetables, whether grated, sliced or whole, are the simplest forms of raw food. Fruit which is not cooked comes into this category, so do the seeds like sunflower and pumpkin and the natural herbs and plants like parsley, mint, thyme, dandelion, nasturtium, nettle etc. Some cereals, such as oats and bran can be consumed raw. All nuts and even mushrooms can be taken in the raw state.

Raw Food

The advantage of raw food is that there is no loss of the essential vitamin and mineral content and nourishment of the body's cells is therefore increased. A further advantage is that when the food has a high water content – lettuce, melon, etc. – the water content is of the highest quality. (The exception is where these foods – salad foods, in particular – are grown with the aid of a fluoridated water supply.)

Raw food is also beneficial in that it contains more fibrous matter and so requires more chewing. While it is very easy to over-eat 'pappy' foods like white bread and mashed potato, raw food, because it requires more chewing, readily satisfies hunger.

Precise knowledge of the loss of food value has not been accurately determined in all cases, but it is obvious that cooking methods which involve the use of water in particular, account for considerable wastage. Heat of any sort is damaging, but boiling water is the worst offender. The main loss of vitamins in cooking processes is that of vitamins A and C. Vitamin B is lost only at higher temperatures, as in a pressure cooker. The greatest wastage due to the boiling of vegetables is of mineral salts and this can range from 10 to 60 percent of the original content. Some examples are given below:

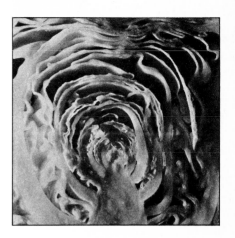

Percentage loss of mineral content

	Minutes boiled	Calc.	Phos.	Magnesium	Iron
potatoes	25	0	1	3	3
spinach	15	0	3	19	9
peas	20	1	6	11	11
cabbage	30	0	15	2	3

It can be seen that the loss of magnesium and iron in cooking vegetables can be serious. This may be reduced dramatically when vegetables are steamed, baked, casseroled or cooked in their skins. The potato skin is one of the richest sources of potassium. Raw cabbage and oats form two of the best sources of silicon. There is a great deal to be said for eating cabbage and oats raw and for adding a little raw spinach to a salad.

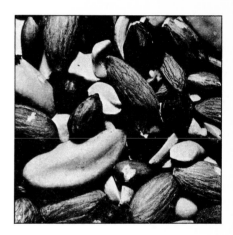

Losses in food value are not confined to cooking processes. Some wastage arises in food preparation. The outer leaves of green vegetables contain more vitamin A than the inner ones. In tomatoes, the vitamin A content of the skin can be around twenty times that of the flesh. Outer dark leaves of vegetables can contain fifteen times as much calcium and twice as much iron as the inner leaves. Vegetables and fruits also lose some nutritional value when stored for a period.

For a complete raw food diet to be reasonably balanced it must contain nuts, cheese, cereals, the seed oils, honey, molasses and herbs. A certain amount of protein is available in fruit and vegetables, but this is insufficient to meet normal daily requirements. The protein content can be increased by nuts, cheese and cereals and the carbohydrate by cereals, honey and molasses. It is recommended that the raw fruit and vegetable content should comprise 80 percent of the total daily consumption, with the protein content 10 percent and the rest made up from 8 percent cereals with honey and molasses supplying the remainder. Fruit and vegetables can have a high sugar content and consequently there is less demand for sugar from other sources.

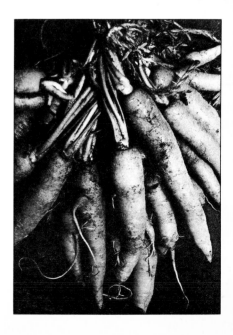

A great many of the body's ills are due to excessive acidity. This is largely accounted for by the excess of acid forming foods in the average diet. The main acid and alkaline food groups are listed under the Hay Diet. A glance at the grouping shows that fruit and vegetables are preponderantly alkaline forming. It is this alkalinity which makes a raw food diet therapeutic. When reduced to half the normal food intake, raw food is the base for a balanced nutritional regime.

Raw Food

There are degrees of acidity and alkalinity which have to be taken into account. Pork, for instance, is more acid than lamb and fruit and vegetables vary in alkalinity. Spinach and lettuce can contain too much oxalic acid for young children and some adults and rhubarb has a high oxalic acid content and should rarely be consumed. In certain cases of arthritis, oranges are not recommended. Acid fruit, however, normally has an alkaline reaction and is therefore classed as alkaline.

Some acid foods are necessary, since practically all protein would be removed if a total alkaline diet was achieved. As a short-term therapy a completely raw food diet would be highly alkaline and cleansing. As a long-term project, it would require some of the acid protein. But any normal balanced diet should contain at least one raw fruit and salad meal each day to achieve a correct acid/alkali ratio. It is the lack of balance in diet which creates a lack of balance (diseased state) within the body.

A preponderantly raw food diet is particularly useful for people suffering from multiple sclerosis and Parkinson's disease. It also assists rheumatic and arthritic subjects and aids respiration in cases of chronic catarrh. It is not suitable except in limited quantities for those with weak digestions and is not recommended for the very young or the very old.

Alan Moyle

Natural Hygiene

Natural Hygiene is described by its arch protagonist, Herbert M. Shelton, as an art and a science. Its purpose is the ascertainment and application of the laws of life in order to maintain or retrieve health and happiness. Hygiene promotes and restores health with reference to the causes of health rather than those of disease. That which is not useful in health is equally non-usable in sickness.

The only certain way to prevent disease is to maintain health by healthful living. For those already sick, the only road to health is through a reform in the habits of living.

There is a unity of causation, of healing, of disease and of care. All so-called disease, accident apart, is occasioned by toxaemia, no matter in which part of the body or mind it is manifested. Care of the patient involves reduction of the toxic state, whatever name is given to the disease. Enervation of the body is likely to reduce its capacity to eliminate efficiently. Efforts must therefore be made to reduce fatigue, not by stimulating treatments, but by resting both internally and externally (see *Fasting*).

It is dangerous to suppress symptoms to remove pain, reduce swelling or lower blood pressure when these may be nature's compensation for faulty function. The causes themselves must be removed. Nutrition, therefore, is not looked upon as a therapeutic modality but as one of the factors that has to be improved upon in order to permit self-healing to take place.

The Hygienic System formulates a number of eating rules, based on physiological law:

1. Eat only when hungry, when the body instinctively desires food.

2. Avoid eating if tired, dull, lazy, listless, in pain or mentally distressed. Digestive power is reduced and putrefaction likely.

3. Eat slowly, chew thoroughly. "Chew and taste your food; your stomach has neither teeth nor taste buds."

4. Food combinations. The ideal rule is don't combine, eat one food per meal. The chart shows how to combine sensibly, if you must.

5. When sick, refrain from eating. (See *Fasting*).

Joseph Goodman

FOOD COMBINING CHART
Scientific Food Combinations
According to the Principles of Natural Hygiene

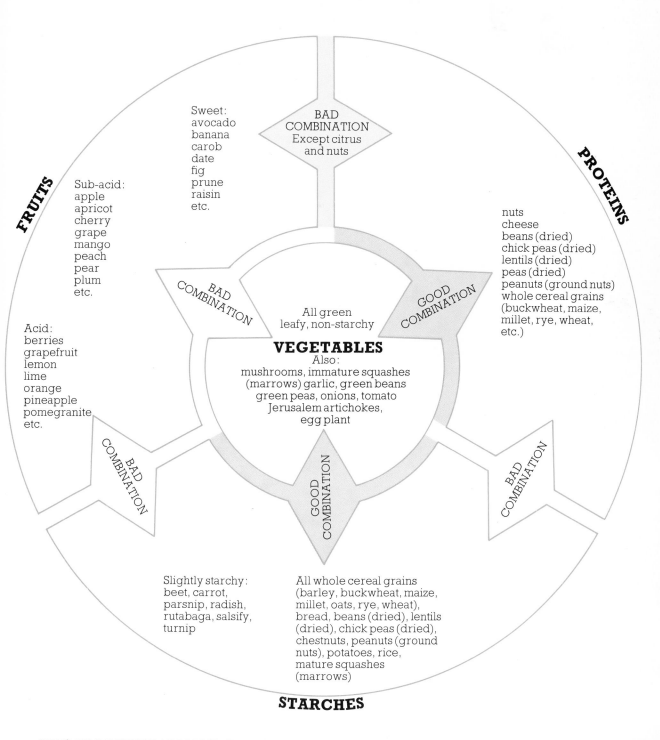

FRUITS

Sweet:
avocado
banana
carob
date
fig
prune
raisin
etc.

Sub-acid:
apple
apricot
cherry
grape
mango
peach
pear
plum
etc.

Acid:
berries
grapefruit
lemon
lime
orange
pineapple
pomegranite
etc.

BAD
COMBINATION
Except citrus
and nuts

BAD
COMBINATION

GOOD
COMBINATION

PROTEINS

nuts
cheese
beans (dried)
chick peas (dried)
lentils (dried)
peas (dried)
peanuts (ground nuts)
whole cereal grains
(buckwheat, maize,
millet, rye, wheat,
etc.)

All green
leafy, non-starchy

VEGETABLES
Also:
mushrooms, immature squashes
(marrows) garlic, green beans
green peas, onions, tomato
Jerusalem artichokes,
egg plant

BAD
COMBINATION

GOOD
COMBINATION

BAD
COMBINATION

Slightly starchy:
beet, carrot,
parsnip, radish,
rutabaga, salsify,
turnip

All whole cereal grains
(barley, buckwheat, maize,
millet, oats, rye, wheat),
bread, beans (dried), lentils
(dried), chick peas (dried),
chestnuts, peanuts (ground
nuts), potatoes, rice,
mature squashes
(marrows)

STARCHES

NOTE ON SEQUENCE OF EATING: Eat the juciest
foods first; then the less juicy. Eat the driest
and most concentrated food last of all.

The Hay Diet

Simple food combinations recommended in the Hay type of diet are:

Green vegetables with protein
Green vegetables with starches
Green vegetables with fats
Proteins with fruits
Starches with fats
Proteins with fats
   To be avoided are:
Proteins and starches
Starches and acid fruits

William Howard Hay first published his book *Health via Food* in 1934. The ideas propounded in it were not just the discoveries of one man, for Hay drew upon the knowledge and researches of many eminent contemporaries, among them Sir W. Arbuthnot Lane, Dr John Harvey Kellogg, Dr J. H. Tilden, Dr V. H. Lindlahr, Dr Valentine Knaggs, A. W. McCann, Hereward Carrington, H. M. Shelton and Arnold Ehret.

The Hay Diet, so called, became very popular in the 1930s both in Britain and the United States. Essentially it is concerned with sensible food combining and an understanding of acid-alkali balance. Many people eat too much acid-forming food, such as meat, bread, grains and alcohol. The result is that the digestive tract becomes progressively acid saturated, leading first to constipation and lassitude and ultimately to positive ill health. The recommended ratio in a balanced diet is 20 percent acid-forming to 80 percent alkali-forming foods. These principles have subsequently been elaborated upon by other writers, of whom the most representative was probably the late Harry Benjamin ND *(Your Diet in Health and Disease).*

The reasoning behind this system is that proteins require acid secretions for digestion, initially in the stomach, carrying over into the intestines, whereas carbohydrates require alkaline secretions, initially in the mouth and more in the intestines. Consequently a mixture of protein and starch (e.g. meat and potatoes) is contraindicated because the one prevents the proper assimilation of the other.

Melons, milk and other liquids should be taken alone, if thirsty, and not in conjunction with solid foods.

Joseph Goodman

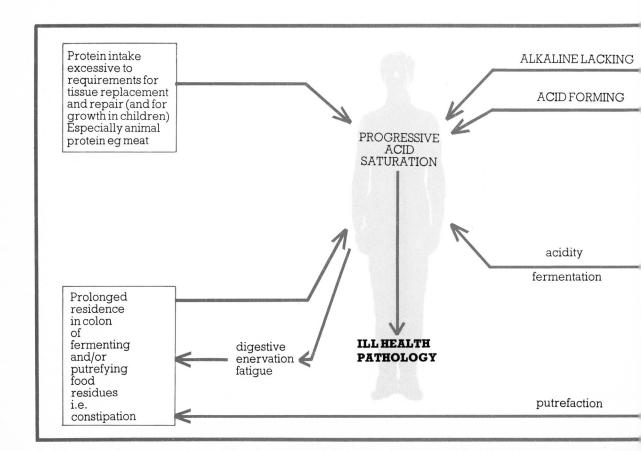

HIGHLY ACID	ACID	NEUTRAL	ALKALINE	HIGHLY ALKALINE	VERY HIGHLY ALKALINE
alcohol	beans,	oils:	apple	almond	beans, dried
artichoke,	kidney	avocado oil	apricot, fresh	avocado	lima
Jerusalem	navy	olive	artichokes,	banana,	string
barley	white	sesame	globe	speckled	bean sprouts
bread	garbanzo	coconut	asparagus	only	dandelion
buckwheat	beef	soy	bean, snap	bean, fresh lima	greens
caffein	Brussels sprouts	sunflower	broccoli	blackberries	dates
honey	cashew	safflower	cabbage,	carrot	figs, esp. black
lentil, dry	coconut, dried	cottonseed	red	chives	prune
millet	egg yolk	almond	white	endive	raisin
oatmeal	fish	linseed	savoy	peach, dried	Swiss chard
peanut	fowl		Chinese	persimmon	tubers
potatoes,	fruit, dried	fats:	cauliflower	pomegranate	
sweet	game	butter	celery	plum	
rice, br. &	milk,	cream	cherries, sweet	raspberries	
white	pasteurized	margarine	& sour	spinach	
rye grain	products	animal fat	chicory		
spaghetti	mushroom	lard	coconut, fresh		
products	mutton		meat & milk		
sugar,	pork		coffee		
cane & raw	poultry		substitutes		
tobacco			corn, fresh		
walnut, English			sweet		
wheat grain			eggplant		
			garlic		
			gooseberry		
			grapefruit		
			grapes		
			kelp		
			leek		
			lemon & peel		
			lettuce		
			melons, all		
			milk, raw,		
			yoghurt		
			onion		
			orange		
			peach, fresh		
			pear, fresh		
			peppers, green		
			& red		
			potato, exc.		
			sweet		
			radishes		
			rhubarb		
			tomato		
			turnip		
			watercress		
			yeast		

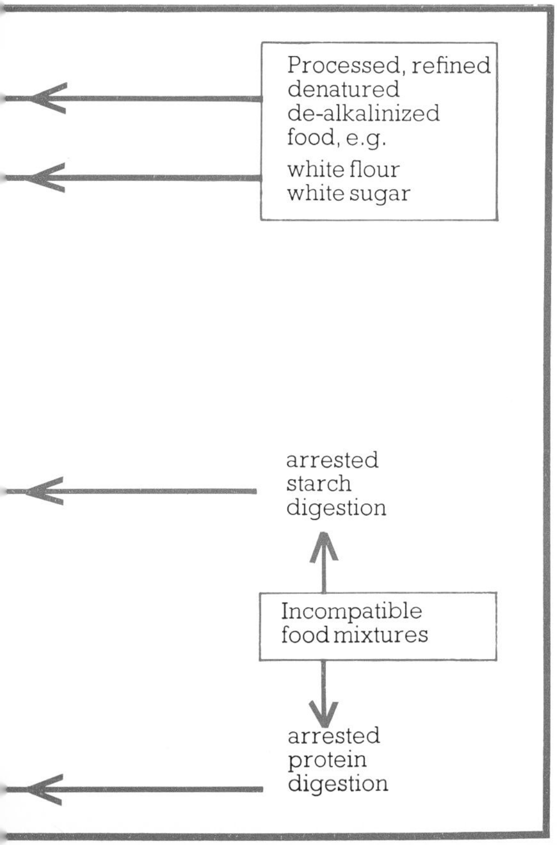

Processed, refined denatured de-alkalinized food, e.g.

white flour
white sugar

arrested starch digestion

Incompatible food mixtures

arrested protein digestion

Supplementary Diets: Introduction

Farming based on chemistry alone will lead to deficiencies. When a soil is depleted of essential elements it may be expedient to add the missing chemicals, but in the long term the soil will become even more impoverished. It is obviously necessary to study the *world* of the soil, something the Soil Association of Great Britain and other such organizations have been actively engaged in for many years.

A healthy soil is one that is alive: changing with the seasons, adapting to transient hazards and responding to natural environmental cycles of weather, animal, plant and micro-life. A healthy human being has equivalent capacities.

The need for supplementation of human diets, therefore, depends on the organic quality of the individual concerned and on the quality of the soil providing that individual's nourishment. If both are low, it may be necessary to give temporary, sometimes permanent support with supplements. Accompanying such supplementation, of course, must be efforts to deal with the underlying problem.

There is a danger inherent in modern eating habits that is often overlooked. As with a muscle or gland that is not used and eventually withers, so will a function that is neglected lose its potency. From every mouthful of food that is chewed, the body extracts those elements necessary for each step of the total metabolic process from digestion through anabolism and catabolism to excretion. Artificially packaging each mouthful into its so-called essential constituents denies the body the exercising of its power of *selectivity*. Even if it takes several generations, the constant use of concentrated, encapsulated or frag-mented substitutes for real food will lose to the human species its power of selection.

Those with already impaired functions will obviously benefit to the extent that the supplement makes good a deficiency, provided it is without detriment to other organs and functions in its short-circuiting sphere of activity. Insulin, for example, enables a diabetic to survive an impaired pancreas but in no way improves the total hormonal integrity of the body. (See *Carbohydrate Metabolism*). High fibre may increase bowel activity but in total body terms will eventually prove counter-productive; the same applies to high protein. What is needed is adequate fibre and adequate protein. Both are usually available in the original, unmolested edible foodstuff.

Joseph Goodman

Food Supplement Therapy

From the very earliest times, mystical qualities have been attributed to certain foods and plants, or they became popular through the applica-tion of the 'doctrine of signatures' – the use of plants which bear a physical resemblance to the whole, or part of, the body. Some of the principles of folk medicine are retained in the popular food supple-ments of the present day, but many have survived largely because of a reasonable degree of empirical corroboration.

Food supplement therapy uses foods, rich in essential nutrients, as an aid to recovery from disorders which may have been due in part to a deficiency of those nutrients. The basis of the naturopathic man-agement of disease is nutritional readjustment. This ensures that the patient is obtaining the best quality of food to rebuild vitality and enable the healing process to operate optimally. Certain foods may be needed in greater quantities because they provide specific nutrients or have other properties which can help in restoring the body to normal health.

Food Supplement Therapy

Apple Cider Vinegar

This is prepared by fermenting the juice of apples and has gained a wide reputation as a preventive of arthritic disorders and many other chronic complaints. Its use was based on the observations made by the American doctor, D. C. Jarvis, who noted the relative freedom from arthritic disorders among the country people of his native Vermont. He advocated the regular use of apple cider vinegar with honey and warm water. This is claimed to normalize digestive secretions and improve calcium metabolism.

Honey

Honey has been hailed as a cure for hay fever and allergic complaints in particular. Its benefits are believed to derive from the concentration of pollens in its composition, as well as the presence of many minerals and trace elements. Its high fructose and glucose content make it a favourite general tonic and energy food, although, being a rather concentrated form of carbohydrate, it is not as suitable for sustained energy levels as taking natural protein from grains and pulses.

Molasses

A byproduct of the sugar-refining process, molasses contains about twelve percent protein and a high proportion of minerals, being particularly rich in calcium and potassium. It is regarded as a good general tonic and often prescribed for its mineral content where the levels of calcium and potassium in particular, need to be increased. It tends to be laxative in effect.

Wheatgerm

The food processing industry has both created the demand for, as well as the supply of this relative veteran of the supplement list. The germ of wheat is removed in the milling process during the manufacture of white flour. It is the most nutritious part, being rich in vitamins B and E, both vital to metabolism. Wheatgerm is easily administered, as it can be sprinkled on cereals, fruit or vegetables and incorporated in cooking as an oil. As with so many essential nutrients, however, some of the vitamins are destroyed by heating. Many of the commercially available wheatgerms have been partially heated to prolong shelf life and these have a poorer biological activity.

Brewer's Yeast

Vitamin B is necessary in larger amounts for a variety of complaints, since it is so intimately involved in many aspects of metabolism. The B vitamins Thiamin, Riboflavin, Pyridoxin and Niacin are found in yeast, which is a popular and reliable tonic for this reason and for its protein content. Brewer's yeast contains at least twenty percent of protein. This is often prescribed in powdered or tablet form and there are savoury extracts which also contain yeast.

Various other high protein supplements are marketed in the health food trade. Their protein content is generally derived from soya.

Ginseng

The newest tonic to gain favour in health-conscious circles is probably the oldest. Ginseng root, grown in China and Korea, is renowned for its general tonic and aphrodisiac properties. It is administered as slices of the root, which may be chewed, or preparations are available in tablet form. As with so many of the tonic foods, its benefits appear to be achieved by a normalizing effect upon the body metabolism, and a restoration of the adaptive processes which help to overcome stress.

Roger Newman Turner

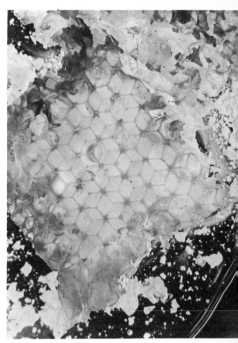

Honeycomb

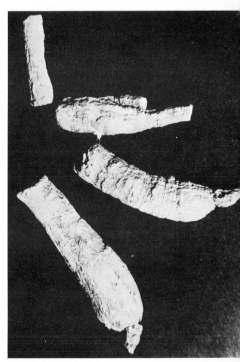

Ginseng root

High Protein

Next to water, protein is the most plentiful substance in the body. It is important for the maintenance of good health and for the growth and development of all the body tissues – muscles, blood, skin, hair and so on. Protein is also essential for the synthesis of hormones in the body and for preventing the blood and tissues from becoming too acid or alkaline.

Probably the first recorded high protein diet was that devised by an American, William Banting, in 1863, to help him slim. The major features of the diet were increased meat, fish and fruit intake, with the exclusion as far as possible of all sugar, starches and fats; liquid intake was reduced and he took an antacid to counteract the natural acidity of protein.

High protein diets have varied little since Banting's time – increased intake of protein in the form of meat and fish and a decreased intake of fats and carbohydrates. In recent years, vitamin supplements are often added to these diets. However, except in genuine cases of protein deficiency, which are somewhat rare in Western countries, a high protein diet can only be considered as a cosmetic device and should be undertaken with caution.

While protein is responsible for maintaining the acidic/alkaline balance in the body, additional protein produces an acidic urine and a decrease in the natural alkalinity of the blood. In addition, a by-product of protein metabolism by the body is the toxic substance uric acid, and increased protein intake leads to increased uric acid production. In young, healthy people the body is capable of eliminating this extra acid, but in older people where the elimination of waste products in general via the lungs, skin, kidneys and bowels is less efficient, uric acid can accumulate along with other acidic waste products. Even in the short term, this can in older people (above about 45) have a deleterious effect on health, particularly in rheumatic or arthritic people. There is evidence that excess protein intake can increase the incidence of rheumatism.

The apparent advantage of high protein diets for slimming is that protein takes longer to digest and is therefore more satisfying than carbohydrates or the cellulose material of vegetables and salads, i.e. if more protein is eaten, then less carbohydrates will be eaten, and it is the carbohydrates that are converted by the body to fat. If used, however, for slimming purposes, it is advisable to stay on such diets for only short periods of time.

High Fibre

Despite the increasing popularity of the 'high fibre' diet, nutritionists agree that there is as yet no satisfactory definition of 'dietary fibre'. While dietary fibre is generally considered to be that part of plant fibre which is eaten but passes through the digestive system to be excreted, it is now realized that some constituents of plant fibre are digested and that these must be considered when evaluating the value of fibre in diet.

Nevertheless, in 1959 a list was compiled of non-infectious diseases rare in rural Africans but prevalent in Western man. Of thirty diseases listed, by far the largest coherent number were diseases of the colon: constipation, diverticular disease, irritable colon, appendicitis, haemorrhoids, ulcerative colitis, cancer of the bowel and so on. In 1960 it was suggested that the high fibre diet of the Africans was responsible for the difference. Evidence accumulated since then tends to support this theory.

High Fibre

By 1975, fibre-containing plant-energy foods, starch and fat contributed 82 percent of the energy to people in developing countries, but had shrunk to 32 percent in the Western world. Certainly, fibre has a part to play in digestion and a shortage of fibre might significantly affect health.

While 'fibre' is popularly thought to mean bran and associated foods, all plant foodstuffs contain different types of fibres in varying quantities. In an age of refined foodstuffs there is certainly a danger of removing too much fibre. Removal of fibre from carbohydrate foodstuffs for instance, leads to overconsumption or over-rapid absorption of the refined end-product; there is some evidence that gallstones can result from a refined carbohydrate diet.

The principle function of fibre is to normalize the transit period of food through the digestive system, allowing complete digestion and efficient elimination of waste products. Bile acids, which are produced by the body to aid the absorption of food, can also be affected by fibre levels. Some fibres have the effect of carrying down more bile acids in the colon, which in turn might help reduce cholesterol levels. Thus there is some evidence that dietary fibre may protect against coronary heart disease by lowering plasma cholesterol; rolled oats and rice seem to have this effect on cholesterol, but there is however, no evidence that all fibre has this effect. The reason for the low incidence of atherosclerosis and low cholesterol concentrations in the African Bantu has been attributed to low fat intake and high fibre content of their diet.

An interesting experiment was recently conducted to examine some of the benefits of a high fibre diet. In a pilot experiment, thirty-eight patients suffering from peripheral vascular diseases were divided into two equal groups, a control and an experimental group. The controls ate a Western-type diet for one month containing 30 percent low-fibre starch foods, 45 percent fat, 12 percent protein, 13 percent sugar and salt as desired. At the end of the month this group showed no improvement in their conditions. The experimental group over the same period ate 80 percent fibre-rich unrefined starch food, 10 percent fat, 10 percent protein and no sugar or salt. Considerable improvement was shown by this group.

Following this experiment, a second test was conducted at the Longevity Research Institute in California. Twenty patients suffering from severe degenerative diseases ate the same high fibre diet and exercised vigorously over thirty days. On discharge, the majority had given up antidiabetic drugs, hypoglycaemic drugs or insulin, while some patients who had been scheduled to have coronary bypass operations felt they no longer needed them. On average, blood cholesterol levels fell by 25 percent and blood pressure levels fell so significantly that those using hypertensive drugs no longer needed the drugs. Despite the apparent success of the experiments, researchers point out the many variables and that the work is very tentative as to the value of high fibre diets.

Clearly Western man eats less fibre than he used to; the role this plays in disposing him to specific diseases is not yet, however, certain. High fibre diets do seem in some cases to lead to remission of certain diseases; bran has been successfully used in the treatment of diverticular disease. The prophylactic effect of continual high fibre diet on the other hand, has yet to be evaluated. Perhaps the commonest affliction of the digestive system of Western man is constipation which can frequently be caused by lack of fibre. As one nutritionist has pointed out, while constipation may not be dangerous, it is certainly uneccessary.

TOTAL DIETARY FIBRE IN GRAMS PER 100 GRAMS OF FOOD

cabbage (cooked)	2.93
carrots (cooked)	3.70
peas, raw	7.75
tomato	1.40
apple (flesh only)	1.42
banana	1.75
pear (flesh)	2.44
plum (flesh and skin)	1.52
strawberry	2.12
white flour	3.45
wholemeal flour	11.00
bran	48.00

Vitamin Supplements

Vitamins may be classified according to their solubility:

Fat-soluble

Vitamins A, D, E, F, K
Insoluble in water.
Impaired by any interference with fat absorption.
Considerable stores in the liver mainly.
Daily intake not essential.
Excess intake can be toxic.

Water-soluble

Vitamins B, C, P
Insoluble in fat.
Impaired by soaking in water.
Not stored in the body to any extent.
Daily intake essential.
Excess intake excreted, no toxic effects.

Vitamins are organic substances *(amines)* other than the macro-nutrients, minerals and salts that are essential for normal metabolism, growth and development of the body (*vita* = life). They are effective in minute quantities as regulators of metabolic processes; whilst they are not energy sources, they act as co-enzymes in enzymatic systems in the processes of energy transformation.

There is controversy as to whether or not vitamin supplementation is necessary or even desirable given that the individual is eating a diet of whole foods well-balanced in their macro-nutrient content and compatibility. On the one hand, evidence is presented as to the poor quality of foods grown and reared; the inevitable contamination in all stages of planting, growth, preparation and presentation; the stress factors of modern civilization making mock of previously accepted minimum requirements. On the other hand it is pointed out that vitamins are co-enzymes only; they act as part of the metabolic processing of food. Supplementation, therefore, of vitamins without an increased intake of appropriate food transforms their role from that of nutritional substance to that of medicinal drug, especially if taken in mega-doses.

The chart shows the functions that the body is enabled to perform because of any particular vitamin, as well as the symptoms it will manifest if any group is in short supply. The purist will claim that any deficiency must be made good by careful selection of those foodstuffs rich in the missing vitamin as well as the avoidance of those elements that interfere with its availability to the body. Protagonists of supplementation are of the opinion that in some cases barrow-loads of foodstuff may have to be consumed in order to get to the quantity of vitamin necessary. (See *Orthomolecular Medicine*).

Joseph Goodman

VITAMIN	Food Source	Function	Deficiency Symptoms
Vitamin A (carotene)	Green vegetables, milk, cream cheese, fish liver oil, liver, kidney.	Essential for growth, health of the eyes, structure and functioning of the skin and mucous membrane.	Night blindness, low resistance to infection. Infection of mucous membrane, i.e. catarrh, bronchial complaints. Skin and nervous tissue disorders.
Vitamin B1 (thiamine)	Yeast, wheat germ, kelp, soya beans, green vegetables, milk, eggs, oysters, meat and liver.	Essential for growth, carbohydrate metabolism and function of the heart, nerves and muscles.	Nervous disorders, blood disorders, skin and hair problems, depression, beri-beri, gastric disorders, ulcers.
Vitamin B2 (riboflavine)	Yeast, wheat germ, soya beans, peanuts, green vegetables, milk, eggs, meat, fowl.	Essential for growth, health of hair and mouth, general well-being, function of eyes.	Dry hair and skin, retarded or slow growth, mouth and tongue sores, poor vision, nervous disorders, lack of stamina.
Vitamin B3 (pantothenic acid)	Yeast, liver, eggs, brown rice, bran, whole grain products.	Health of skin and hair. Essential for growth of all tissue.	Dry skin and hair.
Vitamin B6 (pyridoxine)	Yeast, wheat germ, melon, cabbage, milk, egg yolk, fish.	Protein metabolism. Health of skin. Function of nerves and muscles.	Skin eruptions, nervous rashes, irritability, insomnia, muscle cramps,

VITAMIN	Food Source	Function	Deficiency Symptoms
Vitamin B12 (cyanocobalamine)	Yeast, spinach, lettuce, eggs, liver, meat.	Health of nerve tissue and skin. Protein metabolism.	Anaemia, tiredness, skin disorders, poor appetite.
Biotin	Liver, kidney, vegetables, nuts.	Probably necessary for healthy skin, function of nerves, muscles and mucous membranes.	Undetermined.
Choline	Egg yolk, liver, kidney, brains, sweetbreads, dried yeast.	Essential for the functioning of the liver. Prevent build-up of fatty acids.	Premature ageing. Build-up of fatty acids.
Folic acid	Green leafy vegetables, liver, brewer's yeast.	Important for red blood cell formation, for growth and division of cells.	Poor growth, anaemia, vitamin B12 deficiency.
PABA (para-aminobenzoic acid)	Liver, yeast, wheat germ, molasses.	Aids bacteria in forming folic acid; aids red blood cell formation.	Fatigue, irritability, depression, constipation.
Inositol	Eggs, meat, liver, kidney, whole grain products.	Essential for the functioning of the liver. Prevents build-up of fatty acids.	Premature ageing. Build-up of fatty acids.
Niacin (nicotinic acid, nicotinamide)	Yeast, liver, kidney, milk, whole grain products; and can be converted by the body from tryptophan.	Essential for growth, health of skin, function of the stomach and intestines and nerves.	Pellagra, skin disorders, nervous and intestinal disturbances, headaches, insomnia.
Vitamin C (ascorbic acid)	Citrus fruits, melon, berries, tomatoes, raw vegetables.	Essential for growth, cell activity, health of gums and teeth.	Sore gums, lack of immunity to infection, pains in joints, scurvy.
Vitamin D	Milk, butter, fish, liver oil, eggs, fresh green vegetables, sunshine.	Formation of bones and teeth, regulating calcium and phosphorus metabolism.	Tooth decay, bone deformities, calcium and phosphorus deficiency, rickets.
Vitamin E (tocopherol)	Seed germ oils, egg yolks, green vegetables, milk.	Normal reproduction. Function of nerves muscles.	Premature ageing, incomplete pregnancies, sterility in males, muscular and nervous disorders.
Vitamin F (fatty acids)	Safflower, soya, corn and cod-liver oil.	Helps regulate blood coagulation and is essential for normal glandular activity.	Brittle hair and nails, dandruff, varicose veins.
Vitamin K	Soya beans, vegetable oils, green leafy vegetables, tomatoes, liver.	Essential for blood clotting.	Prolonged bleeding from cuts and sores – lack of clotting agent.

Fruit and Vegetable Juices

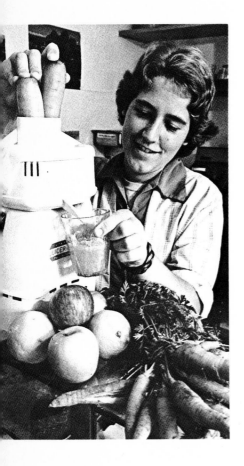

Most commercial and convenience foods are, to varying degrees, deficiency foods, for modern food technology is extremely destructive. The various processes of food refining create deficiencies in vitamins and mineral salts and so cause nutritional imbalance. While a diet of raw food does much to correct such imbalances the inclusion of raw fruit and vegetable juices in a diet has certain advantages.

Locked in the cells of raw fruit and vegetables, particularly if they have been grown in healthy soil, are all the substances needed for human nourishment – carbohydrates, proteins, vitamins, minerals, fats and so on. Many of these nutrients are bound up in the roughage of fruit and vegetables, and while roughage is necessary in a diet, too much is inadvisable. Raw juices provide the answer to this problem.

A second advantage of juices is their rapid assimilation by the body; taken on an empty stomach they will be absorbed by the blood and glands within fifteen minutes or so of ingestion. In this respect juices should be regarded as a food and sipped, not gulped.

Raw juices are divided into two groups, fruit juices which are regarded as cleansers of the human system and vegetable juices which are the regenerators and builders of the body. Juices can be used as either food supplements or for specific therapeutic values. Vegetable juices have particular therapy values: beetroots and nettles counteract acidity, raw cabbage is excellent for gastric and duodenal ulcers, diverticulitis, irritable colon and so on. Celery is useful for arthritis, rheumatism and diseases of the musculo-skeletal system, while both apple and grape juice are recommended for insomnia and nervous disorders. Both fruit and vegetable juices are useful for their vitamin C content.

A good, basic raw juice is equal quantities of apple, carrot and beetroot; to this can be added any of the specific therapeutic vegetables such as those just described.

The preparation of raw juices requires a special electric juice extractor – ordinary blenders are not sufficiently powerful for the purpose. Fruit and vegetables should be used as fresh as possible and all bad or brown parts should be cut out. A little lemon juice squeezed into the juicer before use helps retain the original colour of fruit and vegetables.

Alan Moyle

Mineral Supplements

Minerals are the body's inorganic nutrients, which, since the body cannot synthesize them, need to be frequently replenished. Minerals are fundamental to the normal physiological processes of the body, maintaining normal nervous, muscular, lymphatic systems and so on. For many of these processes, minerals act as catalysts, without which the body processes would simply fail.

All of the minerals known to be involved in body processes must be supplied in the diet, though except for calcium, phosphorus, iodine and iron the normal requirement levels of minerals has not been established. Minerals are divided into macro-minerals, those minerals present in fairly large amounts in the body, and trace minerals or elements, which although present only in minute amounts are essential to normal functioning. The various mineral functions are all interrelated and changes in the amounts of one mineral will affect the functioning of all the others.

SOME ESSENTIAL TRACE ELEMENTS IN THE BODY AND THEIR IMPORTANCE

Mineral	Importance	Deficiency symptoms	Suggested dietary allowance per day	Source
Cobalt	Is part of vitamin B12. Maintains red blood cells.	Pernicious anaemia.	Average daily intake is usually 5.0–8.0 mcg.	Liver, kidney, oysters and milk.
Copper	Necessary to formation of red blood cells. Is part of many enzymes.	Weakness, skin sores.	2 mg for adults.	Liver, whole grain products, green leafy vegetables.
Iodine	Necessary for proper function of the thyroid gland. Prevents goitre. Regulates body metabolism.	Enlarged thyroid. Loss of energy, dry skin and hair.	Men – 130 mcg. Women – 100 mcg.	Plant and animal seafoods.
Iron	Necessary for haemoglobin production. Promotes growth.	Anaemia, weakness, constipation.	Women – 18 mg. Men – 10 mg.	Leafy green vegetables, liver, dried apricots, walnuts.
Zinc	Necessary for insulin synthesis and male reproductive fluid. Aids healing process.	Retarded growth, delayed sexual maturity.	15 mg.	High protein diets, brewer's yeast, wheat bran, wheat germ.

THE MACRO-MINERALS OF THE BODY AND THEIR IMPORTANCE

Mineral	Importance	Deficiency symptoms	Suggested dietary allowance per day	Sources
Calcium	Necessary for strong bones and teeth. Helps normal blood clotting, muscle, nerve and heart functions.	Soft or brittle bones; back and leg pains.	0.8–1.4 grams depending on age.	Milk, dairy products, bone meal, calcium lactate.
Chlorine	Regulates acidity/ alkalinity of the body. Helps produce digestive acids.	Loss of hair and teeth. Poor digestion.		Salt.
Magnesium	Helps the body to use fats, carbohydrates, protein and other nutrients.	Nervousness, tremors.	Men – 350 mg. Women – 300 mg.	Fresh green vegetables, soyabeans, corn, apples, almonds.
Phosphorus	Helps with calcium to build bones and teeth.	Loss of weight and appetite.	800 mg.	Fish, eggs, poultry, whole grain, nuts, meat.
Potassium	Helps control the activity of the nerves, kidneys and heart muscles.	Respiratory and heart failure.	Probably about 2 grams.	Leafy vegetables, oranges, whole grain, mint leaves, potato skins.
Sodium	Necessary for functioning of nerves, muscles, blood and the lymph system.	Weak or shrinking muscles. Loss of appetite, nausea.	6–18 grams, as sodium chloride (salt).	Salt, seafoods, beets, kelp, meat.
Sulphur	For the formation of body tissues.		Sufficient sulphur is obtained from normal protein intake.	Meat, fish, nuts, eggs, cabbage, Brussels sprouts.

Biochemic Remedies

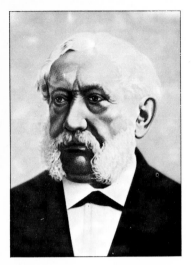

Wilhelm H. Schuessler.

Millions of cells go to make up our bodies. To function correctly, these cells require a constant supply of chemical substances – some exceedingly complex, and some which are much simpler and occur in nature as mineral salts.

The theory that an imbalance or deficiency of certain mineral substances in the cells could cause a disturbance of function and health in the whole organism, was the life's work of a German doctor – Wilhelm H. Schuessler who lived from 1821–1898. He isolated twelve mineral salts as essential cell nutrients, calling them Tissue Salts, and his form of treatment became known as Nutritional Biochemistry, since it deals with the chemistry of living things (bios, Greek = life).

Schuessler put forward five principles in support of his studies:
1. disease does not occur if cell activity is normal;
2. cell activity is normal if cell nutrition is normal;
3. the human body requires both the complex organic compounds and inorganic (mineral) substances as cell nutrients;
4. a mineral salt deficiency will impair the ability of cells to assimilate and utilize the organic compounds;
5. cell nutrition and metabolism can be revitalized by supplying the deficient mineral salts in a readily assimilable form.

It may be thought that few people living in the Western world today are undernourished and that it is not possible for body cells to be lacking in their essential nutrients. Certainly, a balanced diet of proteins, fats, and carbohydrates should provide everything the body requires for growth, maintenance and repair, but it is still possible for a localized deficiency to occur. This can be due to injury, fatigue, medicinal drug poisoning, and other causes not yet fully understood.

Fundamental to Schuessler's biochemistry is the principle of assimilation. This can be achieved by the administration of a micro dose that can pass rapidly into the blood stream through the mucous lining of the mouth and throat. The homoeopathic principle of trituration – a controlled mixing and grinding process – is used to incorporate the mineral salts in micro dose amounts into a milk sugar base. From this, small moulded tablets are prepared which, when placed on the tongue, allow instant assimilation.

Selecting a Remedy

In biochemic therapy, the predominant symptoms point to the tissue salt or salts needed in any given case. Each has its own distinctive symptom picture which is the surest guide to the tissue salt required.

Clinical experience indicates that some ailments respond better to the use of two or more tissue salts taken together. To meet this need, various combinations are available, some in proprietary form, such as *Elasto* tablets, recommended for the treatment of circulatory disorders, aching legs and feet, *Nervone* a nerve nutrient, and *Zief* for rheumatism; others are designated alphabetically, Combination 'A', 'B', 'C', etc., and recommended for the treatment of specific groups of common everyday indispositions.

Tissue salt therapy is suitable as a first-aid for the treatment of simple, easily recognized ailments. If the symptoms persist, or if they are in any way unusual, medical advice should be sought.

All the twelve tissue salts are safe; they may be taken alone or with each other without fear of side effects, and they are non toxic and non habit forming. Nevertheless, the instructions on the label regarding dosage and frequency should be followed. The most generally useful strength, or potency, of the tablets is 6x – this form of declaration following homoeopathic tradition.

The remedies are available at health stores and some chemists.

A. J. Ruffhead

THE TWELVE TISSUE SALTS AND THEIR USES

Biochemic No. and Name	Chemical Name	Function	Indication

1. Calc. Fluor.	Calcium fluoride.	Gives elasticity to tissues.	Relaxed condition
			e.g. haemorrhoids
			    varicose veins
			    muscular weakness
			    poor circulation

2. Calc. Phos.	Calcium phosphate.	Aids assimilation of food. Essential for sound bone and teeth formation.	Chilblains, indigestion, lowered vitality and during convalescence.
3. Calc. Sulph.	Calcium sulphate.	Blood purifier.	Spots, pimples, slow healing wounds.

4. Ferr. Phos.	Iron phosphate.	Constituent of red blood corpuscles and plays vital part in distribution of oxygen throughout the body.	All symptoms of an inflammatory nature
			e.g. inflammations of the skin
			    feverishness
			    sore throat
			    muscular rheumatism.
			Use it internally in the early stages of the common cold; externally in powder form; for cuts and abrasions.

5. Kali Mur.	Potassium chloride.	Takes part in the metabolic process in the formation of fibrin from albumen.	Congested conditions, whitish catarrhal discharges.
6. Kali Phos.	Potassium phosphate.	Nerve nutrient.	Nervous tensions, depression. Loss of sleep. Irritability. Nervous headaches. General debility.
7. Kali Sulph.	Potassium sulphate.	Promotes healthy formation of epidermal tissues.	Yellowish exudations and discharges of the skin, nose or throat. Brittle nails, poor condition of hair and scalp.
8. Mag. Phos.	Magnesium phosphate.	Nerve and muscle fibre nutrient.	Relief of darting pains, cramps, acute spasms, hiccoughs, colic. Can usefully be taken in conjunction with Kali Phos.
9. Nat. Mur.	Sodium chloride.	Controls the distribution of water in the tissues.	For both dry or excessive moisture in the system.
10. Nat. Phos.	Sodium phosphate.	Acid-alkaline regulator of the cells.	Acidity, heartburn, indigestion.
11. Nat. Sulph.	Sodium sulphate.	Excess water eliminator.	Bilious conditions, colic, headaches.
12. Silica	Silica, Silicon dioxide, Silicic acid.	Elimination of waste materials.	Toxic accumulations, pus formations, boils, styes.

Orthomolecular Medicine

Orthomolecular medicine is a term originally used by the chemist and Nobel Prize winner Linus Pauling, who describes it as "the preservation of good health and the treatment of disease by varying the concentrations in the human body of substances that are normally present in the body and required for health". At its simplest, orthomolecular medicine would include the use of insulin in the treatment of diabetes – insulin being normally present in the bodies of non-diabetic people. However, although Pauling first used the term in the late 1960s, the method of treatment originated in the 1950s and became known as megavitamin therapy. In 1952, Dr Abram Hoffer and Dr Humphry Osmond began treating schizophrenics with high doses of niacin, a member of the vitamin B complex. According to their results, as many as 75 percent of their patients regained their health. Since then, megavitamin therapy has grown to include the use of large doses of vitamin B6 and B2, folic acid, ascorbic acid and other vitamins, such as B17 (Laertrile), as well as minerals and hormones.

The treatment of mental illnesses with vitamins is now called orthomolecular psychiatry, a term again used first by Pauling to be "the treatment of mental disease by the provision of the optimum molecular environment for the mind, especially the optimum concentrations of substances normally present in the human body". Pauling believed that some forms of mental illness might be due to vitamin deficiencies occurring even with adequate diets. He suggested that some people might be genetically predisposed to idiosyncratic needs for very large doses of vitamins. Depression, anxiety, alcoholism, drug addiction, hyperactivity in children and similar illnesses have all been treated with, principally, megadoses of vitamins. While, however, considerable success rates have been claimed for this form of therapy, there is as yet no conclusive proof that high doses of vitamins are truly effective in mental illness. Certainly no controlled experiments have been performed and the existing results are complicated by the fact that practitioners of the therapy also use other methods in their treatment regimens including tranquillizers, anti-depressant drugs, electro-convulsive therapy (ECT), cereal-free diets and exercise.

The use of therapeutic high vitamin doses is not confined to mental illness. Pauling, for instance, achieved instant fame by claiming that high doses of vitamin C were effective in curing the common cold and was useful as a prophylactic. Several studies have investigated this claim, the majority of which produced negative results. Despite this, there is a common belief among the public that vitamin C may be so effective. Orthodox researchers hold the opinion that there is not sufficient evidence that vitamin C in such high doses (from 3–15 grams per day) is in fact safe. Certainly vitamin C in these doses produces a highly acid urine which may, over a long period, be detrimental to health. Vitamin C has also been claimed to be effective in some cases of rheumatoid arthritis and other connective tissue diseases. This use of vitamin C is based on the theory that ascorbic acid is required by the body for the synthesis of connective tissue.

Dr Atkins' diet recommends megadoses of B-complex vitamins and C and E vitamins to keep blood sugar stable, for, being a slimming diet, Dr Atkins believes that obese people are hypoglycaemic. However, as one nutritionist pointed out, blood sugar remains remarkably stable without the use of unphysiologic doses of vitamins.

Megavitamin therapy is often used today to describe the prescription of high doses, but not necessarily megadoses, of vitamins. There is an increasing trend for people to be encouraged to take higher and higher doses of vitamins as dietary supplements before it is known whether such supplementation is either effective or safe.

Restrictions in diet may be made because of:

1. personal likes and dislikes – physical, mental, emotional or drug-induced;

2. lack of time, lack of teeth, lack of zest for life;

3. religious, economic or fashion dictates;

4. inherited and metabolic disorders with consequent inability to process fats, carbohydrates or protein;

5. organic diseases and surgery physically interfering with food breakdown;

6. the need to prepare for or conclude a period of fasting;

7. the need for a physiological rest whenever a fast is not desirable or possible: this may entail a mono diet or one restricted to raw or non-animal foods, for example.

Restrictions imposed may be of one or more items such as salt, sugar, coffee, gluten or milk because they have come to be associated respectively with conditions such as fluid retention, heart disease, high blood pressure, multiple sclerosis or catarrh.

The restrictions may be of certain classes of foodstuffs such as fats in gall bladder or liver conditions, starches in hypoglycaemia or animal protein in hypertension. In contrast, vegetarianism, veganism, fruitarianism imply abstinence from certain foods as a way of life rather than as a restriction because of lack of health.

Joseph Goodman

Mono Diets

The virtue of a mono diet lies in its simplicity. By eating only one selected item of food for a period of time, the body is able to rest and so encourage self-healing. The omission of all those foodless substances that were probably long term causes of the ill-health itself can only be advantageous. If overeating was one of the basic causes, then by sheer respite of volume the organs of digestion, absorption and excretion will be able to recoup overwhelmed energy. Not least, for those unable to fast, i.e. take water only, either for medical or idiosyncratic reasons, a mono diet is an ideal way of initiating re-balance.

On first consideration, there seems little rationale for the choice of one item over any other: grapes, grapefruit, oranges, rice, potatoes, toast, prunes, eggs, milk, watermelon, wheat grass, carrots, even urine, all have had their exponents, their moments of publicized glory and their faithful adherents. Some choices are obvious: liquid is essential in dehydration, dry foods mop up engorgement.

That health improvements follow is beyond doubt; the belief that a specific change will follow a specific mono diet is, however, irrational. If the justification for the use of, say, grapes is for its potassium content, then grapes could just as well form part of a well balanced diet abundant in potassium foods – highly desirable, for example, in heart conditions; if the justification for the use of grapes is that it 'cured' someone of cancer, the most that can be said for its expectations in another is that the sufferer concerned must be as grape-consciously unique as the originator of the so-called grape cure.

Recovery from illness is the prerogative of the body. It alone has power to respond to environmental factors: those that inspire hope and courage, those that permit undrugged sleep and relaxation, those that make up nutritional deficiencies and those that withhold harmful influences. Abstention from self abuse and mind body orientation towards health are the justifications for mono diet.

Joseph Goodman

Food Allergy and Clinical Ecology

Clinical Ecology is a new science beginning to grow in Great Britain, but it has already been developed considerably in the United States and Canada. Although still regarded by most of the medical profession as unconventional, the people involved with it are almost entirely physicians, a number of whom hold professional positions in paediatrics, medicine, allergy and even cardio-vascular surgery.

Clinical Ecology is particularly concerned with environmental exitants in air, water, food, drugs and environmental chemicals in our habitat. Most medical research is concentrated at the end point of disease processes whereas clinical ecologists feel that many diseases are totally individual reactions to environmental insults. Food allergy, or hypersensitivity, accounts for about 80 percent of the total problem and, in a high proportion of patients, is the only problem.

A very wide range of chronic illnesses appear to be related to food and environmental problems and include depression, alcoholism, schizophrenia, migraine, hypertension, obesity, rheumatoid and osteo-arthritis and bowel disorders such as ulcerative colitis. Some other conditions generally accepted to be allergic in origin, such as asthma, eczema and rhinitis are sometimes treated inadequately as foods and hydrocarbons are not usually considered.

The key to understanding food allergy lies in the concept of masked food allergy described by the eminent American allergist, Dr Herbert Rinkel. He discovered that food eaten frequently will modify or mask the adverse effects of prior ingestion of that food. Hence, if a person is allergic to wheat, each time he has a further dose, he will transitorily feel better. When he leaves off the wheat he will initially feel worse but five days after the last ingestion of wheat he will feel better. A further dose after five days abstinence will cause the symptoms dramatically to recur. Hence, if a patient has three food allergies, he will be suffering a complex mixture of masking effects, withdrawal effects and re-introduction effects and the relationship of his illness to food will be far from clear. However, if the patient follows a carefully structured dietary programme in which initially all the common food allergens are omitted, for at least five days, the problem can be elucidated when the likely foods are subsequently eaten one at a time.

Alternatively, sublingual tests in which three drops of a foodstuff are placed under the tongue can be employed. With these, a very instant reaction can be obtained as there is extremely rapid absorption from the sublingual area. I find these tests less reliable than the full ingestion test, especially in middle-aged people and particularly with cereals.

Ordinarily, skin testing is useless for food allergies, but a very elaborate variation, the Rinkel titration technique, in which varying dilutions of the food are employed, gives good results in expert hands.

The main strength of the concept of food allergy is in its scientific assessability. Hence, not only can a disease be demonstrated to have been cured by the withdrawal of a food or foods, but it can be re-created by the reintroduction of the food. The recreation can furthermore be demonstrated by double blind techniques such as feeding the patient from a masked coded syringe through a stomach tube. With a drug one can only demonstrate a cure rate, part of which might be spontaneous. Consistent multiple recreations of the condition, such as was recently reported by Dr Finn and Dr Cohen of Liverpool University in the *Lancet* has far greater scientific reliability.

When a co-incident inhalant problem exists, the matter should ideally be sorted out in a Clinical Ecology unit, in which all conceivable complicating inhalant problems have been eradicated.

John Mansfield

Carbohydrate Metabolism

The choice of foods relevant to those with disturbances of carbohydrate metabolism becomes evident with an understanding of the physiological and chemical processes involved. Most readily available of the macro-nutrients, carbohydrate (literally carbon oxygen and hydrogen) is cheapest and most easily convertible by the body for energy purposes. There are three main food forms:

1. *Monosaccharides*, simple sugars such as: *glucose* from fruits, vegetables and the culmination of carbohydrate digestion; *fructose* in fruit juices and honey; *galactose* from the breakdown of animal milk lactose.

2. *Disaccharides*, combinations of two simple sugars, such as: *lactose* combining glucose and galactose; *sucrose* in beet, sugar cane, honey, maple – a mixture of glucose and fructose; *maltose* from malt products and germinating seeds – comprising two glucose molecules.

3. *Polysaccharides*, a complex of glucose units, insoluble in water, of high molecular weight, chiefly: *starch* the food reserve of plants protected in granular envelopes that may need to be split by cooking in order to permit the penetration of digestive enzymes; *cellulose* not digestible by humans but essential as roughage.

Carbohydrates need to be broken down into monosaccharide units before they can be absorbed through the intestines and then assimilated into the blood stream. Wheat, rice, potatoes, sugar cane and beet are examples of polysaccharides whose digestion has to start in the mouth. Salivary enzymes split the starch even as the food is being chewed into a swallowable ball. Some types of carbohydrate are further split in the stomach but the main digestive area is in the small intestine where partly-digested material from the stomach is acted upon by juices from the pancreatic gland.

The resulting glucose readily finds its way into the blood stream where, in a healthy person, it is kept at a constant level. After a meal, for example, the normal circulating level of blood sugar is increased; the increase is transported to the liver where it is stored in an inert form called *glycogen*. As there is a limit to the storage capacity of the liver, saturation is reached if there is constant overeating especially of sugary foods. A new storage place must be found: the fat depots under the skin. These become the repositories of the glucose now transformed into fat by various metabolic processes in the liver.

Underlying these mechanisms of balance is the hormonal system. An increase of sugar in the blood triggers a response in the pancreatic islets of Langerhans. They secrete the hormone *insulin* into the blood stream, a chemical messenger that encourages the organs concerned to transport glucose into the liver. Without insulin, as in *diabetes mellitus*, sugar would accumulate in the blood with dramatic and dangerous effect. Insulin is the only hormone concerned with sugar-level reduction. There are at least five hormones involved in increasing the levels of blood sugar. These are secreted by the adrenal glands, the thyroid, pancreas and pituitary to act as a physiological counter to insulin.

Diabetes, therefore, can result either from underproduction of pancreatic insulin or over-production of its antagonists. Diseased glands may be responsible or the administration of excessive quantities of hormones as drugs, not least the contraceptive pill. In all cases, *hyperglycaemia* is the result.

Anybody suffering excessive thirst and urination, especially if there is weight and energy loss, should have their urine tested to see if it contains sugar which will have 'spilled out' from the blood stream into the urine. A laboratory blood test will also be necessary: after an overnight fast, a specimen of blood is taken and its sugar content measured. This fasting level should read between 80 and 120 mg

Carbohydrate Metabolism

per 100 ml of blood. 50 mg of glucose is then drunk and half-hourly specimens of blood taken for an estimate of their sugar content. The resultant curve plotted on a graph will indicate the tolerance the subject has to sugar intake and the degree of diabetes present if any. As the illustration shows, in diabetes the blood sugar level goes well over the kidney threshold soon after glucose is ingested and all urine specimens would contain sugar. Even after two hours the curve will not have returned to its fasting level.

Hypoglycaemia

The blood sugar coin has two sides. Sustained physical effort or a period of fasting will reduce sugar levels, but, in health, compensatory mechanisms will soon re-balance. In diabetics, over-dosage of insulin will have the same effect and, again, will normalize if insulin is reduced. However, hypoglycaemia is also found in the state of *anorexia nervosa*, (a pathological inability to eat), in malnutrition of the aged and in people with disturbed carbohydrate metabolism. The latter includes a condition called *reactive hypoglycaemia* in which there is a transitory low level of sugar that occurs after the intake of glucose foods.

Persistent starch eating, caffeine and stress are some of the factors leading to such a breakdown of metabolism; heredity also plays its part. Sugar foods and drinks provide the aggravation. The latter offer a welcome pepping-up to the brain and nervous system deprived of nourishment, but they contribute to a worsening of the condition in the long·run: simple sugars go straight into the blood stream and, as the level rises, the pancreas increases its insulin secretion. The more sugar eaten, the more the insulin. The more the insulin, the lower the sugar level drops in response and the more the sufferer becomes aware of the lack of and 'need for' sugar. Eventually, the pancreas over-reacts even to normally safe foods, especially in the obese.

Once again a confirmatory blood test will be needed, of 5 or 6 hours duration this time. A hypoglycaemic curve, as shown, is one that drops well below average fasting level after the intake of glucose.

Nutrition

Those with pronounced diabetes due to non-functioning islets must resort to medical treatment with the possibility of insulin injections for all time. Diagnosed renoglycosurics without diabetes, mild diabetics and hypoglycaemics *must* attend to their nutritional needs if there is ever to be a return to normal metabolism. Even insulin-dependent diabetics will improve in many ways with sensible nutrition especially if obesity was involved in the onset of their disease.

What to eat is no more important that what not to eat: to be avoided for ever are all de-natured, refined foodstuffs that occupy valuable space in the digestive system, maximum starch bulk with minimal food value (see *Wholefood*); sugary foods that satisfy craving or the need for stimulus but leave the system worse off than it was; fried foods that impose a strain on the body's already limited capacity to handle fat; stimulating drinks like tea, coffee or alcohol because of their long-term depressing effect; drinking with meals because the digestive juices become diluted and therefore less effective in food breakdown and, of course, smoking for a variety of reasons.

The liver and the kidneys, the hormonal glands, the digestive and absorptive organs and the nervous system are all involved in conditions of carbohydrate disturbance; nutritional considerations, therefore, must relate to the whole organism and not just to one specific part. What is good for the body is good for its parts. Only when food as a whole has been considered for that individual is it fruitful to look to fragmentary parts of the food or the person. Whereupon,

Carbohydrate Metabolism

The curves shown are examples of faulty carbohydrate metabolism. Individual curves may show considerable variations.

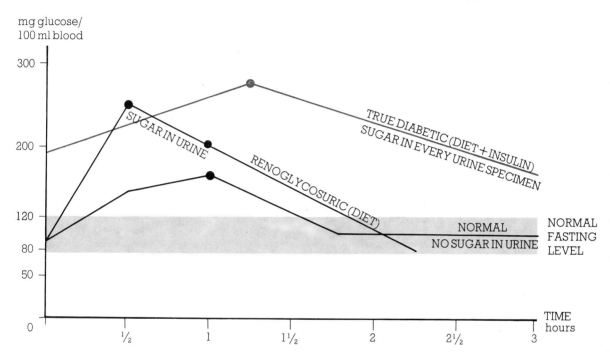

mg glucose/ 100 ml blood

TRUE DIABETIC (DIET + INSULIN)
SUGAR IN EVERY URINE SPECIMEN

SUGAR IN URINE

RENOGLYCOSURIC (DIET)

NORMAL
NO SUGAR IN URINE

NORMAL FASTING LEVEL

TIME hours

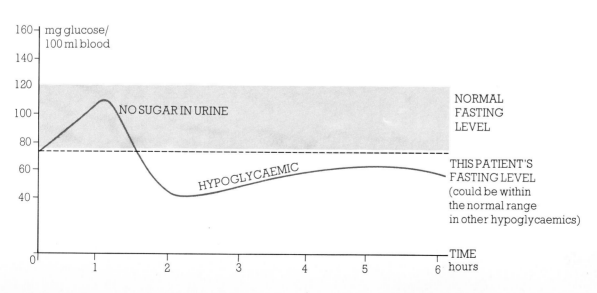

mg glucose/ 100 ml blood

NO SUGAR IN URINE

NORMAL FASTING LEVEL

HYPOGLYCAEMIC

THIS PATIENT'S FASTING LEVEL (could be within the normal range in other hypoglycaemics)

TIME hours

Carbohydrate Metabolism

there is reason to believe that:

1. pancreatic insulin production is impaired in the absence of foods rich in Vitamin B6, in magnesium, in first-class proteins (those containing all the essential amino acids) and in essential fatty acids;

2. the liver that is deficient in Vitamin B2, in protein, in pantothenic acid is less likely to secrete the enzymes necessary to inactivate insulin at hormonal request;

3. stress produced by low blood sugar leads to a retention of sodium and water and a consequent loss of potassium; frequent small meals may therefore be preferable for a time, high in potassium and low in sodium;

4. the body's ability to make use of its food intake is affected by emotional and structural factors;

5. there is no diet for either diabetes (hyperglycaemia) or hypoglycaemia; there *is* a right way of eating for each individual concerned.

Joseph Goodman

Fasting

As the chart on page 127 indicates, abstinence from food can be voluntary or imposed; nutritionally, religiously or politically expedient; productive or destructive. Hygienic fasting is a voluntary act concerned with improvement of the quality of the faster's life.

It is important to distinguish fasting from starvation which is a pathological state; fasting means doing without food but not air and water and occurs entirely within physiological limits. In the state of emptiness that ensues, the phenomenon demarcating the two activities is the return of genuine hunger; it is only if a fast is continued after natural hunger returns that starvation takes place. Fasting therefore is beneficial; starvation hazardous (from the Anglo-Saxon *steorfan*, to die).

Abstinence is a process instinctive in all animals not spoiled by domesticity, essential to survival when the organism is overloaded with undischarged toxins. A toxic overload accumulates when:

1. more food is habitually eaten than is required for the body's needs;

2. food of a poor quality imposes a strain on the digestive and assimilative functions of the body;

3. enervating habits reduce the eliminative detoxifying capacities of the liver, kidneys, lungs and skin and the excretory efficiency of the bowels, bladder and uterus.

To fast is to rest the body physiologically so that energy normally expended in dealing with food is diverted to healing purposes.

The wasted appearance of a famine victim will make evident the fact that a fasting or in this case a starving person is still eating – eating the body's reserves. When all the food reserves are consumed and the essential organs affected, fasting becomes starvation. The accompanying tables provide a reassuring illustration of the degrees of loss during abstention, vital organs being preserved to the point of death.

The economy of nature is such that reserve stores are available in the body for stress situations when food is either not available or better left uneaten. Every cell and every organ has its private reserve and is also able to call on stores of glycogen in the liver, protein in the blood and lymph, fat in the fat depots (even of thin people) and assorted food elements in the bone marrow and the glands. In the people most in need of fasts, there are additionally the accumulations of easily convertible material lodged in watery swellings, tumours, rheumatic joints, congested lung tissue, fatty walls, catarrhal cavities and engorged or impacted intestines.

Vital organs and tissues, therefore, receive their nourishment during a fast from:

a. food stocks within the body;

b. less important structures;

c. the salvable portions of dead and diseased tissues.

An obese individual may take up to forty days or more to relinquish his excesses. Fasts have been known to last ninety days. In the average naturopathic practice, ten days is a useful period of abstention but as no two people are the same in their responses it is rare for a fasting timetable to be arranged beforehand. It is recommended that newcomers to fasting do not exceed three days except under the supervision of someone experienced in conducting fasts.

Fasting does not cure disease. It is often the first step in the direction of the body healing itself:

a. it halts the intake of what have generally been the causes of the disease itself;

b. it enables the vital organs to rest by reducing their work-load: heart, kidneys, lungs, spleen, liver;

c. storage organs such as the stomach and gall bladder are permitted to empty and so cleanse themselves of obstructive impurities and infective or putrefactive organisms;

d. organs of elimination such as kidneys, bowels, lungs can deal with backlogs without having to deal with new waste matter;

e. physiological chemistry and secretions are normalized;

f. diseased and abnormal accumulations are broken down.

As a result of an initial fast and subsequent care in nutrition and other aspects of daily living there is usually:

1. a rejuvenation of cells and tissues;

2. a revitalization of bodily energies;

3. improved digestion, absorption and assimilation of foodstuffs;

4. normalization of weight;

5. increased breathing capacity;

6. an improved clarity of thinking and a strengthening of the mind.

Fasting is safe if all sensible precautions are taken; for example, it is dangerous for a fasting person to take any drugs. The newly-tuned nervous system with its heightened awareness may react to defend itself with dramatic consequences.

It is important to break the fast with care. Because the stomach will have shrunk in its emptiness, single items should be consumed at first, gradually increasing during following days. A good rule to follow is: take as many days returning to a full diet as has been spent in actually fasting.

Finally, let the newly educated body indicate when not to eat in the future; never when fevered, or so-called infected, or following shock or serious injury or in any acute illness. The body will be appreciative.

Joseph Goodman

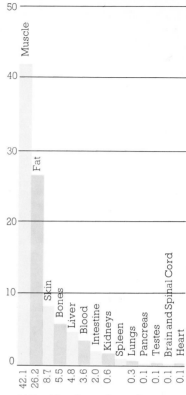

% Total loss borne by each organ

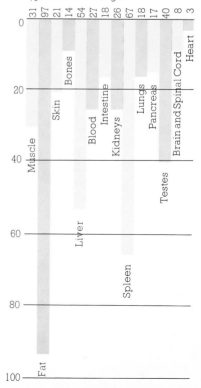

Charts showing weight loss after death from starvation.

Cymatics

Modern physics regards matter as being composed of energy that when apparently moving proceeds in waves, and when apparently stationary exhibits fields of force. Matter can, however, still be manipulated by the laws of mechanics and geometry. Nevertheless, the existence of such diverse phenomena as psychokinesis, water divining and healing, in fact, the odd events that cannot be explained by the mechanical approach to matter, make sense when relativity theory is used. Einstein said: "There is no place in this new kind of Physics for both the field and matter, for the field is the only reality".

It follows that mind is matter and matter is mind. So, in spite of the incredible apparent diversity of human beings, we are one with a conscious universe. Following up this idea of unity, we can use the new physics and the older mechanical sciences to produce new therapies.

An approach that has considerable possibilities is Cymatics – the study of the relationship between waves (vibrations) and matter, the two-way reaction between free vibration and the solid state. In the eighteenth century, Ernest Chaldni showed that sound produces patterns in sand spread on thin metal plates. Recently, Hans Jenny demonstrated the effect of sound in three dimensions. His tonoscope can be used with the human voice as the source of sound. When the letter O is spoken into the microphone a spherical pattern is produced. The sound OM is widely considered in the East to be the source of everything. The Mandukya Upanishad says "All that is past, present and future is truly OM. That which is beyond the triple dimensions of time is also OM." This holistic concept which modern physics has adopted is very ancient.

The human voice is widely used in the East and Africa in healing – and influencing emotional states. Magnetic tapes can be looped to provide repetitive cycles of low frequency sounds vibrating a microphone placed over areas of the body it is desired to influence. Alternatively, sound or music baths can be used. Mechanical vibrators of variable frequency are also effective. At present, these treatments are mostly used on painful conditions of bones, muscles and joints; the wider effects of these forms of therapy have yet to be explored. The heating effect of very short wave electro-magnetic radiation has many applications from cooking to physiotherapy. Colour therapy is another form of vibration which influences mind and body.

A static pattern can affect vibrations proceeding from its sphere of influence. Many buildings, for example, influence the emotional states of people in them. Recently some of the principles involved in constructing such buildings have been worked out by Jay Hambridge and Matila Ghyka. They are based on manipulating the Golden Mean (1:1.618) which, by simple geometric constructions, can produce a growing series of harmonious spatial relationships. The principle is one of symmetrical logarithmic growth. All living things increase in size according to this formula which is easily demonstrated in plants, shells and crystals. The Golden Mean can be used to analyse harmony, and Kayser's monumental work *Harmonia Plantarum* demonstrates that the growth of plants follows the laws of music. The Ancient Egyptians understood these principles, hence the pyramids, which have a complex harmonic structure, but also the peculiar property of preserving living tissues from decay. From this observation Pyramid Energy and Psychotronics have developed, in which forms respond to the human gaze by revolving. Dr Aubrey Westlake's pattern therapy has had considerable success. The production of homoeopathic potencies by Malcolm Rae's magneto-geometric method suggests that radionics and homoeopathy may also be part of cymatics.

Alec Forbes

Psionic Medicine

Historical Introduction

Psionic medicine is a new approach to medicine, in that it has been found that the inclusion of the paranormal, in diagnosis and therapy, is essential to a truer understanding of the nature of health and disease, and the future development of the art and science of healing. It seeks to determine by the use of the dowsing or radiesthetic faculty the cause of the imbalance and disharmony in the vital dynamic forces resulting in disorder and disease, and to discover what will eliminate the causal factors and restore balance and normality, in particular by the use of radiesthetically determined homoeopathic remedies.

Psionic medicine is a direct development of the pioneer work of the French priests, notably Abbés Bouley and Mermet, in the early years of this century in the employment of the radiesthetic faculty for medical purposes. Their work was further developed in England by Dr Guyon Richards – a general practitioner – who, in 1922, had originally studied the theory and practised the techniques of Dr Albert Abrams. He gathered round him a distinguished band of qualified medical men, and together they founded the Medical Society for the Medical Study of Radiesthesia in 1939, and published a journal, *Radiesthesia*.

Unfortunately, the majority of the original medical group died between 1946–52, but one of its members, Dr George Laurence, has carried on the work up to the present time. By his researches in the between 1946–52, but one of its members, Dr George Laurence, has carried on the work up to the present time. By his researches in the 50s and 60s, he has shown that the use of the human reflexes in conjunction with the dowsing faculty can indicate not only the physical lesions but their basic constitutional causes in the individual as well.

The Principles of Psionic Medicine

Dr Laurence found that his radiesthetic work corroborated a good deal of McDonagh's unitary theory of disease, particularly his postulate that all diseases are merely aspects, in various ways and forms, of imbalance or abberration (to use McDonagh's term) of the protein of the human body, and that no disease can be cured unless balance is restored; the main aberration being over-contraction and over-expansion of the protein as a whole or in many of its parts. This seemed to make such sense that Laurence adopted it as the basis of his radiesthetic work, and interpreted it to mean "that any toxic factor, although its incidence may fall more heavily on one system or organ than another, must affect the whole organism to a greater or lesser extent".

He found that besides the toxic factors there were others of a more profound nature first postulated by Hahnemann, the founder of homoeopathy, in his *Miasmic Theory of Chronic Disease*. Hahnemann had sought the answer to the question "why do so many chronic ailments remain uncured in spite of the incontrovertible truth of the homoeopathic doctrine?" His conclusion was that it was due "to an unknown primitive malady which owed its existence to some chronic miasm".

Laurence found that Hahnemann's miasmic theory in the light of our modern knowledge was indeed true beyond any doubt, and that the detection, recognition and elimination of the miasms has proved of inestimable value both in the treatment of chronic disease and in the field of preventive medicine.

But he found that in addition to these hereditary miasms there were also acquired miasms or, as he prefers to call them, "retained toxins of acquired infections". These "toxins" or "hang-overs" can themselves be responsible for many ailments and, when present together with an hereditary miasm, can cause very serious departures from

Psionic Medicine

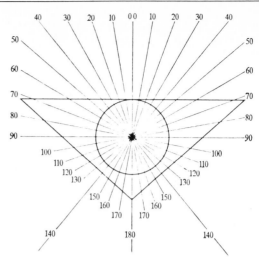

The W. O. Wood Chart, as used by Dr Laurence in the development of psionic medicine and now employed as an essential part of the psionic dowsing technique. The concept on which psionic diagnosis and treatment is based is that health is a state of balance and harmony on all planes, or, in radiesthetic terms, a balanced harmonious behaviour of energy patterns constitutes health. Any loss of balance, however slight, constitutes ill-health; gross and chronic imbalance is disease. If health is now represented as 0, or zero on any diagnostic chart or rule, then ill-health and disease are represented by a deviation from the norm (zero) by a plus or minus reading, the pendulum registering this in degrees on the chart.

The technique both of diagnosis and treatment, when using this diagram, is based on the establishment of an equilibrium of forces between three factors: the patient's witness, usually a blood spot (but this can be hair or a saliva or urine specimen) which is placed in the right-hand corner of the triangle; the diagnostic witness or witnesses placed in the left-hand corner, and the radiesthetically indicating remedies, usually homoeopathic, are placed in the apex of the triangle. These together should establish a state of dynamic balance, registering as zero on the diagnostic pattern, and recorded by the pendulum swinging up and down the zero line.

normal health. A very common combination, for example, is the hereditary T.B. and T.K. miasms together with the acquired toxin of measles, which is particularly protean and devastating. It is just as important to eliminate the acquired toxins as it is to get rid of the classical hereditary miasms if the symptoms and manifestations of any disorder – sub-acute or chronic – are to be dealt with fundamentally and adequately.

But what was of even more importance was that Laurence had found the solution to the problem which had defeated Hahnemann, namely how to get rid of the miasm both hereditary and acquired. This he found could be done by the use of potencies of protein, and later by potencies of DNA and RNA.

He also found that homoeopathy in general was the treatment of choice, when determined radiesthetically, for correcting protein imbalance, in view of the fact that it works by virtue of the specific 'vital essence' – the *vis medicatrix* – of each remedy (liberated by the act of potentization) and is thus able to work therapeutically on supersensible levels. The spiritual science of Rudolf Steiner has moreover provided an understanding of the true nature of the healing force – *vis medicatrix naturae* – as being an aspect of the etheric formative forces.

Summary

1. Psionic medicine is essentially simple both in theory and practice and requires a minimum of equipment and apparatus.

2. Accurate assessment can rapidly be arrived at or fundamental causal factors, environmental, hereditary, internal, supersensible.

3. The very earliest departures from health can be detected, thus providing a true preventive medicine; and this is especially so in the detection and elimination of hereditary miasms in children, thus breaking this etheric hereditary chain for the first time in history.

4. There is hope for chronics, as the cause of a chronicity can be diagnosed and eliminated, so that further degeneration is arrested and restoration made possible. Experience in very many cases has proved conclusively how important it is to eliminate causation before treating symptoms.

5. Treatment is entirely individual and consists essentially in stimulating and cooperating with the healing forces of the body.

6. The course and results of therapy can be monitored radiesthetically during the whole series of treatments, and necessary adjustments made with confidence.

Aubrey T. Westlake

The word 'Radiesthesia', literally translated, means sensitivity to radiations. One practitioner in the medical field has defined it as the faculty of radiation-perception, a term describing the innate ability in people to detect vibrations or waves of force which emanate from all objects in the physical universe, and from levels of consciousness that lie beyond the range of physical sense perception. These waves or radiations can be detected by any person who is sufficiently sensitive to record their impression, or who is prepared to take time to develop the ability. It is a fact that some people are sensitive enough to simply use their hands to pick up the energy fields of various objects, but most practitioners use a pendulum which amplifies the neuro-muscular response to provide a clear set of signals. These signals provide data relevant to the search that the radiesthetist is carrying out which may be for water, oil or mineral prospection, missing objects or persons. In the medical field, a simple example would be the identification of the correct medicine for a patient. This can be done by placing a box of remedies within easy reach of the left hand and then gently swinging a pendulum over a witness of the patient. The witness or *témoin* as the French call it, can be a photograph of the patient, his blood spot, a lock of hair or even a signature. Mentally asking which remedy the patient requires, the practitioner moves the index finger of his left hand from remedy to remedy until his pendulum swings into a clockwise movement which indicates the suitability of the remedy for the patient's health problem. This process may be repeated until a suitable group of remedies is found. These are then prescribed for the patient. Various practitioners interpret the signals given by the pendulum in a variety of ways, but by far the most common and generally agreed format is that a clockwise rotation means yes, an anti-clockwise one signifies no, and an oscillation is neutral. To make it even simpler, many practitioners drop the anti-clockwise movement and just use the neutral and clockwise swings of the pendulum for their work.

Medical Radiesthesia

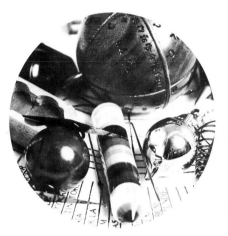

Various pendulums used in radiesthesia. The large wooden sphere is the Chaumery & Belizal Universal pendulum. Next to the spiral pendulum is one designed by Abbé Mermet. Central is a colour pendulum designed by David Tansley and used in 'spun pendulum technique' for treatment at a distance. Next to it is a Turenne pendulum with rotating magnetic needles. There are many different types of pendulum which have specific uses in radiesthesia.

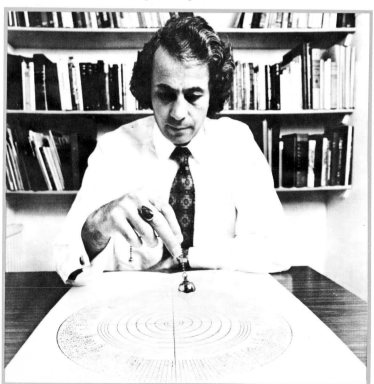

David Tansley using a radiesthetic chart which contains the fundamental rays of many homoeopathic remedies. With the patient's witness suitably positioned, the pendulum (in this case the type used by Abbé Mermet) will swing along the line of the remedy indicated.

Medical Radiesthesia

A typical diagnostic chart used in radiesthesia. The base of the triangle is oriented to the north and the practitioner sits facing point C. The patient's blood spot is located on point A and the appropriate disease or organ witnesses of Turenne singly at point B. Deviations from normal health or the presence of specific diseases are read off in degrees on either side of the zero line (C–D). The effectiveness of any remedy can be determined by placing it at point C. If it moves the pendulum back along the zero line it will be of help in healing the patient.

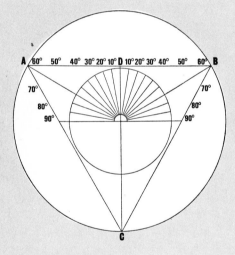

It is generally agreed that the physical senses are not employed in radiesthetic work, but that a super-sensible faculty or extrasensory perception is brought into play. This ability to detect radiations does not spring from some vague and mystical sensory apparatus, but is simply the natural expression of a faculty that everyone has. Basically it is the use of psychometry or the psychic sense of touch. Man has used it for centuries to enable him to delve into areas of knowledge and information that his physical senses cannot relay to his conscious mind. In this way he was able to bring his life into conformity with those energies and forces that play through the universe and make their impact upon man and his environment. There is an ever-increasing body of evidence to show that ancient megalithic sites and the early churches in this country were placed at specific geographical locations which related the flow of energies through the earth at certain times of the year. The Chinese used divination of this kind in order to site their houses in areas that would be healthy, and pendulums found in ancient Egyptian burial chambers suggest that they too used a form of radiesthesia to probe the mysteries of their environment and perhaps to search for appropriate sites for their monuments.

Radiesthesia first gained popularity in Europe at the turn of the century, and then mainly due to the activities of French priests, particularly the Abbés Mermet and Bouley. The word radiesthesia comes in fact from the French, Radiesthésie. The Abbé Mermet was probably the most remarkable practitioner of all time, with an almost infallible ability accurately to find what he was looking for. It was not unusual for him to be able to pinpoint a source of water in a country some six thousand miles away, and, while he was at it, reel off correct information as to depth, types of geological strata the drillers would have to penetrate, the potability of the water, its temperature and flow in gallons per minute. In looking for a missing person he could describe their movements from the time they were lost. If they met certain people, he could also gain a description of them and ultimately he could say where they were if alive or where the body was hidden if they had been murdered. The Abbé Mermet used his gift in all phases of radiesthesia including treasure hunting and prospecting. For amusement, it is said, he would, while sitting in his study in Switzerland, use a pendulum to count the number of cars crossing any bridge over the river Seine in Paris at a given time, and do it accurately. It is not unusual then that this man whose vocation it was to help people through radiesthesia, would turn his talents to the medical aspect.

His ability to diagnose the ailments of people using a pendulum was as dramatic as his ability to prospect for water or look for missing persons. In doing diagnostic work, he pointed out that the body of a person was no different basically than the body of the earth. Each had its cavities and each had streams of fluid flowing beneath its surfaces. If it was possible to detect what lay under the surface of the earth, it was just as simple to determine if disease had invaded an organ, and this could be done on site or from a distance. One doctor, who had irately condemned the Abbé as a "dowsing quack", confronted him with a photograph of a young man connected to his family. Within two minutes an accurate diagnosis was given and the doctor, quite taken aback, said: "I would not have believed it possible but I do now for I can't ignore the facts. Everything you have told me is absolutely correct. You have even pointed out two things to which I had not paid much attention, but which I know to be perfectly true". From time to time, Abbé Mermet would use radiesthesia to determine which homoeopathic or herbal remedies would help a patient get well, pointing out that in the Bible it states "The Lord hath made medicines out of the earth; and he that is wise will not abhor them". (Ecclesiasticus,

Ch. 38, v. 4.) Although a pioneer in this form of treatment mentioned in the Bible, he did very little work along these lines. Other members of the Church, especially those doing missionary work in tropical countries, made a great study of it and became famous as phyto-therapists, among these were Father Bourdoux and the Abbé Kunzle.

By the 1930s radiesthesia had become popular in England and in 1933 the British Society of Dowsers was founded to study the field in general. By 1939 Dr Guyon Richards had started the Medical Society for the Study of Radiesthesia and so great was the enthusiasm that almost all of the founder members made significant contributions to the field of medical radiesthesia; physicians like Dudley Wright, Ernest Jensen and Winter Gonin and Richards himself gave much in those early days. Later Dr Aubrey Westlake wrote *The Pattern of Health*, a classic in the field of medical radiesthesia and Dr George Laurence developed the theory and practice of Psionic Medicine.

As has been suggested above, medical radiesthesia is concerned with detecting the hidden causative factors of disease that do not lend themselves to identification by means of standard clinical tests, and to the finding of those medicines that will eliminate the disease. Now what of the apparatus used for this work and its method of employment? The practitioner will normally use a specific kind of rule or a geometric pattern or both, for diagnostic purposes. Importance is placed upon the alignment of the rule or pattern. There are, of course, variations in

Medical Radiesthesia

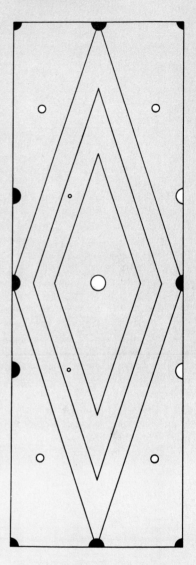

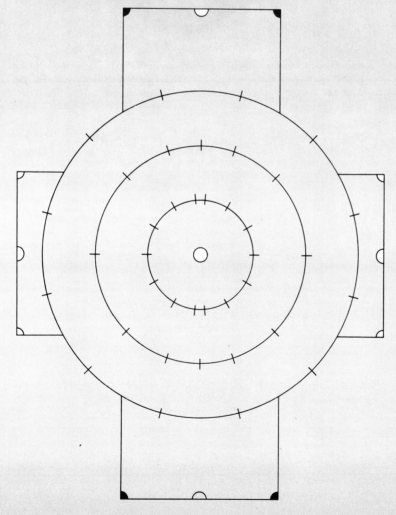

Dr Aubrey Westlake's patterns. The Static Diamond is used for treatment at a distance and specifically:

a. as an energizer of Bach and Biochemic remedies.

b. as a stabilizer in conjunction with the Celtic Cross.

c. for Colour therapy.

The Static Celtic Cross used specifically to treat at a distance with the Bach Flower Remedies and Biochemic tissue salts.

Medical Radiesthesia

Various patterns used in medical radiesthesia for diagnosis or treatment at a distance.

this, but normally the pattern is oriented with its top end to the north and the practitioner faces that direction when working. Rules are often oriented east to west. Certain points on the chart or along the rule will indicate health or diseases of different types. Placing a patient sample on the west end of the rule, the practitioner can for example determine the vitality level of the patient. A certain point on the rule will represent optimum vitality, and if the pendulum begins to swing into a clockwise or anti-clockwise direction before it reaches this point, then this will indicate the lowered point of vitality. Some practitioners will amplify the radiations from the patient sample by placing a magnet or a device known as a 'radium block' at one end of the rule, thus enabling them to get readings more easily. Vernon Wethered, a well known practitioner in this field, often employed a phial of liquid adrenalin to stabilize the energy fields along his rule.

Witnesses of various diseases and organs, or for that matter any substance, are used both with the charts or rule. Their purpose is to serve literally as a sample or witness of the disease or organ that information is being sought about. With the patient sample on the west end of the rule and a disease or organ witness on the east end, the practitioner can determine the state of the health of that organ in the patient or if a specific disease is present. The witnesses most frequently used are an invention of one of France's most famous radiesthetists, Turenne, an engineer by profession who was to make a great contribution to radiesthesia through his research work. The Turenne witnesses are small phials of an inert powder impregnated with the vibrations or frequencies representing a whole range of diseases, organs and elements.

Where the practitioner employs a chart that incorporates a triangle into its design (as in Psionic Medicine), the Turenne witness is placed on the left point of the triangle, the patient's blood spot on the right one. When a specific causal factor has been determined by the pendulum swinging away from the zero or midline of the chart, it is common practice then to introduce certain remedies into the apex of the triangle which faces the practitioner; when the right remedy or group of remedies are thus placed they cancel out the vibratory power of the disease and the pendulum then returns to the midline and swings back and forth.

It is possible, of course, to work without charts or Turenne witnesses if you are a highly capable radiesthetist like the Abbé Mermet. He suggested some of these questions when examining an animal or human subject for disease: 1. Is any organ affected by disease? 2. If so, which one? 3. Which part of the organ, and if possible, where is the precise seat of the trouble? 4. What is the nature of the disease? 5. To what extent has it progressed?

This procedure may be carried out with the patient present or using a photo or blood sample and anatomical charts. Distance is of no consequence in this form of diagnosis. Similarly, distance is not seen as a barrier to treatment and many radiesthetists use a variety of charts or other devices to amplify the healing energies of homoeopathic remedies, colours or herbs in order to project them to their patient at a distance. Readings are taken at intervals to follow and monitor the effectiveness of the healing process, and many quite remarkable results come from such methods.

The use of radiesthesia has been employed to good effect by lay and qualified practitioners alike. Certainly it adds a whole new dimension to the practice of any healing discipline be it medicine, chiropractic, osteopathy or naturopathic healing, and it is sufficiently wide in its approach to stand on its own merit.

David V. Tansley

Radionics

Radionics is a method of diagnosis and healing at a distance through the medium of an instrument using the ESP faculty. In other words it is a form of instrumented radiesthesia through which a trained and competent practitioner can determine the cause of disease within a living system, be it human, animal, plant or the soil itself. The cause of the disease having been established, suitable therapeutic energies can be projected to the patient in order to help restore optimum health.

Radionics as a healing art emerged from the researches of a distinguished American physician, Dr Albert Abrams, who was born in San Francisco in 1863. Despite the fact that Abrams was already fully qualified as a medical doctor, he went to Germany and enrolled in the famed Heidelberg University Medical School as a first-year student. Upon graduation, he was awarded both the gold and silver medals of the University for the excellence of his work. In America, he became Professor of Pathology and Director of the Cooper Medical College (Dept. of Medicine, Leland Stanford University of California). He wrote several medical text books, one of which dealt with spinal reflex therapy and ran to five editions in four years. He eventually became a specialist in nervous diseases.

During the course of his research work, Abrams discovered that specific areas of the abdomen gave a dull note on percussion when particular diseases were present in the patient. In order clearly to identify these disease reflexes from each other, he devised an instrument with calibrated dials to measure disease reactions and intensities. From this work, which Abrams called the Electronic Reaction of Abrams or ERA for short, came radionics as we know it today. Abrams' pioneering work created much interest amongst the more perceptive practitioners of the various healing disciplines, but it also came in for a great deal of criticism from those who had no wish to seek out and try new methods of healing.

In 1924 his instruments came to England and a Committee under the Chairmanship of Sir Thomas (later Lord) Horder investigated his claims. To the amazement of the medical profession, the Committee, after they had run exhaustive tests, admitted, though reluctantly, that Abrams' claims for the diagnostic value of his methods were valid. Later, Lord Horder said, "The fundamental proposition originally announced by Dr Albert Abrams must be regarded as established to a very high degree of probability". Abrams died before these findings were made known.

By the 1930s, Ruth Drown, a chiropractor in the United States practising in Hollywood, had developed new and more sophisticated forms of radionic instrumentation along with new diagnostic and treatment techniques. In the course of her work she found that it was possible not only to diagnose the diseases of a patient from a distance, but also to treat that patient from a distance using a sample of blood from the patient as a linking agent. Abrams himself had actually diagnosed disease from a distance of one mile, but Drown found that any distance could be instantly spanned and presented no barrier to proper diagnosis and treatment.

During the late 1940s and particularly the 1950s, a great deal of research into radionics was initiated by George and Marjorie De La Warr at their laboratories in Oxford. Once again, instruments and techniques were refined and improved and a lot of work was done in the field of radionic photography, a field which Drown had opened up in the 1930s. By the early 1970s, Malcolm Rae had come to the forefront of radionic research, adding a whole new dimension through the use of magnetically energized geometric patterns and electronically pulsed distant treatment. During this period, chiropractor David Tansley, well versed in the Eastern concepts of the chakras and subtle

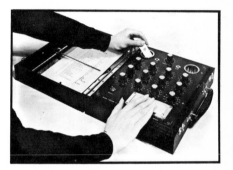

Standard Delawarr diagnostic instrument. The operator offers the patient's sample (blood spot in this case) to one of the two wells of the instrument with the left hand, while stroking the detector pad with the right hand to elicit a response or 'stick' which indicates whether the sample is being offered to the appropriate well.

Radionics

anatomy of man, introduced these ideas into radionics and made them a part of everyday practice in order to simplify diagnostic and treatment procedures and give them a deeper value and effectiveness.

It is a basic tenet of radionics that man, as well as all life-forms, share a common field of energy, and that each individual has his own particular surrounding energy field, some aspects of which are electromagnetic. If this field should become sufficiently distorted, then ultimately disease will manifest itself in the organism at a physical level.

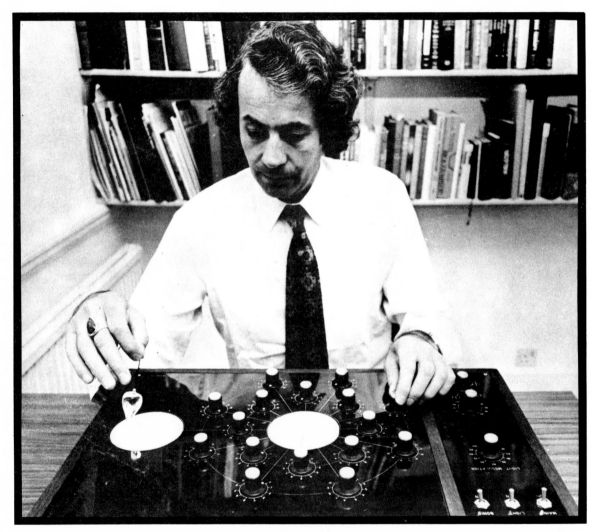

David Tansley using the Mark 3 Centre Therapy radionic instrument which he designed and built for the purpose of diagnosing and treating at a distance, the chakras and subtle bodies of man.

In radionics, all diseases, organs and remedies are seen to have their own special frequency or vibration. These can be expressed in numerical values known as 'rates'; hence the calibrated dials of the radionic instruments upon which the frequencies or 'rates' can be placed for diagnostic or treatment purposes.

When a radionic practitioner makes a health analysis for a patient he utilizes the principles of dowsing by applying the faculties of extrasensory perception (ESP) to the process of detecting disease. This is done in much the same way that a dowser detects the location of minerals, oil or water. This type of ESP is frequently referred to as the radiesthetic faculty through which the practitioner, by means of a series of mentally posed questions, obtains data about the health of his

Radionics

patient which is not normally available to the conscious mind. In other words, the conscious mind of the practitioner mentally asks the subconscious mind of the patient if specific diseases or conditions are present in him. From the resulting mind-to-mind feedback, the practitioner builds a picture of the patient's health problem and thus pinpoints the causes of disease that underly the outward symptom pattern.

It is standard practice when a radionic practitioner is consulted for the patient to send a blood spot or hair sample, accompanied by a case history and a description of present symptoms. If it is at all possible, some practitioners like to see the patient in person for the initial consultation, but in actual fact this is not at all necessary. To make an analysis or diagnosis the practitioner places the patient's sample on his radionic instrument, then attunes his mind to the patient and adjusts the dials of the instrument in a way which is analogous to the tuning of a radio to receiving a distant transmission. He is then ready to go through a series of mentally posed questions, the responses to which will give him a picture of the patient's health and a guide to treatment.

Strictly speaking, a radionic analysis is not a medical diagnosis, but a means of identifying and clearly assessing the underlying causes which give rise to pathological states and their symptoms. These findings may or may not relate to current medical opinion, but this is only to be expected when the radionic practitioner's approach is along paraphysical lines and dealing as it does with causative factors which may not be clinically identifiable or measurable.

Once the radionic analysis is complete and the major causative factors of disease have been accurately determined, the practitioner ascertains what form of treatment is required to restore health. As all pathological states have their own particular frequency or vibration, he selects those 'rates' which will counteract the imbalance or dis-ease in the patient. These 'rates' which are in fact a digitization of radiation (waves) are then projected or broadcast to the patient by means of a radionic treatment set, once again using the blood spot or lock of hair as a link. In order to augment the beneficient effect of the 'rate', some practitioners will add the appropriate homoeopathic medicine, colour, flower remedy, vitamin or mineral sample to the treatment by placing it on the treatment set near the blood spot.

For some it may be hard to accept that such treatment can be effective at a distance. However, the weight of clinical evidence leaves no doubt as to the efficacy of this form of therapy. Should there be any indication that the patient needs other forms of treatment, the practitioner may suggest dietary changes or refer them for osteopathic or chiropractic treatment or, should the case warrant it, homoeopathic or orthodox therapy.

One of the advantages of a radionic diagnosis is, of course, the fact that it is often possible to detect potentially serious conditions at an early stage and, by appropriate radionic treatment, prevent them developing to the point where they become organic and thus clinically identifiable. Of vital importance too is the fact that because radionic treatment takes place at a subtle non-physical level, it cannot harm living tissue or produce any untoward side effects.

Radionics, by its very nature, is an holistic approach to healing; it is above all concerned with the total man, with his mind, his emotions and with the subtle force fields and energies that govern the functioning and well-being of his physical organic systems. The purpose of radionics is to single out the causative factors of disease, and, by removing them, help the individual to re-establish his optimum state of health.

David V. Tansley

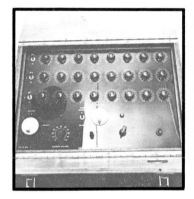

The Base 44 radionic instrument designed by Malcolm Rae. The calibration of the dials from 0 to 44 enables the operator to obtain finer tuning for purposes of diagnosis and distant treatment.

Radionic Photography

Right
Post-surgical photograph by Ruth Drown of a patient's abdomen. The incision lines run from the bottom centre of the picture up to the right-hand corner. The clearly defined dark oblong areas running left from the incision are blood vessels severed during the operation. This photograph was made from a blood crystal of a patient while the patient was within one city block of the office. Dr Drown was the first to obtain photographs of the internal organs of patients by means of her instruments. As others have since found, this form of radionic photography depended on an elusive personal quality in the operator.

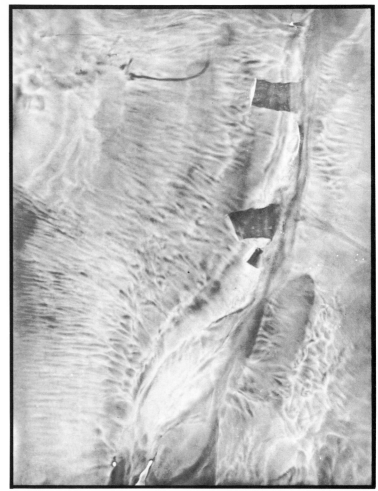

Right
Dr Ruth Drown's radionic camera, or Radio-Vision instrument, made in the 1930s. The photographs were made by directly attaching the patient to the instrument by wire leads or by placing a blood spot at a point in the circuitry. The patient's energy then flowed into the instrument, rates were set up on the dials in order to select the area to be photographed and the selected energy from the patient then flowed across the emulsion of the film.

Far right
Radionic photograph taken with Delawarr equipment showing a diseased heart.

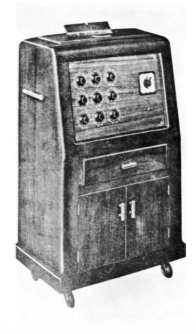

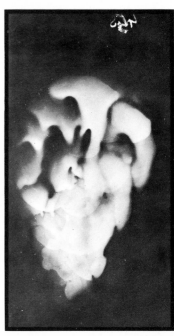

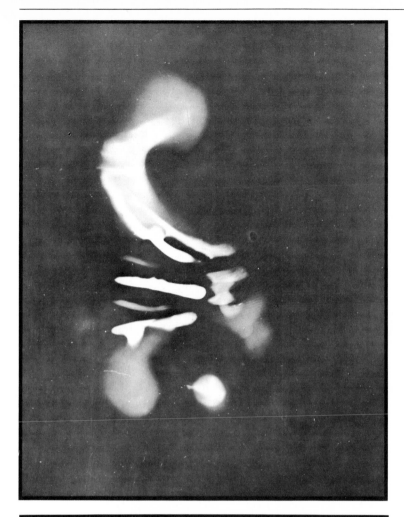

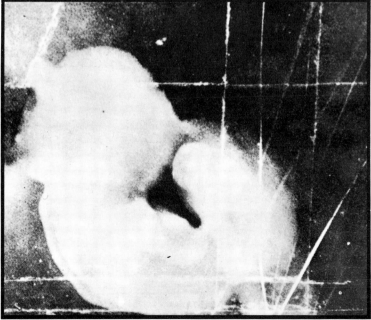

The Delawarr Camera was developed in the 1950s by the late George Delawarr at his laboratory in Oxford. Delawarr and his assistants found that energy radiations from a patient's blood specimen could produce an image on a photographic plate. Two conditions were necessary: firstly, that there was an operator standing beside the camera; secondly, that the instrument was tuned to the disease of the patient. It could therefore be used to affirm a Radionics diagnosis already made. Delawarr wrote in 1958, "The explanation as to why we should be able to get a photograph at all is still a mystery to us. But we do know that this is largely due to a rare personal ability in the operator himself". The camera obtained 'repeatable' results when operated by Delawarr and his colleagues, but when this personal element was missing it did not produce results. It could also be jammed or neutralized by the thoughts or personality of someone present in the room. These limitations were a bitter disappointment, and because of lack of financial support, further experiments on radionics photography were abandoned in the 1960s. Some 12,000 radionic photographs had been taken at the Delawarr laboratories.

Top left
Delawarr radionic photograph of the etheric energy pattern of Dr Bach's Honeysuckle Remedy.

Left
This radionic photograph of a three-month foetus in the womb was taken by the Delawarr Laboratories in the 1950s. The image was produced from the blood spot of a pregnant woman living some 54 miles from Oxford who asked for a check on her pregnancy and to be told when to expect the child.

Lakhovsky Oscillatory Coils

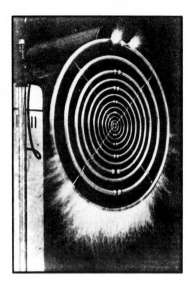

One of the large coils of Lakhovsky's apparatus.

A modern multiple wave oscillator developed by Dr Bruce Copen.

During the 1920s, Georges Lakhovsky, a French engineer, developed a theory which regarded all living organisms as systems of high frequency oscillating circuits, every cell being a simple oscillator 'vibrating' at a particular frequency. He believed that the tiny twisted filaments visible in the nucleus of every cell were the source of this electrical oscillation and were capable of both, transmitting and receiving radiation.

Health, he believed, is the harmonious, dynamic equilibrium of all cells while disease is the oscillatory disequilibrium of cells.

Lakhovsky's theory led him to evolve a new therapy with the object of restoring the cellular oscillatory equilibrium when it is disturbed by disease. This meant inducing the diseased cells to oscillate at a different rate by giving them brief electrostatic shocks that would not harm tissues by inducing heat, yet allow the disturbed cells to find their previous healthy frequencies.

In practical terms, this meant devising an electrical device that would produce an electromagnetic field which oscillated on as many different wave-lengths as possible in order to affect all possible types of cell.

In 1931 he made the first successful apparatus, which he called a multiple wave oscillator, and though almost unmanageably large and very expensive it was nevertheless rapidly adopted by several French hospitals for the treatment of organic diseases, including cancer.

The apparatus consisted of two large coils, one a transmitter and the other a receiver. When turned on, an electromagnetic field was created in the area between the coils. The patient was placed in this field so that it passed through his tissues, restoring cells to a healthier vibratory pattern. Treatments were performed for roughly fifteen minutes a day until the disease had cleared.

In recent years, advances in electronics have enabled the equipment to be reduced both in size and cost.

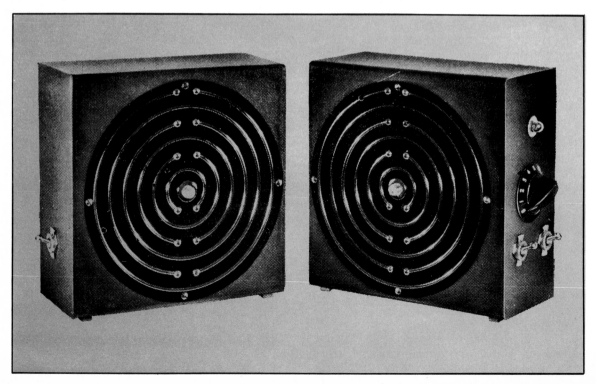

Orgone Therapy

Orgone therapy was developed by Dr Wilhelm Reich, the well-known scientist and psychiatrist who began his career as an analyst in Freud's circle in Vienna. Reich's work on character-disorders and their effects on the body led him, while working in Oslo in 1939, to discover a new form of energy which he called orgone energy. Orgone energy is identical with the life-energy that the Hindus call *prana* and which is known under a variety of other names. Experiments by Reich and by many others has put on a firm basis the view that biological energy is a distinct form of life-energy with unique bio-electric properties. Russian work on 'bio-plasma' over the past twenty years strongly supports this view.

Reich also discovered that life-energy in the body responds directly to atmospheric energy and that atmospheric energy itself can be accumulated. Research in six countries on atmospheric medicine has confirmed this crucial finding.

The 'orgone accumulator' is a cabinet whose walls are filled with alternating layers of organic and inorganic materials, usually glass wool and steel wool. The inner surfaces of the cabinet are of sheet iron and the outer surface of wood or selotex boarding. Reich and a team of some two dozen doctors used the accumulator for a period of fourteen years for treating a wide variety of organic and functional illnesses, until the American Food and Drug Administration made it illegal on the grounds that since orgone energy did not exist, the treatment was fraudulent.

Many biological changes – in blood pressure, breathing rate, rate of healing wounds and burns and recession of cancer tumours – were reported on by these doctors. They duplicate the effects noticed by others who work with atmospheric energy but under the name of 'ionization therapy'.

Reich's work with the orgone accumulator was an important feature of the Second World International Cancer Congress held in Rome in 1968. In spite of the FDA action, the clinical evidence for the effectiveness of the accumulator remains impressive. It is likely that as the fear of using alternative forms of medical treatment lessens, more doctors will find the courage to use orgone therapy for conditions which do not respond well to conventional treatments.

Because the orgone accumulator counteracts illness by increasing the biological charge of the tissues, it works to augment the natural resistance of the body and to strengthen the immune system. The accumulator promotes a response of 'lumination' or expansion to overcome the tendency to contract or shrink which is a prominent feature of many diseases. In other illnesses, where there is inflammation, the accumulator works to restore the body to a more balanced state. It was for this reason that Theodore Wolfe, a well-known specialist in psychosomatic medicine, wrote that the accumulator is one of the most important discoveries ever made in the history of medicine.

The theory and practice of orgone therapy are inseparable from Reich's earlier work on emotional stress, muscular tension and disturbances of orgasm. He found that disturbances in sexual rhythms which prevented deep satisfaction capable of nourishing the whole organism, caused interferences with the balance of pleasure and anxiety in the body. This led to stress responses from the involuntary nervous system which sent out a shock wave of reaction through many different organ systems of the body. Illnesses such as high blood pressure, gastric ulcers, asthma and rheumatism, could be seen as long-term sequels to prolonged disturbances in the rhythmic pulsatory functions of these organ systems; emotional and sexual tension was a prominent cause of the malfunction in pulsation.

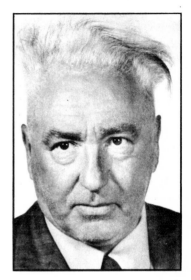

Wilhelm Reich.

Orgone Therapy

Reich distinguished between physical and psychiatric orgone therapy. In the former the accumulator is used to raise the charge of the blood and combat the illness directly at source, while in the latter the therapist worked interpersonally to free the expressions of emotional energy and recover the spontaneous rhythms of the body. 'Bio-energetics' as developed by Alexander Lowen, and 'psycho-peristalsis', developed by Gerda Boyesen, are both offshoots of earlier forms of psychiatric orgone therapy.

Reich did not believe that the orgone accumulator would be helpful in combating ordinary neurotic conditions, nor, in spite of popular belief does the orgone 'box' act in any way like an aphro-disiac and give people better orgasms. On the contrary, Reich pointed out repeatedly that many diseases were the end product of disastrous human and social conditions of life, and he insisted that the orgone accumulator was only one tool in the fight against human misery, which needed at all times to be accompanied by active work to change the emotional blockages that people developed and to overcome the life-negative features of their environment which were responsible for generating those blockages. It is these revolutionary bases of Reich's work that has led many orthodox doctors to prefer to ridicule his achievements rather than study them at first hand, learn from his impressive clinical results, and move on to practise the humane and life-affirmative style of medicine that orgone therapy makes possible.

David Boadella

The basic design of an experimental orgone accumulator. Thermometer (T) measures room temperature, T_1 the temperature above the box walls, and T_2 the temperature inside the accumulator. Reich discovered that the temperature inside the accumulator, as well as close to its outside walls, was higher than the room temperature by an average of 1°C. Reich also said he observed a diffuse bluish-grey light and rapid yellowish rays which are typical of orgone energy. This accumulator is built from layers of metal and wood separated by a layer of cotton.

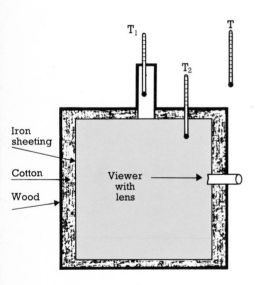

An orgone accumulator for therapeutic use. This box is made from alternate layers of wood and iron, with iron on the inside. The lid of the box with a flexible tube attached allows the patient to breathe accumulated orgone energy.

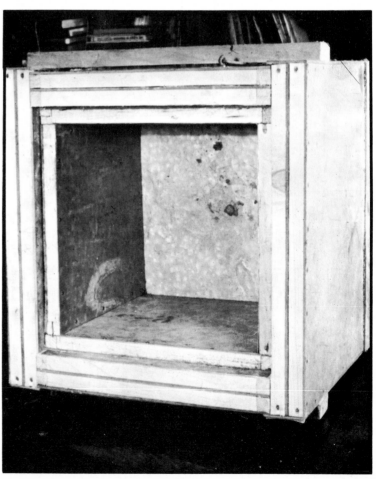

Pyramid Energy

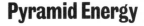

During the 1930s, a French radiesthetist, Antoine Bovis, while exploring the Great Pyramid of Cheops, noticed that the bodies of animals which had become trapped in the King's Chamber and died had not putrified but had become mummified. On his return to France he built a perfectly scaled model of the pyramid and placed a dead cat in the position of the King's Chamber – about one third the distance from the base to the apex. The cat mummified.

Bovis's work attracted no interest until the 1950s, when a Czech engineer, Karel Drbal, decided to investigate further. After a series of successful experiments, Drbal came to the conclusion that there is a relationship between the shape of the space enclosed by the pyramid and the physical and biological processes which occur in that space. Drbal's most famous discovery was that the pyramid will sharpen a razor blade provided the sides of the pyramid are aligned with the earth's magnetic field and the blade aligned at right angles to the side facing north.

Since the 1950s, the claims made for the powers of the pyramid have rapidly multiplied:

Cuts, wounds and bruises apparently heal faster under a pyramid, while sitting under a pyramid will reduce the pain of migraine or toothache.

Water placed under a pyramid seems to take on healing and tonic powers. The water can reduce the inflammation from bites, burns etc and act as a natural aid to digestion.

Sitting under a pyramid improves meditation and produces an increase in the amplitude of alpha brain waves.

Polluted water has been purified by placing it inside the pyramid for several days.

Meat, vegetables and fruit will dehydrate rather than turn bad – in the case of fruit, the skin will wrinkle while the inside stays fresh for weeks.

So far there has been no adequate explanation of these results. A particular drawback to serious scientific experiments with pyramids is that many of the claims are not repeatable in the laboratory – at least on a predictable basis. Another drawback is that lacking knowledge of what is actually happening inside the pyramid space, no instrument has been devised which can detect or measure the apparent energies. Many dowsers however say they can detect particular areas inside and outside the pyramid where the energy seems to concentrate.

Recent research, particularly in Czechoslovakia, has shown that many of the results obtained with the pyramid can also be obtained with certain other shapes, notably cones.

Providing a model pyramid is constructed as nearly as possible to scale based on the Cheops pyramid, it can be constructed of almost any material. Recent work has shown that only the framework of the pyramid is necessary, and that it can be used to stimulate the growth of plants, preserve foods and so on.

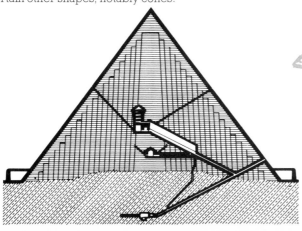

This cross-section of the pyramid of Cheops shows the location of the King's Chamber, roughly one-third the distance from the base of the pyramid to the apex. Experiments with scale models suggest that this position in a pyramid is a focus of the pyramid's energy.

Healing

Healing, like herbalism, must have been one of the earliest therapeutic discoveries of man. It does not take long to observe that some people have the ability to make an emotional relationship with their fellows and help them when they suffer. Healing is a natural human attribute – every mother heals her children daily if she has a close bond with them. Healing is indigenous to all countries throughout the world, and since there is evidence that it existed for at least 4,000 years, it cannot be considered to be the monopoly of any one religion. If there has to be a descriptive adjective put before healing, it should be *natural* healing.

To understand how healing works, it is necessary to look into the nature of man and the physical world. There is only one energy – Mind, the Self, God, Tao, Great Spirit, Sugmad, call it what you will. When this energy is apparently moving, it travels in waves; when apparently still, it exerts fields of force. Mind patterns the force and forms its own reality of particular energies and forces. So does the human mind, but not realizing that there are no limits, accepts its given reality and feels distressed when this and its belief systems are disturbed.

One condition of human life in the physical world is that we must become unique individuals. Because of this, we all manufacture a personal reality, and this accounts for the widely differing views which people hold on the nature of all things, especially healing. The trouble is, if we confine ourselves just to our personal view, we will never see the true nature of anything – the wonderful underlying unity behind our apparent diversity will pass us by. Our realities are limits to be transcended, for we all derive from and are part of one energy "in whom we live and move and have our being". This life-bearing energy obeys cosmic laws, and if the individual mind and physical world conform to them, everything proceeds harmoniously. But when the individual mind builds behaviour patterns not in accordance with those laws and the physical world from which the body is built is polluted, disharmony results and disease follows. Now if the limits imposed by disease are to be transcended, the need for change must first be felt. Then the idea of what kind of change is needed must be formulated. The necessary action can then be taken, and this requires both effort and willingness. At the human level, will directs energy. This corresponds to the reaction of Mind with force to produce the patterns of form at a higher level. The trouble is that the human personality is so deformed by the society it inhabits that we all fall into disharmony and no one escapes disease. But we do not see this and seek to patch ourselves up with therapeutic systems, rather than change the disharmonies which produce our disorders. Healing is not a therapeutic system; it restores the soul to harmony with cosmic laws.

For healing to come about, there must first be *need*, the real desire for change – this can be brought about by someone on behalf of another. Then there must be the *idea* of healing. The healer must have a bond of empathy with the person being healed and be able to hold in his mind the idea of being a channel for the energies of Mind to flow into and change the other person so that he can evolve in accordance with cosmic laws. Next he must *will* the healing to come about. But the healer does not heal – this is done by the *will of Mind*.

Some people who are natural sources of energy and sympathetic by nature are unconscious healers; more people are unconscious drainers of the energy of others. Few who are natural healers, or who suddenly develop the faculty of healing, are unaware of it, though some do not disclose it and remain secret healers. Therapists of all persuasions quite often develop the power of healing. They are usually successful because their patients do well and feel better just for being in

The famous Spiritual Healer, Harry Edwards.

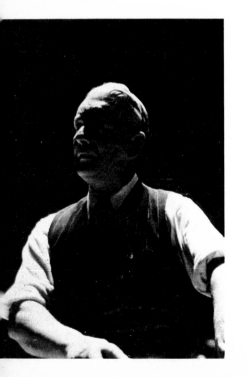

Healing

contact with them. Many do not realize this, attributing their success to the effectiveness of their therapeutic system. Others, especially when they are orthodox doctors, fear the publicity and do not disclose their ability. Most people can learn to heal, though of course not everyone will have a talent for it. We can also learn to heal ourselves, if we realize that our whole life, including its illnesses, is for us an act of learning, whose limits we can transcend, using the principle that *will directs energy*.

Healing is not miraculous. It is a natural law-abiding process. A person has little faith if his beliefs need to be bolstered by miracles, and neither understanding nor love if he can accept only one religion. We may not know exactly how healing comes about – but that it does we can be sure, for healing does work. It is instantaneous for only a very small proportion of people – probably less than one percent. It will fail with about a third, and with the other two-thirds it will work completely for the majority and only partially for the rest. The improvement comes about at varying speeds. Even though the disease may not be altered after healing, real healing harms no one; everyone feels better and is able to meet his disability in a new way. Healing primarily affects the soul and mind, not the body.

Failures in healing may come about in several ways. Sufferer and healer may not be compatible, and a proper channel for the healing force may therefore not be established. The answer here is to try more than one healer. If all fail, the condition may have gone too far, or the karma or fate of the sufferer may be fixed and impossible to change. Some other forms of therapy should then be tried, and if they fail, acceptance is the only course. If the illness is fatal, there is nothing to be frightened about in dying; there is only transitory discomfort and a passage of consciousness to another form of life.

There is some confusion about the words Spiritual and Spirit Healing. Spiritual Healing is the use of the umbrella term 'spiritual' to cover the higher aspects of man's mind and Mind. Actually, man's consciousness is divided into seven levels, but in this short article I have avoided using this classification. The ability to establish quickly, deep empathic relations is frequently associated with clairvoyant and mediumistic powers. Many healers are aware of benign spirits who are attracted by the healing process and who may make helpful suggestions. This is Spirit Healing, another natural, normal phenomenon. But it is not the only way that healing comes about. It is not, indeed, the essential basis of healing, which is the channelling of harmonizing energy through the healer to the healed. The frills lie in the mind of the healer. It is time people gave up thinking exclusively about this or that form of healing and began to study the essential basis of healing itself.

When being healed, a person mostly feels heat, sometimes where the healer's hands are held, sometimes in the disabled area of the body. Instead of heat, there may be cool feeling or a tingling more like the sensation from drinking a slightly sparkling wine than the pins and needles of an irritated nerve. Occasionally, a sensation like an electric shock will run along the limbs to the extremities or along the spine. Mentally, a state of peace or joy is experienced, sometimes slight, sometimes nothing, occasionally a peak experience, or a period of transcendence or a revelation may occur.

The disadvantage of therapeutic systems is the amount of equipment they need. This reduces their ease of application and puts up their cost. Nowhere is this more clearly shown than in orthodox medicine. The proliferation of its machinery is rapidly pushing it further into a situation of diminishing returns, where its virtual monopoly in Western civilization has already placed it. Contrast this with healing, which needs no apparatus, only two people and time. These two people

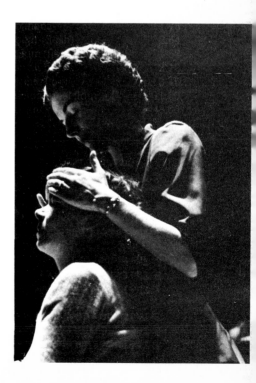

Healing

need not even meet, for it can be performed at a distance. Healing can even take place out of time. When a healer is asleep, he or she may, consciously or not, travel to a sick person and perform an act of healing, appearing to the person being healed as if present. Moreover, one healer can conduct group healing sessions so it need not even be a one-to-one relationship.

The simplicity, effectiveness, cheapness and easy application of healing is leading to its increasing use. This will bring with it the dangers of popularity and exploitation. For while nothing but good can come from true healing, like all effective processes it can be misused. The energy transmitted by a disturbed individual may be distorted and produce additional disharmony. The energy may be directed, say, towards the relief of a symptom or outward manifestation of a disease and not towards the correction of the disharmony of the whole person. This can produce greater suffering. It is, therefore, essential that all those aspiring to heal or who know they have healing ability should undergo a period of training from an experienced healer and be accepted by a panel of healers before he or she begins to practise.

An important recent advance in the study of healing made with a British invention used in biofeedback, the 'Mind Mirror', is the observation that healers produce an unusual symmetrical bilateral pattern of electrical brain waves and that the people they heal are induced to share this pattern during the act of healing. This suggests the possibility of using biofeedback techniques to train healers and a quick way of finding potential healers, as well as testing them. Nevertheless the presence of the pattern of brainwaves found in healers does not mean that such a person is fit to heal. Training is also essential.

Healing is accepted by all levels of society in Britain and openly practised. Most large towns have a healers' association or fellowship. At the moment, most healers do not charge for their services because they feel that *they* do not heal and that a natural gift should not be exploited. This attitude does them credit. Nevertheless, consulting rooms cost money to run and sparetime occupations erode family life as well as carpets and furniture. The labourer is worthy of his hire in any field, and there can be no bar to a healer receiving reasonable payment for his services and expenses.

In Britain, the General Medical Council states that a doctor may suggest to his patients that they should have healing, provided he feels sure that the healer is competent and remains responsible for them. In the hospital service the situation is not so clear-cut. The medical staffs and management committees of over 1500 hospitals have agreed that healer members of a national organization may treat patients in hospital. In 1973 the British Medical Association asked the Department of Health and Social Security to put a stop to healers treating patients in hospital, but the Minister refused to intervene. Even today, a consultant who wishes to have his patients treated by healing can find his alleged therapeutic freedom restricted by the administration and colleagues in a hospital, although both may have previously agreed to allow healers to be admitted at his discretion. The medical profession and its administration seem divided among themselves.

In the USA, the law forbids manipulation of a person's body for therapeutic purposes by everyone lacking a recognized qualification. This has restricted the development of Natural Healing and has led to many healers gravitating towards a church in order to practise healing with some degree of protection, since the laying on of hands is a recognized religious procedure. The Spiritual Frontiers Fellowship, the Association for Research and Enlightenment, Life Energies Inc., the Academy of Parapsychology and Medicine and the Foundation for

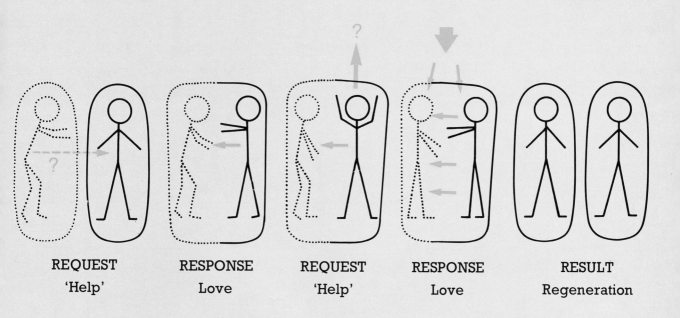

REQUEST RESPONSE REQUEST RESPONSE RESULT
'Help'   Love   'Help'   Love   Regeneration

Parasensory Investigation have been long in the field, yet not wholly devoted to healing. However, the enforcement of that law is now relaxing in several States and the American Spiritual Healers Association was founded in 1976. In 1978 a New York hospital began training selected nurses to heal. In this respect, the USA is in advance of Britain.

Healers greatly outnumber the practitioners of all the other alternatives to orthodox medicine in Britain. There are, at a rough estimate, and including those who only practise occasionally, about 20,000 healers compared with probably less than 2,000 practitioners of the other alternative therapies and 55,000 medical practitioners. The leading organization is the National Federation of Spiritual Healers, with regional branches all over the country and over 2,000 healer members. Other large organizations with many healers are the British Alliance of Healers' Association and the Spiritualist National Union. Organizations, some of whose members are healers, are the Churches' Fellowship of Healing, The Spiritualist Association of Great Britain, the World Federation of Healing, Greater World (Christian Spiritualists), the Aetherius Society, The Atlanteans, White Eagle Lodge, Christian Scientists and others. There are also some well-known individuals who run small schools of healing.

It will, therefore, be clear that there is no single organization controlling healing and that attitudes, standards and methods all differ. This is an administrator's nightmare, a Jeremiah's delight, but what potential it has! There is, however, a need for caution – a healer needs not only natural talent, but dedication, purity of motive and training – so choose your healer carefully.

Alec Forbes

Diagram showing the basis of healing.

Metaphysical Healing

Metaphysical healing is a very real therapy which benefits millions of people throughout the world. Like Christian Science, it derives from the teaching of Phineas Quinby, who was born in New England in 1802, and who numbered amongst his pupils Emma Curtis Hopkins, who made a vast impact upon the early New Thought teachings and Mary Baker Eddy, the founder of Christian Science.

All of the early founding men and women who created the New Thought movement, now centralized in the International New Thought Alliance, were students of Mrs. Holmes's Christian Science Theological Seminary, which she founded in 1887 in Chicago. Mrs. Holmes taught that "the remedy for all defect and all disorder is metaphysical, beyond the physical, in the realm of causes which are mental and spiritual . . . it stands for the practice of the presence of God reduced to a scientific method; of living a selfless life through union in thought with a power that is Love in action".

In the Declaration of Principles of the International New Thought Alliance (INTA), which embraces the whole movement of the School of Practical Christianity (known around the world as UNITY, a great body of hundreds of churches and schools), the Religious Science movement, Divine Science, Churches of Truth, Churches of Christian Philosophy, Churches of Divine Metaphysics and countless independent churches, institutes, colleges and centres, all affirm the fifth point: "that we should heal the sick through prayer and that we should endeavour to manifest perfection even as our Father in Heaven is perfect."

It is believed that about thirteen million people accept the basic idea that healing can be achieved through metaphysical prayer. They vary from group to group throughout the world, but all invoke the actual presence of the power of God working within the human body to eliminate ill health and restore well being. In most groups, the element of thanksgiving for health is an essential part of the process. Some seek the actual induction in the mind of harmony with the spirit, and thus the body of the sufferer may be restored to health.

Thousands of people are authorized to practise as healers by their respective religious organizations. The act of healing is achieved through spoken or silent prayer, either in the presence of the sufferer or from a distance. Healers also work in conjunction with orthodox medicine, attending clinics and visiting hospitals.

The INTA, the leading body recognizing practitioners of metaphysical healing, celebrated in 1977 the 65th annual congress, although the movement has existed since the 1850s.

George Hall

Psychic Surgery

In 1935, Harold S. Burr, professor of anatomy at Yale University, announced that he had discovered the energy body – a second body possessed by human beings which provides a blueprint for the physical body, controlling and determining the function of cells and organs, and the shape, size and colour of the physical body. This energy body is in turn affected by the emotions and mind of the individual. For example when someone feels well, there is a high level of energy whereas when there is feeling of lassitude or tiredness, the level is low. Burr thus became the first scientist to demonstrate what mystics throughout history have known.

Psychic surgery, which has stirred more interest and controversy than any other form of healing, utilizes the energy body to produce its remarkable results. Whereas orthodox surgeons work solely with the physical body, psychic surgeons work with the energy body to alter the blueprint, whereupon changes takes place in the physical body.

One of the most famous physic surgeons was a Brazilian, J. P. de Freitas better known as Arigó. In common with many psychic surgeons, Arigó had a spiritual guide. His guide, Adolphus Fritz, a deceased medical student, whispered in his ear to give instruction for each healing. Fritz told Arigó how the surgery was performed, "We disconnect the energy body from the physical body, so that the tissues become an amorphous, jelly-like mass. Then we remove the diseased tissue, which is no longer connected to the body, and reconnect the fields".

The surgery itself and the conditions under which it usually takes place violate all the principles of orthodox surgery. It is equally effective in a village church, in a room, a house or in the open air. There are no sterilization procedures or preoperative preparations. The patient is in everyday clothes which are rolled back to expose the site of the operation. No anaesthetics, hypnosis or suggestion are used or required, and it is unusual for the patients to feel pain even with open heart surgery or an operation for the removal of a tumour on the brain or stomach. No infection occurs – with many healers there are even no scars after the operation. The time for an operation varies from half a minute to ten minutes and afterwards the patients walk away having suffered no shock at all. The healer may be in a deep trance, fully conscious or somewhere between these two states.

The phenomena which occur are at times incredible, sometimes amusing, but always remarkable. For instance, tissue anywhere on the body is parted using only the bare hands of the healer; tissue or strange objects may be removed from the opening – egg shells, broken glass, old plastic bags, pieces of seaweed, a live shrimp. Cotton wool, dipped in oil, may be dematerialized into the chest of the patient and a few minutes later rematerialized from the neck, minus the oil, or it may be dematerialized in one ear and later removed from the other.

A healer may point his own forefinger or that of a bystander from a distance of about eight inches at the spot on the body where he wishes to make an incision, whereupon a clean cut oozing a few drops of blood appears almost instantaneously.

Some healers have been seen to remove an eyeball, remove connective tissue from the rear and then replace it.

A healer may also use a knife, sharp or blunt, or scissors, which he wipes on his sleeve before manipulating around the eye of a patient whilst he removes a small growth without causing any pain or damage. These phenomena satisfy the human need for 'seeing is believing'.

Psychic Surgery

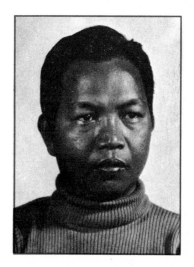

Tony Agpaoa, a leading Philippines healer. He runs a forty-bed clinic for Europeans and North Americans.

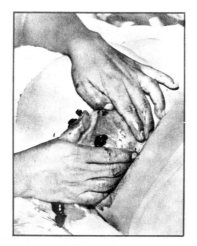

Far left
Psychic surgery in the Philippines. The right hand of the healer is penetrating the stomach, while in the left hand he holds a piece of tissue removed from the body. The black spots are coagulated blood.

Left
Materialization. In this picture the overlay of materialized tissue is clearly visible and the fingers do not penetrate the stomach.

Psychic Surgery

Psychic surgeons are often simple, barely literate, but sensitive people, who are using natural abilities. Many are devout Spiritualists or Spiritists who believe they are helped by Guides or Protectors or a group of discarnate Doctors who guide them or their hands. They are extremely dedicated, warm and wonderful people who are devoting their lives to helping others. Many will accept no payment. They undergo years of training and practice – for instance, the Filipino Tony Agpaoa, probably the best known psychic surgeon in the world, started healing at the age of seven or eight, and is now nearing forty. He underwent many years of training, fasting, prayer and meditation. He has a clinic in a rebuilt Dominican Monastery, which equals the standards of any Swiss clinic.

The numbers treated by the best healers are extraordinary. It was estimated that Arigó in Brazil helped a million or more individuals before his death at the age of forty-nine, though not all of these underwent surgery. Psychic surgery takes place daily in the Philippines, in Brazil and in Britain, and has been reported in North Africa, the Himalayas and the Andes.

Psychic surgery would repay close study by a team of specialists over a long period of time to understand what takes place, and how it could be used to benefit all mankind. Anyone who is sufficiently dedicated and open-minded can develop this ability.

Marcus McCausland

Human Cybernetics

Human Cybernetics is concerned with creating a receptive state of mind to the healing process. As a psycho-therapy it operates at three levels: as a direct healing therapy for a sick person, as a powerful support therapy when a patient is being treated by another practitioner and as an aid to the healthy person in thinking and staying well.

The concept of Human Cybernetics was first proposed by Norbert Wiener, who in his early writings describes the presence of God, the Infinite Power in man, as the foundation of all action and reaction. This idea was later developed by Professor Prescot Lecky in his self-image theory. However it was Dr Maxwell Maltz, one of the world's leading plastic surgeons, who brought wide public attention to the therapy with his book, *Psychocybernetics*.

Human Cybernetics is based on the idea that the human mind and the human brain are interdependent. Further, the human brain must transmit the idea of wellness (health) into the cell tissues of the body before the state of unwellness (ill health) can be dissolved and give way to healthy tissue. Maltz realized that if a damaged body is to be successfully repaired, the patient must be convinced that the repaired tissue is a good and effective replacement for the damaged one.

A positive state of mind is essential to all healing processes, and it forms one of the basic tenets of Human Cybernetics. The therapy embraces seventy-seven essential points in its healing programme. The first concern is to remove from the patient's consciousness any notion of ill health. The therapist then invites the patient to become receptive to the infinite power from without, which can create new growth. Gradually, the patient learns to acquire a positive mind and body. A further step is creative thinking, so that the body and nervous tissues can be rebuilt and the patient starts to look for healthy signs in himself. A good climate for complete recovery is established through sensible dietary habits, meditation and a state of thankfulness. Thus the patient eliminates ills and assumes the mantle of health.

Within the Human Cybernetics educational system there is specific teaching of the techniques of healing outlined above. They are described in detail in the organization's publications and casettes.

George Hall

Psychosynthesis

Stages in Psychosynthesis

In the overall process of psychosynthesis, we can distinguish two stages – personal and transpersonal psychosynthesis. In personal psychosynthesis, the integration of the personality takes place around the personal self, and the individual attains a level of functioning in terms of his work and his relationships that would be considered optimally healthy by current standards.

In the transpersonal stage of psychosynthesis, the person learns also to achieve alignment with, and to express the energies of, the Transpersonal Self, thus manifesting such qualities as a broad sense of responsibility, a spirit of cooperation, altruistic love, a global perspective, and transpersonal purpose.

Often the two stages overlap, and there can be a considerable amount of transpersonal activity even in the early phases of personal psychosynthesis.

Method Employed in Psychosynthesis

To be maximally effective in our own psychosynthesis or in helping others, we need to have at our disposal a broad range of methods. As each person is a unique individual, it is important to choose, out of the range of methods available, the ones that are best suited to each person's existential situation, psychological type, specific goals, desires and path of development. A few of the techniques commonly used are guided imagery, self-identification, meditation, development of the will, symbolic art work, journal-keeping, ideal models and development of the intuition, though a complete list would be much longer. The emphasis is not on the techniques, but on fostering an ongoing process of growth that can gain increasing momentum.

The Will

As this process goes forward, it entails developing one's personal will – the will of the personal self. Through this development, we acquire the ability to regulate and direct our many personality functions. We gain the freedom of choice, the power of decision over our actions, and become increasingly able to follow a path in accordance with what is best within each of us.

And as we reach toward the Transpersonal Self, we liberate more and more the synthesizing energies that organize and integrate our personality. We can make increasing contact with the will of our Transpersonal Self, which provides ever clearer meaning and purpose in our lives. We become able to function in the world more serenely and effectively, and to relate to our fellows in a spirit of cooperation and good will.

Synthesis and the Psyche

Psychosynthesis, in its fundamental nature, is synthesis of and through the psyche. Here psyche is understood to be not only the human personality, as usually implied by conventional psychology, but much more inclusively, the Psyche or Soul of the ancient Greek philosophers: the Higher Self. Therefore *psycho*synthesis is that form of synthesis which expresses the will of the Higher Self, and is achieved through wisdom and love – the two fundamental qualities of the consciousness of the Higher Self.

In its broadest sense, psychosynthesis is a point of view and an attitude, from which to act with wisdom and love. As such it is well suited to psychology, education and medicine, and also to religion, the social sciences, philosophy, and all other aspects of society in which *the consciousness of the individual human being* plays a role.

Psychosynthesis Institute, London

Auto-suggestion

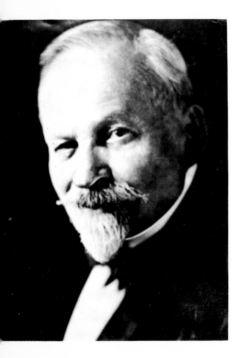

Emile Coué (1857–1926)

Auto-suggestion is a self-administered suggestion meant to bring about either a psychological or physical change without any subsequent conscious effort and involvement. More frequently the reference is to a psychotherapeutic system developed by the Frenchman Emile Coué (1857–1926) – *Couéism*. Coué believing that by the skilful application of auto-suggestion, the majority of patients seeking to overcome their presenting symptoms, and he put the success-rate as high as 97 percent, would benefit.

Immediately following World War I, 'Couéism' was at the height of its popularity, and was heralded by many as a psycho-physical methodology that bordered upon being a panacea. Its reputation was occasioned by three basic factors. The first of these was the profound effect the work of the French philosopher, René Descartes (1596–1650) had upon Western thought, because it was Descartes who postulated that man could be and should be the "master of himself". This was summed up in his dictum, "I think, therefore I am" – *Cogito, ergo sum* – which has been interpreted over the centuries to mean that through applying logical thought to any problem it could be resolved without external assistance. A present-day legacy of this Cartesian philosophy can still be heard when people suffering from psychoneuroses are told: "All you have to do is adopt a more positive mental attitude instead of your present negative one" or "Pull yourself together". To the millions who accepted this concept in relation to emotional disorders, and saw their symptoms as a sign of *weakness* and themselves as *weaklings* because they could not master how they felt, Couéism seemed to be the most acceptable answer, for auto-suggestion was presented "as an instrument for self-mastery".

The second factor in its wide acceptance was that it not only offered a means of self-help to those suffering from psychological disorders, but also showed a way to bring about organic changes and the remission of various physical illnesses that had hitherto failed to respond to orthodox medical treatment.

Finally, it appeared to be so simple and did not involve the person wishing to use it in any arduous regimen. All that many thought they had to do was to follow the instructions Coué gave to his patients at his clinic in Nancy, France; that each night, immediately before going to sleep, and each morning upon waking, they were to repeat to themselves, silently, 15 to 20 times, the suggestion: "Each day, and in every way, I am getting better and better". And it was the apparent simplicity which more than anything else led to Couéism falling into disrepute, as those using it in that simplistic manner disregarded what Coué personally did with each patient, and sometimes more than once, before instructing them to repeat the night and morning suggestion pattern.

In order to understand auto-suggestion as a therapeutic system it is necessary to trace its development. During the years 1885–86, Coué followed the work and experiments undertaken by one of the founders of modern hypnosis, Dr A. A. Liebault, who founded what has become known as the 'Nancy School' of hypnosis, and it was Liebault who stated that the success of hypnosis was entirely due to suggestion. Earlier, Alexandre Bertrand in his books published in Paris in 1823 and 1826 had asserted that the hypnotic state and the effects resulting from hypnosis were brought about through the patient's own imagination acting upon him or herself. Aware of these views, it seemed logical to Coué that if all hypnosis in the ultimate analysis was 'auto-hypnosis', and that all results of hypnotherapy stemmed from a patient accepting a suggestion, then it must be possible to devise a method which dispensed with the hypnotist. The idea of obtaining the benefits of hypnosis without a hypnotist being involved was popular, for many people then as now saw a hypnotist as being a form of Superman endowed with the unique gift of being able to take over the mind and thought-processes of lesser mortals, and naturally had a fear of being hypnotized.

Although Coué discarded the use of the word 'hypnotism', the method he used with every patient he saw, and it is estimated he was seeing 40,000 per year prior to World War I, was hypnotic.

Each patient was initially put through a series of hypnotic suggestibility tests to ensure they were amenable to suggestion, and only when each experiment, as Coué preferred to call them, had been successfully completed did they become "ripe for curative suggestions". Then, with a patient in an altered state of consciousness, identical to hypnosis, he would instruct the patient to close his eyes and suggest that every word he said from that moment onwards would be permanently engraved upon the patient's mind. He would then proceed to give a series of suggestions meant to promote psychological and physical well-being.

Writing about his work, Coué explained it was necessary for the suggestions he gave to each patient to be repeated periodically until there was a marked improvement in the condition, after which the length of time between the sessions with him could be extended and finally discontinued.

He also instructed the patient that the time spent with him was not sufficient; that they too had an important part to play in their own return to good health by repeating each night and morning, while in bed: "Each day, and in every way, I am getting better and better".

To deny that auto-suggestion can be helpful in helping some people would be fallacious, but to ignore the fact that, even with auto-suggestion, external help is frequently necessary to assist in its application can lead to failure and despondency. Moreover, it has to be recognized that if a person has unresolved conflicts existing below the level of consciousness, then hours of daily auto-suggestion will not ameliorate the condition, but rather activate the psychological law Coué is credited with discovering, the 'Law of Reversed Effect', which means the more one tries, the harder the goal becomes to achieve!   *Peter Blythe*

Auto-suggestion

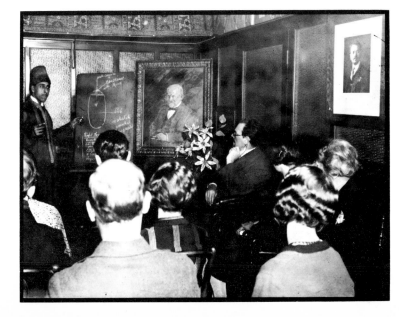

Sirdar Ikbal Ali Shah, brother of the King of Afghanistan, lecturing on Mind Healing and Auto-suggestion at the Coué Institute in London in the 1920s.

Hypnosis

Hypnosis is most accurately defined as being an altered state of consciousness usually combined with physical relaxation which a person allows themselves to enter. In this consent state of hypnosis, the critical factor of the mind – the left cerebral hemisphere of the brain – is by-passed to a greater or lesser degree, thereby allowing suggestions to be accepted uncritically and subsequently acted upon, or alternatively permitting repressed (forgotten) memories to be recalled into consciousness.

Although the origins of hypnosis are lost in antiquity, mention of it being recorded in ancient Egypt and Greece, the title of 'Father of Hypnosis' truly belongs to a Scottish physician, Dr James Braid, MRCS (1795–1860) who practised in Manchester, England. After Dr Braid saw a demonstration of 'animal magnetism' in Manchester on November 13, 1841, conducted by a Swiss mesmerist, Charles Lafontaine, he commenced a series of experiments which led him to reject the theories of Dr Franz Anton Mesmer (1733–1815) and the practice of 'animal magnetism', and to form new concepts and new techniques.

In 1842, Dr Braid offered to read a paper on his findings to the Medical Section of the British Association which was holding its annual conference in Manchester that year. The paper was refused.

The following year, 1843, his book, *Neurypnology; or the Rationale of Nervous Sleep*, was published in which he postulated that the combined state of physical relaxation and altered conscious awareness entered into by patients should be called *Hypnotism;* the derivation of the word being the Greek word *hypnos* meaning sleep.

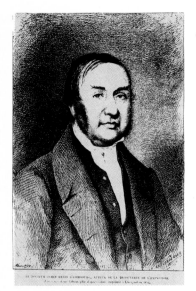

Dr James Braid, founder of medical hypnosis.

Despite interesting work undertaken in the United Kingdom, the United States of America, and Europe, the mainstream of orthodox medicine continued to regard it with open scepticism. Accordingly, in 1891 the British Medical Association (BMA) appointed a committee "to investigate the nature of the phenomena of hypnotism, its value as a therapeutic agent, and the propriety of using it". Two years later, the committee's unanimous report, which contained the paragraph, "The Committee are of the opinion that as a therapeutic agent hypnotism is frequently effective in relieving pain, procuring sleep, and alleviating many functional ailments . . .", was accepted by the BMA, but the majority of medical practitioners still rejected it as unscientific 'fringe medicine'.

A small number of medical practitioners and laymen continued to use hypnosis to alleviate 'dis-ease', and in the 1950s a sub-committee of the British Medical Association conducted a further investigation into its usefulness. Some sixty-two years after the earlier report, in 1955, the new report was published and, like its predecessor, approved the use of hypnosis for the treatment of psycho-neuroses and for the relief of pain. It also recommended that all doctors and medical students should receive adequate training in its application. These recommendations have largely been ignored!

The British Society for Medical and Dental Hypnosis conducts three separate weekends of training for members of the medical and dental professions and has approximately 1,000 members, although it is admitted that additional doctors and dentists are using hypnosis without being members of the British Society.

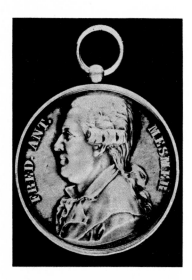

Medallion portrait of Dr Franz Anton Mesmer, practitioner of animal magnetism.

In the United States of America, in 1958, the American Medical Association (AMA) issued an equally favourable report with the recommendation that training in the use of hypnosis be given to all medical students. Three years afterwards, the AMA issued another favourable report which called for 144 hours of post-graduate and graduate training in hypnosis. As in Britain, little has been done to implement either AMA report, and although the American Society for Clinical and Experimental Hypnosis has the largest society member-

Hypnosis

ship in the world, it is small when compared to the number of doctors, dentists, and clinical psychologists practising in the USA.

Currently, members of the medical profession appear to be divided into three categories:

1. Those who consider it to be 'mumbo-jumbo' with no place in medical practice, and who do not wish to consider any of the evidence which is contrary to their own pre-judgement.

2. Nearly as large a number who cautiously admit that hypnosis might be helpful in certain cases, but they have little or no knowledge of the subject and do not use it themselves.

3. A small vocal minority who advocate its usage and practise it.

What has led many doctors to reject hypnosis has best been summed up by one of the world's leading authorities on the subject, Dr William S. Kroger, MD, in his book *Clinical and Experimental Hypnosis*, where he has written: ''However, it is true that hypnosis has been hurt more by the extravagant claims of its ardent proponents than by its opponents''.

The most extravagant claim for hypnosis has been implied rather than boldly stated, and that has been the strong suggestion that it borders upon being a panacea, a wonder, one-session cure-all. It is far from being that. A therapeutic session may well require one hour, and many one-hour sessions may be necessary before the presenting symptom or syndrome remisses. General medical practitioners simply have not got this amount of time to devote to many of their patients who may benefit from hypnosis, even if they had previously received adequate training.

On the other side of the coin, hypnosis is still regarded by a large section of the general public more with fear than scepticism, and these fears, engendered for the most part by the old-time stage hypnotists – banned in the United Kingdom by Act of Parliament in 1952 – can be subsumed under four headings:

1. The fear of being unconscious – asleep – while in hypnosis, and not aware afterwards what they had done during the session.

2. Fear of loss of verbal control while in hypnosis and revealing secrets.

3. Having their mind taken over and dominated by another human being.

4. Not returning to a normal state at the end of a hypnotic session.

The facts about hypnosis are that no one can be hypnotized against their will; it is a consent state rather than a subjective one, and while in hypnosis the patient/subject is aware of what is happening at all times; hence no one will talk while in hypnosis unless they wish to do so. Finally, as it is only an altered state of consciousness, there is no danger of a patient/subject remaining in hypnosis like a latter-day 'Sleeping Beauty' waiting for a hypnotic 'Prince' to give them the kiss of life.

As more and more people are becoming concerned about internal pollution through the over-use of pharmaceutical drugs, and iatrogenic illnesses (illnesses caused by drugs), the demand for hypnosis has increased. Hypnosis can be extremely useful in the treatment of certain psycho-neurotic conditions; helping people to overcome learned, behavioural patterns; and in childbirth, etc., but it will not be suitable for everyone and is only as good as the practitioner. Keeping in mind that the majority of practitioners in the fields of both orthodox and heterodox medicine have not received adequate training either in the application of hypnosis or the psycho-dynamic factors possibly underlying a presenting symptom, it therefore still has to be treated circumspectly.

Peter Blythe

Autogenic Training

Autogenic training is a technique of medical therapy designed to exert a normalizing influence upon mental and bodily functions. The method was founded some forty years ago by a Berlin neurologist and psychiatrist, J. H. Schulz, who based his original research on the earlier work of the renowned brain physiologist Oskar Vogt. During the years 1890 to 1900, Vogt had observed that some of his patients, having undergone a series of hypnotic sessions with his guidance, were able to put themselves voluntarily into a state similar to the hypnotic state. The patients subsequently reported that these 'auto-hypnotic' exercises had considerable recuperative effects. Stress problems like fatigue and tension could be avoided by this method and his patients felt that their overall efficiency had been improved.

By the late 1920s, Schulz had evolved the six standard psycho-physiological exercises of autogenic training which he called the autogenic standard series. These exercises involve a series of verbal formulae upon which subjects passively concentrate, while lying with their eyes closed in a quiet room. Each exercise is practised several times a day until the subject is able to voluntarily shift from a high arousal state to a wakeful low arousal state.

After the standard exercises have been successfully mastered, (which can take several months), other procedures can be taught to deal with a number of functional and organic disorders such as bronchial asthma, writer's cramp, brain injuries and so on.

Another important type of autogenic training which can be practised after the standard exercises have been learned, is meditative training. This begins with passive concentration on a number of visual phenomena and proceeds to a personal interrogatory exercise which leads to deep personal insights. As well as reinforcing earlier physiological training, this method brings with it all the benefits that can be gained from long practise of other kinds of meditation.

Exercise 1 focuses on a feeling of heaviness in the limbs.
Exercise 2 focuses on the cultivation of warmth in the limbs.
Exercise 3 deals with cardiac regulation.
Exercise 4 consists of passive concentration on breathing.
Exercise 5 cultivates the sensation of warmth in the upper abdomen.
Exercise 6 is the cultivation of feelings of coolness in the forehead.

Neuro-physiological

Neuro-physiological psychology is the study of the relationship between the brain, the body, behaviour and emotions; an attempt to see the individual holistically rather than as a collection of separate functions. It is the name given to the research work and remedial programmes undertaken by Peter Blythe and David McGlown at the Institute for Neuro-Physiological Psychology, Chester, England.

Neuro-Psychologists try to isolate those areas of the brain which are involved in certain modes of behaviour, i.e. anxiety-neuroses, depression, phobic states, problem solving, etc., in the hope that when the brain mechanisms are understood this will provide a key to understanding exactly why certain people react or over-react to what would be normally non-noxious situations.

The term Neuro-Physiological Psychology as used by Blythe-McGlown refers to their discovery that for many patients suffering from psychoneuroses there is an organic basis which makes them more prone to emotional, stress disorders. This they have called Organic Brain Dysfunction (OBD). Since OBD – a cluster of small physical difficulties resulting from poor neurological organization – remains undetected and uncorrected by psychiatrists and clinical psychologists this, according to Blythe-McGlown, accounts for the number of people who appear to be resistant to the recommended therapy of choice, be that drug therapy, psychotherapy, behaviour therapy or hypnotherapy. Blythe-McGlown assert that OBD is also the cause of many intellectually 'bright' children having educational problems, but they maintain that once it has been diagnosed both children and adults can be given a remediation programme, based upon 'Reflexive Developmental Patterning', which will restore neurological organization and thereby permit a resolution of their problems to occur.

Biofeedback

The usual attitude to illness is that medical intervention is required to reverse this state, whereas the alternative therapies believe that the body is capable of curing itself, with a little encouragement. Both ways have their validity at the appropriate time, though one should add a third requirement; that we actively cooperate with our body in order to stay healthy.

The biofeedback principle is this: if one can learn to be aware of some body function of which one is not normally aware, then one can learn to control that function. The principle is in essence very simple, but it does demand that the subject shows a respect for himself. The bathroom scales are an example of a feedback device, which requires that one responds to the indication. The bathroom scales cannot cure overweight; they only indicate the success or otherwise of one's efforts to do so. It may be that success will not be achieved unless one considers all the possible reasons for the overeating. Alternatively, the original effort may be reinforced by positive feedback from one's friends about the new slim look, thus helping the change to become permanent.

If it is understood that the biofeedback principle requires more than just simply responding to the readings on an instrument, then we can begin to appreciate why there have been so many conflicting reports from America about the efficacy of the technique.

Biofeedback techniques were pioneered in the 1960s by Dr Joe Kamiya in San Francisco, whose original experiments were concerned with brain activity. The brain is known to generate electrical rhythms which can be detected using an electroencepalograph (EEG) machine. These rhythms occur in four principal groups, each of which can be approximately correlated with a particular brain activity or state of awareness: *beta* waves which have a frequency of 13–30 Hz. (Hz. is the symbol for frequency measured in cycles per second) and are the normal waking rhythm of the brain, though the inference of beta is alarm, a very relaxed person will show very little beta; *alpha* waves (8–13 Hz.) have very little meaning on their own, but in conjunction with other rhythms, seem to be the building block for all the higher levels of awareness. In conjunction with theta, they indicate a calming down or emptying of the mind, usually with physical relaxation; *theta* waves (4 to 7 Hz.) which occur during creative inspiration and meditation; *delta* waves ($\frac{1}{2}$–4 Hz.), the rhythm of sleep, but found in many people in response to new ideas. They are also found in healers and those with paranormal abilities.

Kamiya began his work by monitoring a subject's alpha rhythms with an EEG device. When alpha rhythms were being generated by the subject, a pleasant sound would be produced which would no longer be heard when the alpha fell below a certain level. In this way, Kamiya found that most subjects could learn to 'turn on' or suppress alpha rhythms and that the alpha seemed to be related to a feeling of well-being. Recent studies have shown though, that production of alpha waves in the laboratory does not necessarily help the subject in any way; the alpha wave can only be related to new understanding if there is something new to understand. Again, the biofeedback difficulty manifests itself. If we can aid a subject to achieve a new insight, perhaps by a Sufi teaching story, then he may show high levels of alpha. The phenomenon is not reversable; training the subject to produce alpha by means of biofeedback will not produce new insights.

In the few years which have elapsed since these first experiments, research has blossomed and biofeedback is finding increasing applications in many hospitals, particularly in the USA, to supplement or replace other forms of treatment. It has been used effectively to teach subjects to control abnormal heart rhythms; to indicate stomach

Biofeedback

acidity in the cure of ulcers; to control migraine and tension head-aches; to aid epileptics; for Reynaud's disease; to help in the retraining of muscles; plus assistance in a wide range of nervous diseases.

Sometimes though, the results may have depended as much on the excellence of the therapist as on the biofeedback technique. Dr Kenneth Pelletier of the Langley Porter Institute in the USA had a patient who successfully cured her migraine headaches with an incorrect biofeedback signal. In error, she had been given feedback of the beta signal which one would have supposed would have increased tension. Though this result seemed contradictory, Dr Pelletier had come to have great respect for the wisdom of the body, just as yogis have had for thousands of years. He felt that this particular patient gave herself, as he put it ''time to sit down, to become sensitive to what her personal dynamic was vis-à-vis her migraine . . . and she gave her body the time to have the wisdom to cure itself''.

It is this 'wisdom of the body' which we believe is the important factor in any therapy. If we can ally this 'wisdom of the body' to biofeedback instrumentation, we have perhaps one of the most powerful techniques ever invented towards self-realization.

Measuring Electrical Skin Resistance

Let us now examine one of the very simple but most effective tools – the electrical skin resistance meter (ESR) which indicates physical arousal and relaxation. Connected to the palm of the hand, this electrical measurement is possible because the meter readings are related directly to the behaviour of the autonomic system. The rate of blood flow varies with the body tone and this causes changes of polarization of the sweat gland membranes. The changes of meter readings are not caused by the apparent wetness or dryness of the hands – except when the hands are very cold and dry – but by this polarization which varies according to how tense or relaxed we are. The reactions which make us tense or relaxed are reflected in the 'fight or flight' response and its mirror image, the relaxation response – the responses from the sympathetic and parasympathetic branches of the autonomic nervous system.

The first table illustrated shows the body changes which occur. From this one can see that 'fight or flight' response is inappropriate when talking to the bank manager, since usually one can do neither. If we stay in such a state habitually, then we will suffer high blood pressure, causing strain on the heart; unused cortisone is not easily readsorbed and reduces the body immune response to disease; partially closed down digestive systems lead to ulcers and continuously tensed surface muscles lead to fibrositis.

Our ability to cope with stress depends on whether these responses are free ranging so that we can react appropriately to a situation, or whether we let one situation build up on top of another, so that by the end of the day we are totally unable to relax. The relaxation response is the very opposite of stress and can be learned through the biofeedback principle of monitoring these inner changes – learning how to relax by invoking the parasympathetic system and helping it to work as it should.

The effect of ESR biofeedback training is to normalize the readings. Under-aroused people become more alert and active; those who are over-aroused become more calm and relaxed, while the normal person can increase his range both up and down.

BODY CHANGES

EFFECT OF STRESS	BODY FUNCTION	EFFECT OF RELAXATION
up	HEART RATE	down
up	BLOOD FLOW TO MUSCLE	down
down	BLOOD FLOW TO SKIN	up
down	BLOOD FLOW TO ORGANS	up
up	OXYGEN USAGE	down
up	CORTISONE OUTPUT	down
down	FOOD & ENERGY RESERVES	up
up	BLOOD PRESSURE	down
up	MUSCLE TENSION	down
RESULT Action		RESULT Proper Function of Organs

1. These are general changes. They can be localized to one organ or system.
2. Prolonged "Stress" leads to permanent changes and may lead to disease.
3. Immune Mechanisms and Antibodies are also affected by stress because of the raised Cortisone output.

The effects of stress and relaxation on body functions.

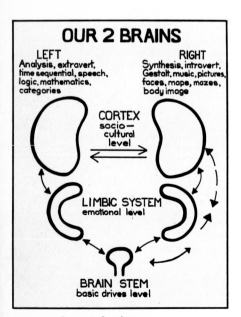

OUR 2 BRAINS

LEFT
Analysis, extravert, time sequential, speech, logic, mathematics, categories

RIGHT
Synthesis, introvert, Gestalt, music, pictures, faces, maps, mazes, body image

CORTEX
socio—cultural level

LIMBIC SYSTEM
emotional level

BRAIN STEM
basic drives level

Our two brains.

EEG Brain Rhythms

Having measured physical arousal with the electrical skin resistance meter, we can now look at mental arousal and relaxation as reflected by the electrical rhythms of the brain. (*See* the Two Correlate Graph.)

Hopefully, the two measurements will relate to each other, in that beta rhythms and a low skin resistance will accompany panic states, while in a relaxed state alpha rhythms and a higher electrical skin resistance will be seen. However, we do not need to respond in this way; it is no use being physically aroused when talking to the bank manager though it is advisable to be very alert mentally.

This separation of the physical and mental states is the desired end of relaxation and Zen training.

To understand this better, we now have to ask the reader to use his brain to consider how that brain functions. Throughout history, man has always been aware of two different ways of knowing; some situations or objects are best understood by detailed analysis, while we shall find out nothing about the 'flowerness' of a flower by pulling off its petals.

There is the way of the scientist and the way of the mystic and yet these ways are not so sharply divided as it would sometimes seem. Our physicists at the frontiers of particle research are apt to make strangely mystical statements, while you can find no one more empirically scientific than a yogi following very complex meditative exercises to produce a desired end result.

The two halves of our brain operate in different modes, though without any precise division of function. It is nevertheless convenient to label as 'left' brain such operations as analysis, logic and speech; and as 'right' brain modes such as artistic appreciation, recognizing faces and holistic ways of understanding. The 'left' brain is outgoing and sympathetic nervous system dominant while the 'right' brain is inward looking and related to the parasympathetic system.

Biofeedback

Two Correlate Graph showing physical arousal and relaxation vertically and mental states horizontally. When the different states are matched, four quite different possible states of consciousness become apparent:
1. Tense body-tense mind. Low ESR-beta EEG = panic states.
2. Relaxed body-relaxed mind. High ESR-alpha, theta brain rhythms = meditation.
3. Aroused body-relaxed mind = mediumistic trance.
4. Relaxed body-aroused mind. High ESR-alpha, beta and theta brain rhythms = Zen meditation.

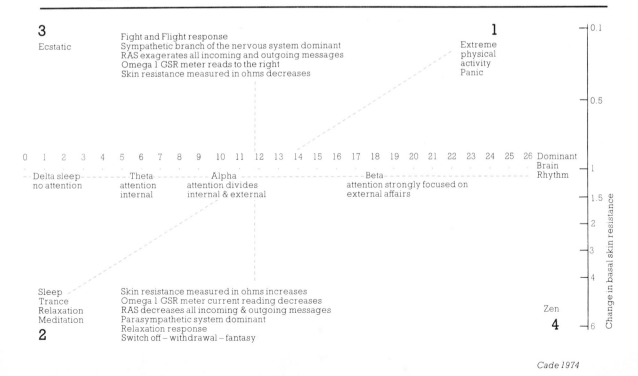

Cade 1974

Biofeedback

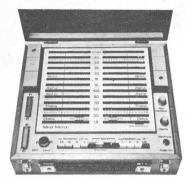

The Mind Mirror is a special type of encephalograph which shows, by means of twelve rows of light-emitting diodes, a frequency analysis of subjects' brain rhythms from both sides of the brain, as they are actually happening. The Mind Mirror differs from standard hospital encephalographs because the latter show the pathological responses of the brain as well as the brain's response to mood, thought and so on. For medical purposes, the reflection of mood and thought is considered a nuisance since it interferes with the readings for pathological responses. For biofeedback purposes, however, such knowledge is an essential guide to the subject's development on the path to self-regulation.

Research with the Mind Mirror has shown that different levels of human consciousness are characterized by certain combinations of alpha, beta, theta and delta brain rhythms. The chart shows these patterns as they appear on the Mind Mirror when subjects' are in these states. Levels four and five are basically states in which the level of consciousness associated with meditation is carried into daily life. By the time this is fully realized (state five) subjects will have achieved the state that Cade calls 'the awakened mind'.

The diagram 'Our 2 Brains' shows the links between the various levels of the brain. Note especially the link from the right brain to the brain stem which contains the reticular activating system (RAS). We shall return to this very important function later. The 'left' half of the brain tends to be dominant since it is concerned with survival, but this is especially true during this period of man's development of technology. Hopefully this same technology, through biofeedback types of technique, will now help to reverse this imbalance, by showing for example how meditation aids the integration of the hemispheres.

There is an instrument, the first of its kind in the world, the Audio Ltd., Mind Mirror, which measures the rhythms from each side of the brain and displays a frequency analysis of them in a form which allows relationships between them to be seen as a pattern – a 'right' and 'left' brain instrument. With such an EEG as the Mind Mirror, one can easily monitor the patterns of different meditations, or indicate to a subject the changes which may occur in the rhythms as a result of exercises designed to aid brain integration.

These exercises can be chosen to produce an increase in the alpha wave and this leads one to speculate on the purpose and importance of such waves. Nature seems rarely to produce such phenomena without a purpose; in this case one could surmise that the alpha waves help to synchronize various centres in the brain, levels of awareness on the point of becoming manifest from various constellations of neurons, so that a more complete experience is realized. It has often been stated that we only use ten per cent of our brain, sufficient for day-to-day living.

If, though, we try to imagine what it might mean to use more of the brain, then this must mean a more complete, in-depth and greater appreciation of both the detail and the whole. The guess is then, that the brain rhythms are perhaps like the clock frequency which would be required for a computer which was both analogue and digital, if such a device could be imagined.

Electrical Brain Rhythms of Different Levels of Consciousness

LEVEL		MIND MIRROR PATTERNS
8	Cosmic Consciousness	?
7	Psychedelia - Gowan Illumination - Bucke Self-remembering - Gurdjieff	?
6	Active Creativity	
5	Fifth State - Goleman Afterglow - Maharishi Illumination - Fromm Lucid Awareness - Cade	β α θ δ
4	Fourth State - Wallace Meditation - Traditional	α θ δ
3	Waking Waking Sleep - Gurdjieff	β
2	Hypnagogic State	α
1	Dreaming Sleep	θ
0	Deep Sleep	δ

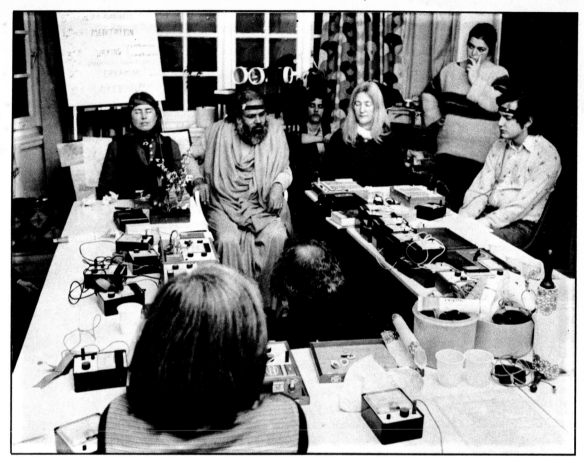

Returning to the illustration 'Our 2 Brains', showing the connection of the right hemisphere to the reticular activating system in the brain stem; Carl Jung called the properties inherent in this control system the 'transcendent function'. It is at this level that we can mediate how we shall use the higher cortex. The RAS is like the starter motor of a car, except that it also controls the level of consciousness; this is the area of the brain where damage can lead to a permanent coma.

Biofeedback training with ESR and EEG develops at this level of the brain the ability to hold a more constant level of awareness, so that the cortex is not driven towards hysteria at the slightest provocation or alternatively lapsing into a bored state when there is no input.

There are many biofeedback techniques, such as feedback of muscle tone to aid reduction of tension; exercises in temperature control of hands and forehead by visualization leading to a reduction of migraine attacks; use of heart rhythm to show arousal, and many others. It was thought that by concentrating on just two ESR and EEG it would be possible to justify, even in a short article, the claim that "if we ally the wisdom of the body to biofeedback instrumentation, then we have indeed a very powerful technique towards self-realization". In case the purist should think that it is being suggested that meditation can be mechanized, please understand that the claim is only that biofeedback instruments can help to clear the path.

However, if we can learn to drop the barriers towards full development, then one of the side effects is that we shall be healthy, since we will have let go those attitudes which lead to the psychosomatic and stress related diseases.

Geoffrey Blundell

Investigating the effects of a Divine Love meditation which is being lead by Swami Prakashanand Saraswati. The experiment was conducted by C. Maxwell Cade.

Meditation

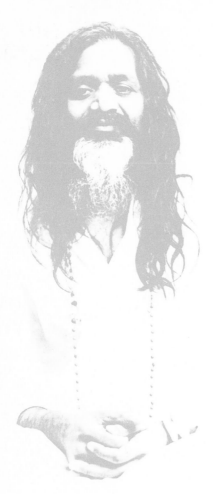

Maharishi Mahesh Yogi, the originator of the mantra meditational method called transcendental meditation, popularly known as TM. Of all the meditation systems, TM has been the most successful in the West and today claims millions of adherents.

It is very much easier to say what meditation is not than to say what it is.

Meditation is not relaxation, though it cannot happen when one is tense. In 1971, Benson and Wallace showed that Maharishi's Transcendental Meditation produced many measurable physiological effects, mental and physical relaxation, slowing of the breath, reduced oxygen consumption etc. A carefully chosen mantra is given to the TM initiate, but Benson later claimed that the word 'bananas' would have been equally effective as a mantra. Certainly, Benson was correct if one considers meditation to be only 'the relaxation response'. Such a relaxed person will be far less likely to suffer from today's hypertension complaints, but this is not meditation.

Most people keep their cars in a better state than they keep their mind. Samsara is the Sanskrit word which means going round and round in circle. We repeat the same mistakes over and over again until we hardly notice the frustration. We want to slim, give up smoking, move out of the city or whatever. The past is memories of family squabbles, business politics and opportunities missed. The future is winning the pools. The present is frantically filled with mundane activities, rather than in the quietness come face to face with our inner self. The 'flight into reality' is how some psychiatrists describe it. We can all recognize ourselves somewhere in this picture as we try to clear the muddy waters of our mind by stirring more and more.

One cannot see into the depths of the lake unless the surface of the water is still and calm.
When the surface of the water begins to clear, then many qualities will be awakened in the meditator. Daniel Goleman in *Meditation as Meta-therapy: a hypothesis towards a Fifth state of Consciousness* claims that:

1. Meditators should have less discrepancy between the real self and the ideal self.

2. Performance in learning and perceptual tasks will be improved.

3. Wallace has called meditation a Fourth state of Consciousness (1–sleep, 2–dreaming, 3–waking). Goleman suggests that in the meditator all these levels may permeate the waking level – this being a Fifth major state of consciousness.

4. People in the Fifth state will function on the level of Meta-needs not pathology, creativity rather than negativity.

Meditation is not restlessness, difficulties, visions, levitation or any psychic phenomena.
Meditation begins with relaxation, but it is possible to relax the body and mind out of step with each other into a condition called 'fixed parasympathetic tone'. The novice finds himself shivering, perhaps unable to move. In olden times this state would have probably been called possession. The remedy is to walk the person around the room until he is fully restored. This is one reason why it is considered advisable to choose a guide or teacher, rather than begin meditating alone. The novice may also experience lights and sounds or telepathic phenomena. In older traditions these events are known as the *siddhis* and are thought of as psychic traps on the road to full development. There is a story about a Japanese monk who one day, while meditating in his cell, saw the heavens open with the Buddha in all his splendour seated on a celestial throne. As soon as possible he had an appointment with the Abbot who listened patiently. "Don't worry" he said, "concentrate on your breathing, it should go away".

Meditation

The meditative mind is a silent mind.

Let us listen for a moment to Krishnamurti's attempts to go beyond the words. Firstly, there is silence, a silence that goes beyond belief and dogma. Meditation is only possible out of a silence in which evaluation and moral values have come to an end. It is not the way of thought, for the invitation can only be given in a still mind. It is not an escape from the world but rather the quality of mind and heart that no longer needs to judge, so that action may begin which is not the outcome of tension, contradiction and search for power. The mind can never become innocent through experience. It is rather the scars of experience which prevent the flowering of meditation. Wander by the seashore and allow the stillness to enter and if it does, do not pursue it, because what you pursue can only be the memory of what was – this is the death of what is. To the meditative mind, division ceases in a state of love.

The mind freeing itself from the known is meditation.

Bhagwan Shree Rajneesh defines meditation as an effort to jump into the subconscious. You cannot jump by calculation because all calculation is of the conscious and the conscious mind will caution 'don't do it, you will go mad'. The problem cannot be solved by facing it rationally and saying 'I shall not allow thinking'. This is the dilemma to which every seeker comes; that one cannot meditate without planning it and thinking about it closes the door. A device is therefore needed to allow the mind to flow around this difficulty. The device may be concentration on the breathing, or the use of a mantra or it may be the attention on the inner sounds as in Surat Shabd Yoga. None of these devices will guarantee on their own that meditation can happen; for some people the grace which flows from a Master is a necessary initiation.

Meditation is not a technique.

There is story of a seeker who had been around all the different groups. He came to yet another – the Master listened to him for a while, then picked up a glass phial containing layers of coloured sand. "Shake the phial" the master requested. The seeker did so and a dirty grey colour resulted. "This is the effect on you of all those teachings" the master said. "Each of them in their own way is pure, but look what has happened to them inside you".

"You must remember to love Godhead more than you love meditation."

These are the words of Swami Prakashanand Saraswati. Let us listen to a few words from his followers about their experiences in his presence during a meditation. "I felt a softening in the heart that I had not experienced before". "I felt some spiritual energy coming from the outside and entering my heart". "There were tears in my eyes, then a very happy feeling". "When Swami-ji touched my head, I lost the feeling of my body and became part of the chanting". "I became contentlessly aware – just aware of being aware, then aware only of brilliantly pure white light".

Geoffrey Blundell

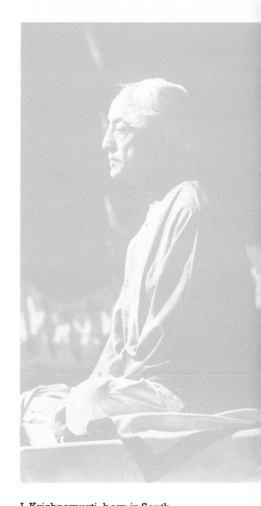

J. Krishnamurti, born in South India in 1896, was originally groomed as the new World Teacher by the Theosophist, Annie Besant. In 1929 he disbanded the organization surrounding him, declaring that he did not want disciples. Throughout his life, Krishnamurti has been opposed to any formal meditation system.

Arica

HUMANITY IS ONE SPIRIT

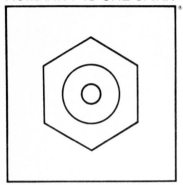

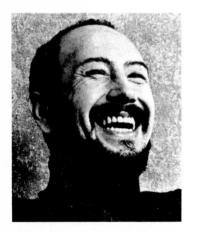

Oscar Ichazo, founder of Arica.

Arica is a contemporary pragmatic system of philosophy central to which is an intensive practical training course. The goal of Arica is unity within the individual, between individuals and in society. The Arican concept of unity is identical to that expressed throughout mystical tradition.

The founder of Arica is Oscar Ichazo, who was born in Bolivia in 1931. In 1964, after many years of studying and experiencing the enlightenment techniques contained within the traditions of esoteric schools in the Far East and South America, Ichazo finally formulated the method that is now known as the Arica System. In 1968 he founded the Instituto de Gnoseologia in Arica, Chile where he developed and taught the system. In 1970 a group of fifty Americans joined him in Arica to take a ten-month intensive training course. The forty-four who completed the course decided to go with Ichazo to New York to found the Arica Institute so that the method could be taught to a wider public. The purpose of founding Arica, according to Ichazo, was out of a ''need to understand that if there is going to be unity among human beings, it will occur because we have achieved that unity by means of reason, by means of science, and not by means of good will. Although good will is a strong and positive quality, it is not enough, as human history has proved ad nauseam. We must agree about our spiritual reality, and about what our psyche is. This agreement is what we need for producing understanding''.*

Both the Arica philosophy and its training methods are the result of a synthesis of Eastern esoteric traditions and mind/body disciplines, and aspects and techniques of Western psychology. Despite the spiritual emphasis in its teachings, the Arica philosophy does not require faith and the system is in fact described as 'scientific mysticism': ''The Arica Theory is the explanation of the *Unity* by the discovery of a new logic that describes the *process and the Unity of the Whole*. With this, we have the tool for systematizing the description of all the human psyche. Since we know the entire territory, and since we have the correct maps and measurements, we can approach the human process with complete knowledge of all the parameters and the possible variables. With this knowledge the *human process* is understood for the first time completely and scientifically, and is scientifically systematized and delineated''.*

The process of training in Arica is viewed as the communication of technical information. The function of the trainer in this respect is to impart information clearly, precisely and without personal interpretation; the responsibility of the trainee is to participate openly, alertly and with an attitude of curiosity. While some stages of the Arica System can be learned individually, considerable emphasis is placed on the fact that the process of learning can be rapidly accelerated in a group situation ''where people give and accept support readily, where the group is a reflector and monitor of each individual's progress''.

Only some five percent of the Arica training system is devoted to imparting the theory, the remaining time being spent in certain types of exercise and meditation, which are seen as giving support and experiential depth to the theory. Since an aim of Arica is mind/body balance, the training focuses from the outset on getting and keeping the body in good condition. Breathing and movement exercises, relaxation and a system called *Psychocalisthenics* are used to this end. Psychocalisthenics is a series of twenty-six breathing and movement exercises derived from several sources, including hatha yoga and pranayama breath control, which are designed to restore the human body to its natural elasticity, balance and strength. There are five stages of Psychocalisthenics: learning the movements, muscular conditioning, emotional conditioning, kinesthetic movement and 'breathing nine colours'. The entire series is designed to provide, in thirty minutes, enough exercise and vitality for the day.

There are nine levels of training in Arica, each one leading to a successively higher state of consciousness. Every level is seen as a further step on the path to developing and unifying the physical, emotional and intellectual aspects of the body; specific exercises and meditations support each level. For instance, a central feature of level one is the *Nine Ways of Zhikr* ritual, a one-hour group exercise done to specially composed music, rhythms, movements and song repetitions combined with precise breathing patterns. Zhikr is derived from the Sufi tradition and is seen as a way of achieving a state of liberated consciousness and ecstasy.

Part of the object of level two is the removal of both physical and psychic tensions "through a process of deep body work called *Chua K'a:* "When we liberate the tensions in our body, we also liberate psychic tensions, because every group of muscular cells is connected to our brain. This signifies that the tension that is at the extreme of a nerve ending has actually imprisoned its corresponding cerebral cell which no longer receives any messages. It is closed in a kind of biological anaesthesia. We do not want to use these muscles in certain ways because they cause us pain. Therefore we restrict these movements and start patterning more comfortable movements; as we do this, awareness, cleverness and the most valuable cerebral functions are lost."*

Level two is also devoted to 'Kath Generation' exercises and the 'Fire Exercise'. Kath is seen as the point of equilibrium in the human body and is situated at a point four finger-widths below the navel; kath energy is the vital energy of the body which this exercise helps to generate and circulate round the body. The Fire Exercise is a series of systematized movements of breathing and meditation combined with music and song repetitions.

Other training techniques used include, in level four, *Psycho-alchemy*, the study and practice of how the psyche transforms physical energy into psychic energy. 'Yantras', precise symbols expressed in form and colour, are also used in many different and specific meditations throughout the Arica System to recall the attention of the interior self. The use of a high-protein diet, low in fats and carbohydrates, is advocated particularly during trainings: to this end *Dragon's Milk*, a high energy food, rich in protein and natural unprocessed vitamins, has been developed by the Institute.

The training course for Arica is intensive, attainment of every level being accompanied by a permanent change in consciousness; "With each level of the Arica System we understand more deeply our life as a human process towards unity in ourselves and all humanity as one spirit".

The ultimate goal of Arica is the creation of a metasociety: "A human society starts becoming civilized when it discovers the *Unity*. But when that society discovers its internal unity because it sees we are equal, it is transformed into a metasociety. This is a different society, a society in perfect unity, a scientific unity where we all understand what our psyches are. With this we read one another more completely. A metasociety can go where voice is not necessary for communication. Such communication is deeper than words. We do not hear it with our ears: we hear inside our hearts. This cannot be expressed in words. Once our karma is completely cleaned, this state is natural within us".*

Peter Robinson

Arica

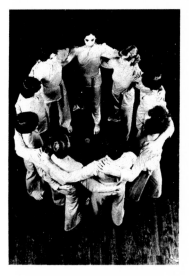

The Seventh Way of Zhikr. To Zhikr is to repeat the name of God. It is a classical method for achieving the state of liberated consciousness and ecstasy.

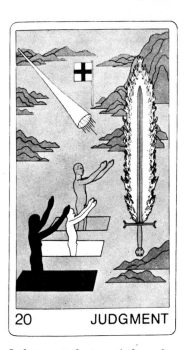

20　　　JUDGMENT

Judgement: the twentieth card of a set of twenty-two cards of the Major Arcana of the Arica Tarot, used in the *Game of Scarab* in level four.

Somatography

Somatography can be described as an auxiliary therapy and training in the field of natural and humanistic therapy. On the one hand it is useful in treating some of the psychosomatic conditions such as neck, shoulder and back pains, gastro intestinal disorders and various states of hypertension; on the other hand it can help educate people to become more aware of their body and how to start listening to the constant stream of informational signals that flow in and out of every part of our bodies; a knowledge of which can help us clarify our thoughts and feelings about ourselves, our situations in life and about our relationships with other people.

Somatography Training is currently available in London, New York and Frankfurt-am-Main, Germany. It appears to date that the work can be useful for both sexes and for persons of most ages.

The whole process originated out of a meeting in London in 1972 between two natural therapists – George C. King from New York City, USA and H. Bryn Jones from Wales. Bryn Jones had been involved for some years in working with the aura – the human aura – whilst George King, a Yoga Master, had built up a successful private practice in massage and physical therapy. Subsequently they jointly developed a framework, called Somatography, for searching into a combination of inner and outer body work – both on the physical musculature of the body and on the, as yet, little known about system of subtle energy that flows through the human body – the energy that acupuncturists call Chi or Ki, as well as the equally mysterious 'field' of energy which appears to envelop the outside of the body – this field is the subject of the techniques of Kirlian photography. The result of this decision is a constantly growing and developing structure which, with only a few years of life behind it, has as yet no systematic theoretical basis capable of withstanding public scrutiny but which is beginning to develop a solid background of information that will it is hoped, one day be synthesized into a cohesive and useful theoretical system or structure. Meanwhile we do have a number of useful and tried body working techniques which are being taught to other therapists and body-workers.

Persons coming for treatment are soon taught that the ultimate answer to their problem lies within themselves. Attention is focused on the need for them to increase (sometimes considerably so) the attention they give to their body, particularly to the muscular aspect of their own self, with its attendant stresses and tensions. Then they are gradually taught how to develop this awareness without the need for the constant presence of the therapist/trainer. We do not look for miracles but for small, sustained increments in the degree of self-knowledge, through the medium of the human body. There is no standardized time-table but the format is usually either a series of individual sessions, each lasting around sixty to ninety minutes at one or two weekly intervals, or through a number of intensive group workshops lasting two or three days each, or a combination of both.

Sometimes the training is linked with guidance from other forms of therapy or training. For instance Bryn Jones, a qualified naturopath, often helps people arrive at a dietary regime that is enhancing to their selves rather than, as is often the case, a diet which often exacerbates their basic problem. Other practitioners may incorporate their knowledge of Yoga, Gestalt therapy and so on.

During the course of therapy some people are shocked to discover the extent of pain and tension which they all the time carry around with them in their own muscular system. The highlighting and subsequent realization of this 'inner pain' seems to be a necessary first step before inaugurating the process of re-training the body-mind to start signalling the approach of inner stress and conflict before it

Somatography

manifests itself too deeply and at a level too far removed from conscious awareness.

Is it successful? In terms of curing serious chronic diseases – well it was never designed for that purpose. In terms of helping people feel a little more able to deal with the stresses of their life, in enabling people to get more conscious pleasure from their bodies and as a prophylactic tool to help guard against the onset of future undesirable states of the body-mind, then the answer must be an unqualified 'yes'.

Since one of the parameters of the work is the resolution of inner and outer conflict it is of interest to note that contrary to some of the so-called alternative therapies, Somatography Training has aroused some sympathetic interest amongst, mostly younger, orthodoxly trained physicians, particularly in the Federal Republic of Germany.

H. Bryn Jones

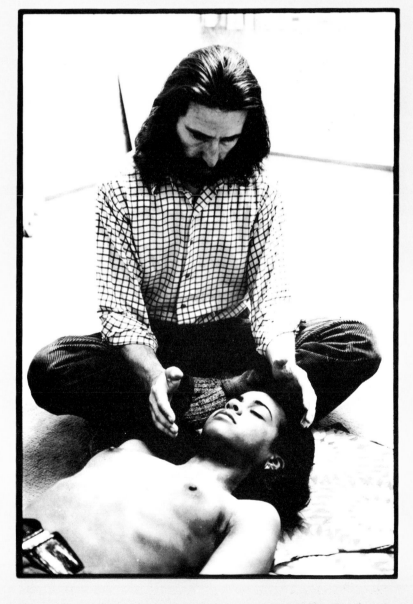

The author, Bryn Jones, using his hands to 'scan' a patient for energy blocks. The part of the aura nearest to the body can often give relevant information about the physical body, whilst areas more distant from the skin sometimes release information pertaining to the mind and the emotions.

Aspects of Bioenergy Work

Bioenergy, (from the Greek: life and force) is the term adopted in latter years for the somatic aspect of Wilhelm Reich's concept of orgone energy – the cosmic energy present everywhere. Reich showed that physical and psychological help is possible only when this energy flows freely in the body. Undischarged bioenergy is bound in the body in various ways, in particular in the muscles, which Reich called muscle armouring. The overall pattern of defensive body armouring Reich called character armouring.

The two therapeutic approaches described here are based on the above premises. Bioenergetics was developed by Alexander Lowen, a pupil of Reich, who particularly uses breathing techniques, body postures and exercises to help people to become aware of their patterns of tension. Bioenergetics differs from Reichian theory in that it is a systematic methodology for dealing with the relationship between somatic functions and psychological trauma.

Biodynamic Psychology, developed by Gerda Boyesen, emphasizes the 'melting' and pleasurable aspects of bioenergy flow, which she relates to Freud's libido concept. Her psychoperistalsic theory – with its concept of visceral armouring – explains how the digestive system functions to discharge tension and stress and to regulate bioenergy flow, thus providing harmony and wellbeing.

BIOENERGETICS

Bioenergetics is a methodology of psychotherapy that has been developed by Alexander Lowen from the earlier work of Wilhelm Reich with whom Lowen was closely associated from 1940.

The Institute of Bioenergetic Analysis was founded by Lowen in 1956 and since then it has developed beyond North America into Europe and elsewhere.

Reich discovered the nature of character armour which is the defensive pattern adopted by the body to protect the person from psychological pain and suffering. This character armour is seen in chronic muscular shapes and tensions in the body, of which the person is largely unconscious. Bioenergetics seeks to bring about the healthy integration of the body and the mind so that the person has the energy to discover pleasure instead of it being siphoned off to maintain the defensive processes. Thus attention is paid to the psychological problem and the physical expression of that problem which is manifested in the body and movement of the client. Bioenergetic techniques attempt to release the physical tensions of the client while dealing with the psychological difficulties. While much is owed to Reich for the understanding of character armour, Bioenergetics is different from Reichian theory for nowhere else is there a systematic methodology dealing with the relationship between the somatic functions and psychological trauma.

There are three major areas of working: 1. Grounding, 2. Breathing, 3. Character structure.

Grounding is to do with one's emotional security and personal authority. All too often, people are dependent on persons other than themselves, or on parts of their body e.g. their brain, rather than their whole person. Grounding is a method of enabling the person to discover his own sense of identity, no mean task. However, it is through our legs and feet that we keep contact with reality or not. For a person to be grounded, they need to be in a particular stance with their feet firmly on the ground and in such a particular position that the energy in the body is able to move in a harmonious flow from the respiratory system that unites with the positive contact with the ground. Where there are problems of insecurity, there will be problems of grounding, of authority. This has to be dealt with in the therapeutic process.

Aspects of Bioenergy Work

Breathing has to do with the oxygenation of the blood which brings vitality, energy and feeling to the body. Where there are defensive blocks in the body, these will be revealed by breathing. Often the breathing patterns which are unconsciously established are caused by chronic muscular tensions due to emotional suffering in earlier years. To develop the breathing is to develop the discovery of feeling and to charge the body with energy and, hopefully, potential for pleasure. In therapy, breathing is developed by placing the body under stress, either by use of the classic bioenergetic breathing stool, or by increasing the charge by kicking the legs on a mattress in a prostrate position, or in hitting the mattress with a racket, etc.

Character structure is important for our understanding of various personality types. No person is one type alone, for most people have all present, which will be manifested under a given set of conditions. Probably one or two may predominate, but no one is likely to be altogether free of them. Bioenergetics has five major structures. These character types are as follows – but first a word of warning: beware of generalizations and beware of the limited amount of information possible in this short space.

The Schizoid character is characterized by muscular patterns of holding the body together against the dread of falling apart. His behaviour is being out of touch with his body and his environment. The task of therapy is to enable the client to confront his frozen terror and fury and to discover his right to exist in the world.

The Oral character is characterized by the muscular pattern of holding on against the dread of abandonment and isolation. His behaviour is an unquenchable thirst for significance in relationships. The task of therapy is to confront this isolation and the consequential rage and enable him to stand without the insatiable demands which he puts on others.

The Psychopathic personality is characterized by the muscular pattern of holding up against the dread of failure if he gives in. He has the need to be superior to everyone in every situation. The task of therapy is to face the fear of submission and to accept interdependency as a valid way of life.

The Masochistic character is characterized by a muscular pattern of holding in against asserting his rights and needs. The task of therapy is to face the fear of admitting he has needs and then to put them before the needs of others so that he can discover his freedom to care for himself before he goes out to others.

The Rigid structure is characterized by the muscular pattern of holding back against exposing the heart to further heartbreak. He has a need to be in control of his emotions and not to be committed within relationships. The task of therapy is to face the terror and fury, to unite the head and genital feelings and to open the longing for contact and acceptance.

To become proficient in understanding character structures is to become proficient in reading the life history of the person before they have said a word. Bioenergetics gives a rapid and dynamic analysis which can be checked or corroborated by the client. Through contact with the body, the client can contact his history and presenting problem, find a way through to the integration of his body and his mind and thus move to a wholeness of self-understanding and awareness.

The way through is by an understanding of the problem – and a willingness to relive the experience of deprivation and suffering. By this means, it is possible to re-evaluate what was an earlier experience of dread and to see it as something that is bearable because it does not cut one off from one's source of well-being. Thus the client need no longer be in a defensive structure, e.g. holding on against

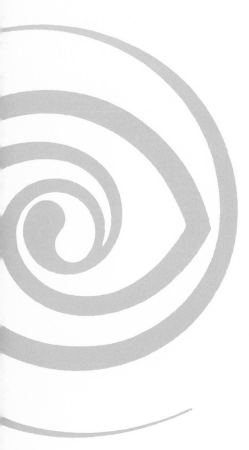

Aspects of Bioenergy Work

abandonment, because he can, as an adult, discover other areas of resources and richness from within himself and outside. So he may relinquish his physical posture and his dread and find a new way beyond fear to pleasure.

Does that mean he is cured? In Bioenergetics, cure is not a word that is used. What is held is that the person becomes able to own what has happened and to absorb the experience into his life for good, and thus be ready for the next step in his growth and development.

Fundamental to the workshops is the concept that in Bioenergetics there is no place for the therapist to hide. Knowledge is an ego phenomenon and one has to go beyond knowledge i.e. the therapist has to feel the flow and sense the course and excitation of the body. One has to know the pain and hurt or the therapist will find it difficult to be patient or reverent with the client. The man who has not wept cannot help another into his loss. The person who has not loved cannot easily help another into his tenderness. Thus he must expose himself to the varieties of human suffering so that, having trodden that ground for himself, he knows something of the ground that others tread.

Geoffrey Whitfield

BIODYNAMIC PSYCHOLOGY

Biodynamic Psychology, developed by the Norwegian psychologist and physiotherapist, Gerda Boyesen, studies and treats psychological processes in the context of the full range of a person's life processes. The processes of 'the mind' and of 'the body' are seen as inter-functioning aspects of the one biodynamic development.

Neurosis Embodied

So, therefore, Biodynamic therapy encompasses much work with the bodily tensions and restrictions – using special massage and movement techniques – and devotes particular attention to a person's bodily expressions. For neurosis is as much a physiological as a psychological development: a person literally embodies his neurosis.

Every emotion, every shock, every frustration, has a direct physiological consequence in a person, as well as psychological. When emotions are repeatedly unexpressed and conflicts unresolved, these consequences become chronic. Stress builds up, layer upon layer, until neurotic symptoms develop – in some cases mainly somatic, in other mainly behavioural. This is particularly distressing in the early years, when it will affect the physical as well as the mental and emotional development of the growing child.

Self-healing and Self-regulation

The healthy organism has, however, the power to express, resolve and digest even severe emotional consequences, given the necessary conditions of peace and security. It is only when a person loses this inherent, natural capacity for self-regulation and self-healing that neurosis develops. Biodynamic therapy seeks to restore this lost or diminished capacity for self-regulation, and to reach the 'alive core' of a person, stimulating and encouraging it to expand.

The 'Primary Personality' and the Muscle Armouring

Only too often this 'alive core' or primary personality gets buried under a 'secondary personality' which the growing child develops, the better to face a not-too-sympathetic environment. This secondary personality corresponds to Wilhelm Reich's concepts of character- and muscle-armouring with which a person protects himself not merely from the onslaughts of the outer environment, but also from his own unwelcome emotions: unwelcome, because the environment cannot accept them. For instance, a child who is often punished for expressing his anger may literally *hold down* his anger by muscular effort. Eventually this holding down process becomes part of the body-structure (muscle-armouring) and the child no longer even feels his anger (character-armouring). Gerda Boyesen has taken this idea further, with her concepts of visceral armour and tissue armour.

Emotional Cycles and Psycho-peristalsis

Central to Biodynamic Psychology is the concept of the emotional cycle, not merely in its psychological aspect, but as a body process.

The rise and fall of every emotion precipitate a vast sequence of physiological changes, right through to the microscopic level and including vasomotoric reorganization (the 'emotional blood circulation'). When the emotional event is past, these bodily processes should – and in a healthy organism will – return to normal. Provided that the bodily effects of the emotion are literally cleared right out of the organism, one can get over the emotional event completely.

According to Gerda Boyesen's theory, the peristaltic processes of the intestines (i.e. tummy rumblings) play a crucial part in this clearing process. As well as playing a role in the digestive process, peristaltic waves will also occur in response to organismic pressure associated with emotional stress. For this aspect of their functioning, Gerda Boyesen has coined the term 'psycho-peristalsis'.

Psycho-peristalsis literally clears out of the body the residual effects remaining from an emotional event. But this psycho-peristaltic phase, by which the emotional cycle should complete itself, can only occur in conditions of peace and security, when the organism is no longer holding itself on the alert.

Visceral and Tissue Armour

When people live in an atmosphere of stress and conflict and can never feel deeply secure, psycho-peristalsis is inhibited. Eventually, the intestinal muscles will actually lose the capacity to respond to the pressures which should stimulate psycho-peristaltic functioning. This loss of response is the *visceral armouring*. When this self-regulating function is lost, the body is never completely clear of stress effects.

With inadequate psycho-peristaltic function, there is also inadequate circulation of the body fluids, and so the tissues are not properly cleansed. Bio-energy then can no longer flow freely to vitalize every cell, and cellular functioning is impaired. This is the *tissue armouring*.

Biodynamic Therapy

Biodynamic therapy follows no pre-determined course: it varies with the needs of the individual client. Often the therapist may work with special massage techniques to dissolve this body-armouring – muscle, visceral and tissue. By using a stethoscope on the abdomen, the therapist follows the peristaltic sounds in detail throughout the massage. These sounds are of an astonishing variety – a complete language in themselves – and come in response to the various touches of the therapist. The sounds indicate that the therapist, touching some particular part of the body tissue where the energy of some past emotion had been suppressed and contained, has now succeeded in setting this energy free for physiological discharge through the psycho-peristalsis. By working to get the maximum psycho-peristaltic sounds, the therapist is progressively clearing the body tissue of the 'stress remnants' from old uncompleted emotional cycles.

Once the body-armouring begins to dissolve, layer by layer, and the bio-energy begins to flow again more freely, there will be a 'biodynamic updrift' of hitherto suppressed energy. When this updrift

Aspects of Bioenergy Work

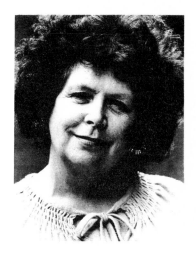

Gerda Boyesen.

Aspects of Bioenergy Work

is strong enough, the therapist may – rather than continuing with massage work – concentrate on encouraging the client to recognize his own 'stimuli from within' and to let them develop and express themselves. These 'stimuli from within' are the stirrings of the person's alive core, now literally pressing for acknowledgement.

The 'stimuli from within' may come in any form, from the tiniest muscular twitchings, or faint shreds of memories, to huge expansive breathing, or to outbursts of deep emotion. Sometimes, old memories and past feelings which had been repressed and buried in the body armour now come back to the surface of consciousness, leading to many insights and profound psychological clearance. Sometimes, the therapeutic process occurs mainly at the organic level.

In either case, Biodynamic therapy is a process of fundamental biological purification; as the neurosis is literally cleared out of the body, the alive core of the organism frees itself from its constrictions, and the non-neurotic, primary personality is uncovered, is redis-covered, and can at last assert and express itself.

Institute for Biodynamic Psychology, London

Psycho-muscular Release Therapy

Psycho-muscular release therapy (PRMT), known in Scandinavia as Release Therapy is a therapeutic system devised by Chester psycholo-gist Peter Blythe, and is based upon the concept that most chronic or persistant psychoneurotic conditions, i.e. anxiety states, clinical depression, phobic states, etc., are due to people being unable to relax certain muscles in their bodies. The muscles which are perma-nently in spasm, it is maintained, act in two distinctive ways. Initially they were tightened up to act as a barrier against intense internal feelings caused by a specific incident or situation, and accordingly use of the musculature in this way, which is normal, can be seen as an 'Adjustment Mechanism' – a natural way of coping with life. However, through continued usage, the muscle tension becomes permanent and ceases to be a purely survival mechanism, instead it begins to habitually transmit, via the *afferent cycle* of the Central Nervous Sys-tem – that part of the nervous system which sends signals to the brain – strong signals which the brain interprets as anxiety.

PMRT aims at helping a patient to release all the feelings which are locked away behind the muscle tension and continually threatening to break through. Release therapists maintain that, in the ultimate analysis, psychoneuroses are disorders of the emotions; a patient cannot feel any differently despite the application of logic, nor can they recognize what the feelings really are as the musculature prevents this.

Blythe claims the system he has developed to assist in the releas-ing of repressed emotions is unique, while readily admitting the fundamental theory behind it is based upon part of the work of Jean-Martin Charcot (1825–93) and his discovery of the 'Hysterogenic' points; that of Sigmund Freud (1856–1939) and his statement that only when a person relives a repressed – buried – incident with emotion will the symptom remiss, and the earlier work of Wilhelm Reich (1897–1957) and his Character-Muscular Armouring.

The difference of PMRT to most other forms of psychotherapy, according to Blythe, is that it concentrates upon releasing dammed-up emotions from the body thus allowing a patient to return to healthy functioning, whereas most other therapeutic systems tend to concen-trate upon helping a patient intellectually to understand why they feel the way they do.

Psychodrama

Psychodrama is an action-oriented therapeutic group method in which an individual enacts problems or conflicts by spontaneously creating those situations in his past, present or future life – real or imagined – which evoke a strong emotional response within him. It is a technique which approaches interactions in a practical, concrete manner by simply looking at a person's life as it is and as they would like to to be.

Jacob Moreno (born 1892) was a Viennese psychiatrist and a contemporary of Freud's. He was impatient with the heavy verbal emphasis of psychoanalysis and its lengthy time period. Moreno searched for a medium that would encourage working on the verbal and non-verbal level with both fantasy and reality, and would facilitate a powerful and total emotional release which he called catharsis. Catharsis is specific to each situation; it cannot be stored for later use, so that an emotional release in one situation (e.g. a conflict with our parents) cannot be applied to another one (e.g. the pain of an important lost relationship).

Moreno suggested that man has problems in life because he must successfully create and live a variety of roles (e.g. mother, wife, lover, teacher, hostess), which sometimes may be in conflict with each other. We all have our 'public' roles, but within us may also be other roles which clamour for expression and freedom. This internal pressure may be a source of anxiety. In the safety of a psychodrama group, one can explore these hidden parts, and perhaps integrate them into our lives so that we move towards integration and balance.

There are five key components to a psychodramatic action (an enactment). The place where the action takes place is the *psychodramatic stage;* it is free from the constrictions of real life and provides a safe place for self-exploration. The action takes place in the present (the here-and-now) as if it were happening for the first time. On the psychodrama stage, there is an attempt to recreate the physical and emotional climate of the setting whether a scene at home, hospital, an office, or perhaps even a fantasied area such as 'heaven', 'emptiness', etc.

The *protagonist* is the person 'working' on their problem; they portray scenes and incidents which they choose, and present them from their individual perspective. The protagonist's psychodrama is facilitated by a *director* who is both producer and therapist. Besides being highly skilled, well-trained and sensitive, he or she must inspire trust and confidence as well as be comfortable working in intense emotional situations. The director has overall responsibility for the psychodrama session. *Auxiliaries* are the necessary others for creating the psychodramatic scene; in a sense the rest of the cast! They will enact other roles; e.g. if a family scene was necessary, a mother, a father, and siblings as well as even the family dog might be required. Auxiliaries can also sometimes be inanimate objects, or a symbolic figure (Prince Charming), or a general role such as 'students', 'the police', 'clients', etc. Finally there are those not directly involved in the psychodramatic action, and collectively they are known as the *audience.* They may give important feedback in the sharing period which follows the enactment, or they may indicate their personal identification with the protagonist's work.

Many techniques are available to the skilled psychodramatist to facilitate the psychodramatic process. A *soliloquy* requires the protagonist to verbalize aloud to the audience what he is feeling and is often used in very tense, emotional situations. *Mirroring* involves other people imitating or even exaggerating the protagonist's behaviour as a means of giving effective feedback as to how others see or experience him. Thus, if he were behaving in a rather whining and obsequious manner, it would become clear through this technique. One of

Psychodrama

psychodrama's better-known techniques is doubling. The *double's* major function (also known as an alter-ego) is to help the protagonist clarify and express feelings. The double is in close physical proximity and becomes an extension of the protagonist. Another frequently used technique is *role reversal* where the protagonist becomes the antagonist and the antagonist the protagonist; in other words they have switched their roles, one for the other. Thus, the husband (protagonist) becomes his wife (portrayed by an auxiliary) and the auxiliary becomes the husband. The husband (now as 'wife') takes on the attitudes, posture, voice, and emotions of his wife and vice-versa.

This technique is often utilized for clarification, or to enable the protagonist to obtain greater empathy and understanding of the situation of conflict 'through the other person's eyes'. Other techniques include working with fantasy material, portraying and 'living' our dreams, or preparing for events which arouse strong emotions such as a crucial interview, a coming confrontation, an imminent death etc.

Often, the utilization of these techniques helps to bring about emotional release, or a reduction in anxiety which leads to the protagonist being clearer about the situation and possible solutions. By participating in psychodrama, it is possible that there will be an increase in self-awareness and one's own sense of aliveness. One may also become more conscious of choices because of increased clarity; and participants may also feel freer of past emotional burdens, and thereby find it easier to discover the joy, creativity and spontaneity in their lives. Psychodrama is particularly effective in facilitating these changes because of the power of enacting a situation rather than just talking about it. Possible solutions to conflicts can be rehearsed in the safety of the psychodrama stage, and participants may develop new and better responses which will contribute to a more satisfying life-style.

Psychodrama is a potent technique to help people restore their inner balance, and move towards harmony and self-fulfillments. But, because of that strength, it is a technique to be employed only by those who have had training in psychodrama and its applications.

Joel Badaines

The New Primal Therapies

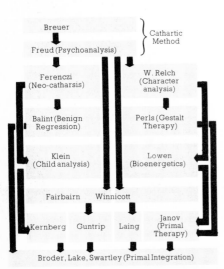

The 'new' primal therapies have a complicated family tree *(see left)*.

'Primal' is defined in Drever's *Dictionary of Psychology* (1952) as "first in time: employed in a special sense by psychoanalysts for a fragmentary recalled experience or scene from early childhood, apparently the first stage in the production of a neurosis".

Freud first used the term 'primal' in 1897, crediting his teacher, Joseph Breuer with the distinction between free, mobile or primary (primal) processes versus tonic, bound or secondary processes. Primary processes express the "pleasure principle", that is, they ignore reality and facts by attempting to satisfy every wish through a simple motor activity in the outer world or by identifying with the source of previous satisfaction in the inner world, e.g., one's mother or her breast. Secondary processes express the "reality principle", finding satisfaction of a wish through taking into account the facts of the outer world. Freud's elaboration of these differences constitutes one of his most fundamental contributions to psychology.

Until about 1895, Freud attempted to work directly with the chaotic, primal processes using his hypnotic cathartic technique. The 'new' primal therapists have yet to describe the theory of primal therapy as briefly as did Freud and Breuer in their *Preliminary Communication* of 1893. However, Freud concluded the release of primal processes was too difficult and dangerous for patient and therapist alike. Likewise, about half the therapists who joined the International

The New Primal Therapies

Primal Association in 1972 no longer practise primal therapy, as it is perhaps the most demanding form of psychotherapy for both patient and therapist. Primal-oriented therapies are often indicated with clients who have had success with more verbally oriented therapies such as Psychoanalysis, Bioenergetics or Gestalt, but who then require a method which allows for deeper penetration into what at first seems to be chaotic feelings.

The new primal therapies, developed since 1965, have learned that the release of primal processes is a natural, organically directed, self-healing process, not dependent upon hypnosis. All that is necessary is that the patient convince himself that it is safe to stop inhibiting the free expression of basic needs, such as the need for skin contact, the need to cry, or hit out when frustrated. Primal processes are like atomic energy, in that the major problem involves releasing powerful energy without destroying both the patient's and therapist's psychological world, either in a great explosion or an insidious accumulation of side effects.

We are learning to integrate primary and secondary processes, using techniques which appear to yield permanent therapeutic change. Our culture, although heavily repressed, will tolerate much more expression of primal processes as a means of producing positive change than did the Victorian era in which Freud practised.

The best known of the new techniques is Primal Therapy, popularized by Arthur Janov, Ph.D., an American psychotherapist who has published such best-sellers as *The Primal Scream* and *The Feeling Child*. On the positive side, Janov has stirred up great interest and demand for cathartic therapy. However, he has been consistently criticized for acting more like a salesman than a professional scientist. He has made exaggerated claims for his product and/or behaved like a high priest of a new religious cult. He claims his form of Primal Therapy is the one and only 'cure' for all mental illness, and suggests that other psychotherapists only harm their patients. Janov's views are not shared by most other primal therapists.

Janov calls the expression of a primary process a 'primal', which has rapidly become part of American slang, and the process of releasing is referred to as 'primalling'.

The role of pain and pleasure while exploring primal processes is a major controversy among primal therapists. Janov describes himself as a dealer of Pain, no more or no less. Many primal therapists disagree with this emphasis on pain, and have confirmed Reich's experiences that, during deep primal regression, patients are more afraid of pleasure than of pain. Our culture teaches us how to handle pain; many people seek pain to sooth their guilty superegos. Janov believes in a 'busting' technique, while other primal therapists feel that such a technique only teaches a patient to reinforce his character armour. On the other hand, 'melting' a patient's armour with tender massage is a natural method of supporting the release of primal processes.

A second major controversy is the depth to which a patient may regress. Freud concluded that the major problem of his patients was the Oedipal complex. Ferenczi began to play with his patients to help them to regress to their pre-verbal childhood. Melanie Klein also used play and artistic activities to penetrate into infantile experiences.

Otto Rank concluded that his patients were traumatized by their experience of birth. Nandor Fodor used dream analysis to resolve not only birth but also uterine traumas. It was not until 1976 that R. D. Laing described an "implantation primal", although Isadore Sadger described "conception traumas" to Freud in 1907.

While some primal therapists are still learning to recognize and

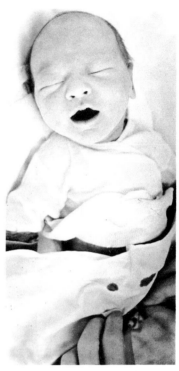

A male child undergoing circumcision.

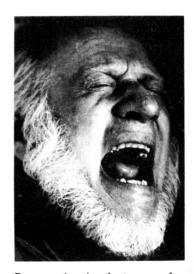

Re-experiencing the trauma of circumcision.

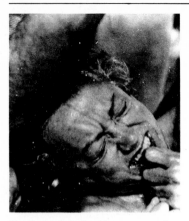

Re-experiencing the trauma of birth in Primal Integration.

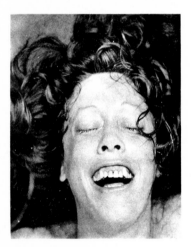

The ecstatic moment of a successful breach birth.

deal with implantation primals, others followed their patients into Jung's collective unconscious. For instance, one of the most therapeutic experiences for a patient suffering from the effects of inadequate mothering involves contacting the Jungian archetype of the 'Great Mother', thereby obtaining eternal nourishment from within.

Occasionally it is necessary to follow a patient 'beneath' the collective unconscious into karmic consciousness, (a Sanskrit word which means 'action', referring to the ethical consequences of actions which do not return within a single lifetime). Penetration of this level frequently produces 'reincarnation primals' which appear to cause equal therapeutic change whether it is fantasy or reality. On this level, therapists and patients are helped by the results of Stanislav Grof's, John Masters' and Jean Houston's distinctions between the various altered states of consciousness produced by the ingestion of LSD. Another model, helpful in understanding karmic experiences, is found in *The Tibetan Book of the Dead* and Jung's commentary on it.

Primal experiences on the 'lowest' or mystical level of transpersonal consciousness are impossible to describe. Any description is limiting, as such experiences are beyond logic, self, beyond gods, beyond words, beyond all dualism. If there is any end to primal exploration, it may be through establishing solid contact with this level, which every mystic and shaman has agreed is underneath everything we think we know.

The new primal therapies are not for everyone. They are most effective when the major psychological conflict involves experiences which occurred before the client learned to talk – that is, usually between conception and the end of the first year of life. The crisis (or turning point) usually involves the re-living of these early experiences, which often includes the admission into consciousness of immense emotional pain and/or intense bodily sensations. The progress of primal therapy is therefore often determined by how much pain the client can tolerate in any given period, and, as a form of treatment, it usually lasts several years. The results are often dramatic and lasting.

Primal therapists have begun to integrate their techniques with other forms of alternative medicine, such as acupuncture and diet. That is what this book is all about.

William Swartley

Gestalt

Gestalt is an experiential learning process. It is used as a therapy and as an educational scheme. The Gestalt attitudes facilitate change in the individual, and thus in any interpersonal situations such as schools, homes, offices. The methods are most commonly used by a Gestalt therapist (guide or leader) in private sessions and in self-discovery groups.

The German word Gestalt has no equivalent in English but means an organized whole, a meaningfully harmonized unity. The 'whole' consists of *figure*, what we see, and *ground*, the constant personality. When these are in positive relationship there is integration and flow. When the formation is disturbed, dis-ease results. To complete the gestalt we begin working with the obvious, the figure. The image suggested is a revolving, floating rubber ball (rather than the analyst's layers of an onion) and we work with the part which is visible above the water, the most easily available. The invisible part has the function of support. All our behaviour patterns, everything in our background that we take for granted and rely upon, acts as a support for our present experience. Change takes place when we realize that we no longer need an aspect of our behaviour pattern once necessary to support us; that it has become an obstacle, instead of a part which enables us to experience more fully.

Gestalt

Dr Frederick (Fritz) Perls is the originator and has provided the principles of our present Gestalt school. He developed his work in America in the late 1950s, since when it has become the third most common psycho-therapeutic affiliation. In England there have been scattered opportunities to experience this self-knowledge process since the launching of the Human Potential Movement in 1970. The first Gestalt Training School in London was established by Ischa Bloomberg in 1974.

Gestalt is a branch of Humanistic Psychology, which addresses itself to positive aspects of personality and living. Each Gestaltist has individual style, and many incorporate other disciplines, such as bio-energetics and guided fantasies in their approach. Many Transactional Analysts have adopted Gestalt as a useful method of incarnating their theories. Art, dance and dreams are often made use of in Gestalt workshops.

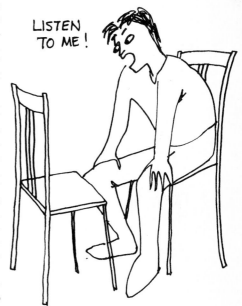

As with most of the New Therapies, analysis and interpretation are avoided. The person is invited to focus on the here-and-now experience in a continuum of awareness. Moreover, in Gestalt, the *content* of the subject's message (story or presenting issue) is subsidiary to the *process*. Body language and voice are brought into awareness to offer a new non-cerebral truth. The work is through sensory awareness, emotional closeness, personal responsibility and spontaneity. Focusing on, repeating and exaggerating what is happening in the moment (for example a gesture, physical tension, a tone of voice) is basic practice. By making explicit blocks and frustrations, a person becomes more expressive and experiences the sense of freedom which follows. Neurosis is built on avoidance, and so we work with the avoidance. Perls said "neurosis is being out of touch".

The philosophy behind Gestalt is existential and largely to do with differentiation and integration. Differentiation alone leads to polarities, which will cause conflict and paralysis. When working with an individual, these polarities are demonstrated by the use of an empty chair (or cushion) which is used to represent the internalized other (perhaps a parent or spouse) or another aspect of the personality. For example, a dialogue between Top Dog (the 'should' side of a person) and the Under Dog (the 'can't' side) clarifies the conflict. By making these polarities more explicit and discovering the needs behind each part, integration takes place.

Gestalt is a powerful method for personal growth and, like any other power, can be mis-used. Along with change comes insecurity, both to the person evolving and to those close to them. Relationships can be rapidly re-vitalized and enhanced. On the other hand, a once-stable intimacy can be outgrown. It is sometimes questioned whether the pain of a broken marriage, especially where children are involved, can justify the flowering of one individual. Distortions of Gestalt are often related to the understanding of what is meant by being responsible. Individuals may develop new self-torture games, blaming themselves for all their suffering. Also the position of autonomy can be distorted into a lack of sensitivity to the needs of others. An inexperienced therapist might discount all but here-and-now data. In groups, focus on the individual is sometimes at the expense of the group process and of a recognition of the group as a larger whole.

Gestalt helps us towards self-knowledge, satisfaction and self-support. It has a Zen flavour in that it values the unfolding of nature through present awareness; growing through becoming more of what we are. It calls forth a creative and free-flowing participation from the therapist, as well as the client. Each is involved in discovering the wisdom and love which lie dormant within.

Ursula Fausset

Co-counselling

Co-counselling is a method of personal development through mutual aid in which two people, who have been trained in both roles, take it in turns to be client and counsellor. The client is the one who is working on himself, the counsellor gives supportive attention and makes occasional interventions to aid the client's work. It is client-directed in the sense that the primary onus is on the client to use his skills to work on himself, but there is a contract that the counsellor will help out with suggestions when the client is missing his way.

One aspect of the client's work is regression and catharsis. This is a healing of the memories, in which the client uncovers memories of early painful experiences and releases the pain through emotional discharge: grief at being unloved is released through tears and sobbing, anger at arbitrary interference through loud sound and storming movements, fear at threats to personal identity through trembling, embarrassment and false imposed guilt through laughter. The client is trained to take charge of this release by always maintaining a focus of attention outside the painful emotion that is being uncovered and unloaded.

The theory underlying this process is that children survive emotionally and socially in our rigid society by defensively occluding and denying the grief, fear and anger produced in them by the inadequate behaviour of parents and others. This hidden distress is displaced outwards in conventional, rigid, compulsive and distorted behaviour of different kinds. It is also displaced inwards in chronic attitudes of self-deprecation, feelings of powerlessness and so on. When the hidden distress is uncovered and thoroughly discharged, there follows insight – a discriminating re-appraisal of the traumatic past and a realization of how its hitherto unidentified effects have been contaminating adult behaviour and attitudes. Armed with such insight, and free of the compulsive pressures of hidden distress, the person is then able to begin to live intentionally, to act within a situation with rational awareness, with a sensitive responsiveness to what is actually going on – rather than compulsively manoeuvering with projected ghosts from the past.

Another aspect of the client's work is the celebration and affirmation of his unique way of being intelligent, loving, of exercising choice and creativity. This complements the way of regression and catharsis and builds up the human centre. And it leads over naturally into goal-setting and action planning for a more worthwhile way of living.

Co-counselling was developed in the USA by Harvey Jackins in the 1950s, and appears to have been influenced at the very beginning by some aspects of dianetics. Jackins called his movement Re-evaluation Counselling and it started to gain momentum in the late 60s and early 70s. It was introduced into the UK and Europe in 1971 and 1972. An independent movement called Co-counselling International was formed in 1974 in order to enable co-counselling to develop outside the theoretical and organizational rigidities of Jackins' approach. It is a federation of co-counselling communities in the UK, Europe and the USA, each of which explores its own way of developing a peer self-help network, while learning from each other.

The purpose of a co-counselling community is to provide basic training in co-counselling (a minimum of 40 hours), ongoing and advanced groups and workshops, co-counselling teacher training, address lists of all local co-counsellors, news letters, theory papers, and so on. Such communities or networks provide an important alternative to established systems of health care provision: they abandon the therapist-client, professional-layman distinction and affirm people-centred values of self-determination and co-operation.

John Heron

Encounter and Humanistic Psychology generally were part of the movement for change which swept America and Europe in the late 1960s. This movement was characterized by a questioning of the traditional values of society, a rejection of artificially imposed boundaries such as 'mind' and 'body', 'mental illness', etc., and perhaps centrally, an acceptance of feelings and emotions as legitimate guides to action and a commitment to exploring the human potential. To some extent, Encounter was a reaction against some traditional forms of therapy which were concerned with preserving the status quo and getting people to adjust to the intolerable psychological burdens of a sick society.

Encounter is a form of group therapy, eclectic by its very nature, being an integration of a wide number of influences and skills stemming from the work of such pioneers as W. Reich, Fritz Perls, A. Maslow, R. D. Laing and others. Below is a diagram showing some of the therapies and schools of thought that have influenced Encounter.

Encounter

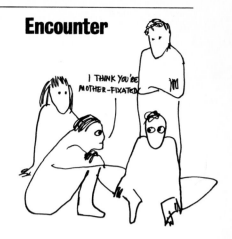

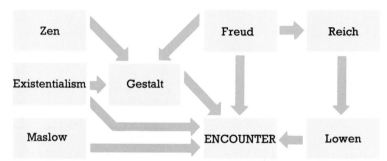

It is often thought that therapy only takes place through suffering. However it has become more widely recognized, as a result of the work of Winnicott and Maslow, that one of the main tasks of therapy is to learn (or relearn) what playing and joy are about. Thus encounter incorporates activities designed to encourage these aspects.

How then do these various influences find expression in the actual process of an encounter group? To begin at its most simple, a group of from 10–16 people sit in a room, on the floor, in a circle, generally although not always with a recognized leader. A session may last one evening, a week-end, or it may be an on-going experience lasting several months.

The aim of the group experience is to encounter each other in real ways; to experience one's own feelings; to be responsible for them; and to relate to other group members honestly. Apart from this there is no formal requirement or structure, although generally groups begin with a variety of exercises to facilitate familiarity between group members. Beyond that, each person is equally responsible for the group activity – total creativity is the ultimate goal.

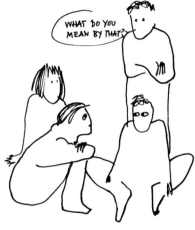

The leader will however generally indicate certain guide-lines. Interpretations are discouraged and people are asked to replace them by a direct expression of their feelings, which may be verbal or physical. For example, one common phenomenon in the early stages of a group is intellectualizing analytical attitudes (see illustrations).
Example: John says to Henry in a tone of annoyance:

"I think you're mother-fixated."

Therapist: "What do you feel about that?" (asking John to make *explicit* his implicit attitude).

John: "I don't like you being so weak. I despise you."

Similarly although memories, dreams, etc. are brought into the group when appropriate, the tendency is to relate narrated experiences to the people in the room (the 'here-and-now').

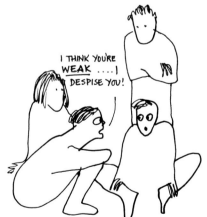

Encounter

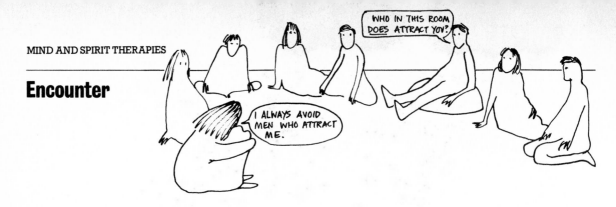

Example: Sarah: "I find when I'm attracted to men, I avoid them."

Therapist: "Could you be more specific? Who in this room are you attracted to?" (asking Sarah to directly experience her attraction and avoidance).

A related principle is the exploration of unpleasant feelings. For example, it is quite common for a group-member working on something to say "I feel embarrassed", "I feel ludicrous", "I feel frightened". The therapist might intervene: "Fine, stay embarrassed, experience what it's like", hoping to encourage that person to explore an area of his experience that he has probably avoided most of his life. Thus we have a process of opening up to new or taboo feelings, including many positive ones such as tenderness, compassion, love.

Another practice is to use movement and the body for self-expression. Whether boredom, grief, love, peace, anger, is the issue, group-members are encouraged to use their voice and their body expressively and actively, to break out of the up-tightness that besets our culture:

Example: Joan: "I really hate my son for making me lose my freedom."

Therapist: "OK, talk to your son directly, imagine he's in front of you. Or we'll get another group member to play him."

In this way the energy of Joan's insight is allowed direct expression, rather than being dissipated in analysis and anecdotal neutrality.

A further aspect of Encounter that is important is feedback. Whenever any person does any extensive piece of work, or is stuck, or in trouble, the leader will often ask for feedback from other members. How do others experience you? Often the answer to this question can begin to free someone from their impasse, or help him or her in future to understand their manipulations and self-presentation to others.

When we turn to the therapist, we find that the degree of directiveness varies from therapist to therapist – but generally involved as a person; communicating his boredom, anger, tenderness, when he feels it appropriate. The Encounter therapist is aware not only of what is being said but also of the form of expression, such as tone of voice, body postures, facial movements, etc.; and pays particular attention to avoidances; demands; repeating situations. A good Encounter leader will have great respect and compassion for the autonomy of the members of the group – they decide to start something; to stop it; to change it, and so on. This is essential for each person's path of self-discovery and growing self-acceptance.

The spirit of Encounter is very positive, even though it may appear to be uncovering many painful and negative feelings. Encounter doesn't give cures; it points a direction of self-exploration and growth in which you can travel for a life-time. You begin in the company of other seekers to learn how to discover yourself and therefore others; how to learn about your being.

Tom Feldberg and Roger Horrocks

Sensitivity Training

Sensitivity training is also known as T-group training, laboratory training or human relations training. It was first developed in the United States in 1947. The central method comprises participation in a T-group (or training group) which has 7 to 15 members and one or two leaders. The task of the group is for each member to learn about the effect his behaviour has on others. This most typically occurs when other members of the group tell the individual how they react to a particular aspect of him or her. T-groups may meet for only a few hours up to as much as 40 hours. Meetings may be intensively focused over a few days or they may be once or twice a week over a period of months. The meetings of the T-group are not planned in advance by the leader, but are at the disposal of all members of the group, who share responsibility for how the time is spent. The leader's task may be to contribute his or her own feelings and reactions to what is going on, to summarize or clarify events or to suggest ways in which the group might work on the goals they have set themselves.

T-groups are most effective in creating learning for their members when participation in them is voluntary rather than coerced; when members are initially strangers and do not have ongoing work or personal relations with each other; when meetings are intensively held rather than spaced out; when the group is protected from the conflicting pressures and commitments of everyday living; when the group is able to create a climate of involvement and trust in one another.

T-groups constitute the major element in sensitivity training but many programmes also include other activities. These may include work in twos or threes or community activities involving members of several T-groups concurrently. The goals of sensitivity training vary somewhat depending on the setting, but typical goals would include:

1. Increased awareness of how others see one.
2. Increased awareness of group behaviour.
3. Increased ability to behave toward others in ways which meet one's goals.

Where the method is employed with participants who have a lasting link with one another, such as work colleagues or married couples the goal is not so much individual change but change in ongoing relationships.

The invention of the T-group occurred in 1947 when Leland Bradford and a group of fellow adult educators met to compare the group dynamics occurring in discussion groups which they were leading. When participants heard of these meetings they asked to sit in on them, and declared them more interesting than the original discussions. Further programmes were organized to include discussion of group processes, which quickly led to the development of the T-group and of National Training Laboratories, which is still the major organization sponsoring sensitivity training in the United States. Since that time, sensitivity training has undergone a process of continuing diffusion and modification. T-groups were first run in England around 1957 and now occur in most countries of the world. The major trend over the past thirty years has been to reduce the emphasis on sensitivity training as a training in interpersonal skills for one's work and increase the emphasis on personal learning and the potentially therapeutic effects of T-group participation. The development of Encounter groups (see separate entry) was much influenced by sensitivity training and some of the key figures in Encounter (e.g. Will Schutz) were previously T-group leaders. The distinction between T-groups and some Encounter methods is at present neither clear nor consistently applied. Most T-groups would more closely resemble basic encounter than other types of Encounter. A second trend has been for sensi-

Sensitivity Training

	Behaviour known to self	Unknown to self
Behaviour known to others	Public	Blind
Unknown to others	Hidden	Un-conscious

Classification of behaviour in the T-group.

tivity trainers working within large organizations to develop methods of 'organizational development' which utilize group participation but are less personally focused.

Various critics have claimed that the 'unstructured' nature of T-groups have harmful effects on some of those who participate, but none of the evidence in support of this claim has shown that the risk of attending a group is any higher than that of numerous other life experiences. Research studies show that about two-thirds of participants experience lasting benefits, including more favourable self-concept, more participative attitudes, more openmindedness, changed behaviour as seen by others and changes in organizational behaviour. These changes were not found among equivalent people who did not attend groups.

The reliability with which groups produce the effects listed above depends on whether the group lasts for an adequate duration, whether the leader has adequate expertise and whether participants have indeed chosen freely to participate. The processes whereby such changes occur are probably best described by Carl Rogers' theory of personal change in counselling and therapy. A simpler model due to Joseph Luft and Harrington Ingham is illustrated. The group's task is to enlarge the domain of publicly-known behaviour by exploring areas which are initially hidden or blind. The trust required to make this a fruitful enterprise arises from the fact that participants control the speed at which it occurs and each individual can also control for him or herself the amount of hidden area to reveal.

Sensitivity training does not typically seek to explore the area in the diagram designated as unconscious. This area is of greater concern to group workers employing Tavistock study group methods and others within the Psychoanalytic tradition.

Peter Smith

Enlightenment Intensive

The Enlightenment Intensive is an interactive group process which was developed in California in the late 1960s by Charles Berner and brought to Europe by Jeff Love. The process derives from a close alignment of the methods of reciprocal co-counselling and the Zen practice of meditating upon a *Koan*, or paradoxical question. It is suitable for groups of between ten and ninety people, depending on the space available. The group is guided by a *facilitator*, and such a person is required to undergo a very thorough training in order to lead the participant through an experience which can produce strong emotional responses.

The basic event usually lasts for periods of three days to a week. People take turns to sit together in pairs for about forty minutes. The whole group is thus divided into *dyads*, and one member of each pair asks his or her companion a Koan, while the other attempts a reply.

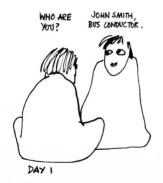

DAY 1

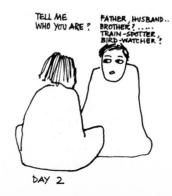

DAY 2

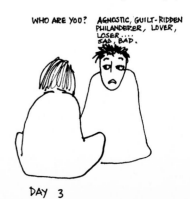

DAY 3

After five minutes, the roles are reversed. At the end of the forty-minute period, there is a break, and each individual selects a new partner. Periods of manual work without conversation, silent meditation and silent meals occur at intervals each day.

The first Koan is "Who am I?" Later Koans are "What am I?", "What is Life?" and "What is Another?" Some facilitators will vary these themes. An extension of the process may allow the use of additional Koans, such as "What is Death?" or "What is Meaning?" When an individual believes that he has solved a Koan (or resolved the paradox), it is presented to the facilitator for evaluation. Thus the trained facilitator takes on something of the role of the Zen teacher.

Recently various types of tantric yoga, drawn from the teaching of Shree Bhagvan Rajneesh, have been included in the programme, or, alternatively, the setting for an event may be within the framework of a conventional Zen retreat.

Theoretically, the participant in an Enlightenment Intensive experiences a progressive relaxation from concern with his own identity. At best there is a release from the excessively tight cognitive structure of the individual and a refreshing sense of discovery and well-being, an event called *satori* in Zen. Obviously some members of the group are more deeply affected by the work than others, but all are helped to understand themselves. It benefits those who are facing a crisis in their lives, people who feel alienated, or who wish to come to terms with their own personality. Whilst being effective as an independent and self-contained process, it is also of use to those who have undergone other group experiences of the gestalt therapy type, for whom a follow-up resource is desirable.

John H. Crook

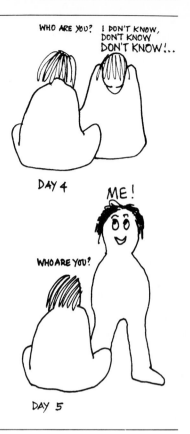

Transactional Analysis is a theory of personality elaborated in the 1950s by Eric Berne, an American psychiatrist. It was evolved originally as a counterthrust to the prevailing psychoanalytic approach and was meant to enable patients to understand quickly and in colloquial language the nature of their transactions without having to engage in a historical exploration of the roots of personality from which they sprang. The essence of the approach is thus to analyse transactions in terms of three possible and mutually exclusive modes of functioning – the Parent, the Adult and the Child. A significant contribution of the theory lies in the analysis of 'Games' which people engage in and which allow them to continue stereotyped relationships with others, relationships which are relatively unproductive but which, being predictably stimulating, offer some limited satisfaction. In therapy the approach is now widely used, not only in North America, but also in India, Japan, Australia, South America and to a growing extent in Europe. It is still largely an insight therapy, though at the same time it lays considerable emphasis on feelings and is also characterized by a 'contract' approach, that is, the patient and therapist will make it a first task to establish a clearly defined behavioural goal towards which they will work together. There is no attempt to establish and resolve a transference relationship, and the work is always face to face; most often in a group setting. In more recent years the theory has been extended to cover in fact some of the developmental aspects (early decisions, existential positions, feeling preferences, behavioural patterns) usually associated with depth psychology. At the same time it has become popular as a means of dealing with and improving 'normal' relationships not only in the therapeutic context but also in education, management and other spheres.

Michael Reddy

Transactional Analysis

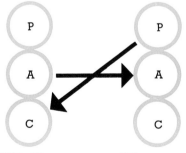

"What time is it?"   "Time you weren't here."

Ego states are sub-systems of the personality between which we shift from moment to moment. As adults (A) we objectively appraise; as children (C) we react more abruptly; as parents (P) we are judgemental and evaluative.

Colour Therapy

The idea of using colour to produce certain psychological responses is very ancient. The sanctuaries of Egyptian and Greek temples were painted, and the choice of colours is thought to have been deliberate. Tibetan teachings, even up to the present time recognize colour qualities in meditation. In India, colour therapy is still practised in a traditional way, whereby water is exposed to sunlight through coloured glass, red light, blue, yellow, green, etc., so that by drinking water after exposure, the patient can be energized, or calmed, or be cured of specific conditions such as acidity. In this century, Rudolf Steiner, in a series of lectures given in Dornach in 1921 suggests that both colour and form can be used as supplementary treatments for certain conditions. The Goethean Science Foundation has taken up Steiner's suggestions in conjunction with their educational work at Clent, Stourbridge, Worcestershire, England. The Hygeia Studios at Avening in Gloucestershire and the Spectro-Chromo Institute at Malaga, New Jersey, research into a particular form of colour therapy combining colour, sound and rhythm.

Human beings, animals and plants are all subject to treatment by light and colour through the very nature of the change from day to night around our planet. This natural process can be so harnessed that it can be used as a supplementary aid in the treatment of illnesses in hospitals and clinics. Colour is the subtle change in atmospheric pressure from the dense red which arises from the infrared (invisible) darkness to magenta which dissolves into ultraviolet, where the pressure is gently lifted. This change in density is registered not only by the eyes, but also upon the skin, or surface of all living things.

This means that blind people can react to colour just as a sighted person does. The reaction varies according to the individual and this variation provides useful guidelines for specific treatments.

Psychologically, it is well known that specific results are achieved by a combination of factors, and not usually through a single ingredient. Colour, therefore, is supported by form. In principle, blue is in harmony with the horizontal and spherical, red with vertical and cubic and yellow with raying out and detaching forms. To have maximum effect, form and colour should be in harmony, but it is also necessary to complement them, so tension is introduced to give increased value to the harmony. The colour therapist therefore adds rhythm which brings with it a time factor.

The colours used in this therapy are those of the natural spectrum: red-orange-yellow; green; turquoise-blue-violet; magenta. These eight colours correspond to the three 'octaves' (or twenty-four vertebrae) of the spinal column, with a further two octaves relating respectively to the sacrum and the skull, the sacrum being below infrared and the skull above ultraviolet. The colour therapist uses the spinal chart (which is also employed by the music therapist and astrologer) to dowse out the problem areas of a patient and thus determine which colour is to be used in treatment. The treatment is then administered under the supervision of a qualified medical practitioner.

The whole human body is a symphony of colour right down to the actual skeleton. Colour therapists also consider the aura. This is the natural area around each living organism which emits a fine electrical current and also receives universal energies from without. Thus the aura manifests strength and also weakness. (The aura should not be confused with the etheric sheath which is much denser and shallower.) The structure of the aura is two-fold. In its perfect state it has a pure, star-like raying out pattern which interweaves with a series of egg-like shells or spheres which lie in fine layers around all natural objects from human beings, through plants, even to stones, although the aura is most alive in humans.

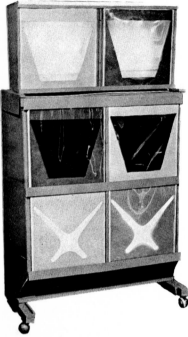

The colour rhythm beamer, developed by Theo Gimbel for use at Hygeia Studios.

THE HUMAN SPINE WITH COLOUR, SOUND AND THE SIGNS OF THE ZODIAC.

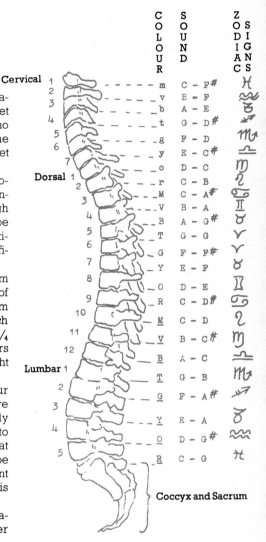

There is no perfect aura, just as there is no perfect spine. Deviations can be detected by experienced therapists who learn to interpret them. So much individual perception is required that there can be no generalization and each case must be considered separately. The therapist must also be aware of his own shortcomings and learn to set these aside when treating a patient.

There are three basic ways in which colour therapy can be applied: (a) through coloured fabrics, walls and illumination (b) by mental image making, counselling and guided meditation (c) through projection, on the spiritual level, to any person anywhere. To be effective, each method requires a specific technique. Hence a scientific study is undertaken, for an intuitive approach might not be sufficiently accurate.

For system (a) an instrument may be used, such as a colour rhythm beamer, a colour level lamp, a colour wall or a colour composer. All of these have been perfected after years of research. The colour rhythm beamer is a carefully constructed colour–form/time instrument which is used in conjunction with music and meditation for a period of 24¼ minutes. No more than three colours may be used within any 24 hours and one of these must be blue. The correct intensity of colour and light are arrived at by the study of light grid patterns.

In system (b) the experienced counsellor can establish a colour image for the patient so that within the patient a healing meditative colour change will arise, working through his mental effort. It is usually necessary to be treated through system (a) before progressing to system (b). Good biofeedback instruments have demonstrated that once the mental image is well established, the same effects can be achieved through system (b) as through system (a). Thus (a) treatment often leads to (b) and the aim is to educate the patient towards this capacity. A refresher course may be necessary from time to time.

Technique (c) requires the therapist to enter into a state of meditation so as to be able to send out a colour image to a person wherever he may be, providing that the name, the face and the place are known.

Finally it is important to understand which colours belong respectively to the animal, plant and mineral kingdoms. Human beings do not belong to any of these realms, but borrow the necessary densities from them. Most experienced meditators are aware of blue arising out of the calm which lowers the brain rhythms.

By further calming and stilling the mind, we arrive at a golden colour which has plant-like designs arising from the deep blue background. Allowing the rhythms to reduce still further, the mind experiences the almost white colour, tinted magenta, making the most exquisite geometric designs floating and continually changing in a flowing, interweaving progression. This colour state is rarely achieved and those who enter it need careful guidance.

Theo Gimbel

COLOUR
M = Magenta
V = Violet
B = Blue
T = Turquoise
G = Green
Y = Yellow
O = Orange
R = Red
Lower case = Light colour
Capitals = Medium colour
Capitals underlined = Dense colour

Music Therapy

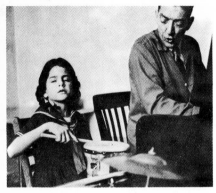

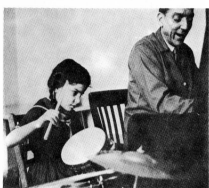

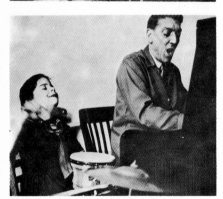

Paul Nordoff working with a seven-year-old autistic girl. It can be seen how uneasiness and detachment lead to engagement and then to internal excitement and pleasure.

Some of the material contained in this article appeared previously in Progress, *the journal of the Disablement Income Group and is reprinted by kind permission of the Publishers*

Music is an expressive art which speaks directly to the emotions, to the feeling life. It is a language which we can all understand, as it encompasses the infinite range of human experience from the superficial to the profound. Music can arouse in us deep emotional responses.

Increasingly, music is being used with handicapped children as part of their everyday routine, as recreation, occupation, maybe to accompany movement or dance, and there may well be some therapeutic benefit in these activities. But the art of music can be used more specifically than this, at a deeper level, consciously directed towards the non-communicating or severely physically handicapped child, to penetrate the barriers set up by his illness, and to motivate him to take part in inter-responsive musical activity. The very form and structure inherent in music can bring a meaningful sense of order and security to the mentally or emotionally disabled.

Handicapped children are isolated children – children cut off by their mental, physical or emotional disabilities from many of the ordinary everyday experiences in life. Frequently they have great difficulty in expressing themselves in speech, and may have only a very limited understanding of language. It is this lack of communication which is the concern of those who work and live with such children.

A particular form of music therapy was initiated during the 1960s for severely handicapped children: some autistic, some mongoloid or aphasoid, some brain damaged. The pioneers were Dr Paul Nordoff, an American composer and Clive Robbins, a special educator in the field of handicapped children. During their practical investigations of music as therapy, they worked in England, Pennsylvania, Scandinavia and Holland. The therapy which they developed has been used specifically at the Goldie Leigh Hospital for severely subnormal children in South London as well as in other centres for children suffering a wide range of handicaps, both physical, emotional and mental.

When working with an individual child the therapist uses a creative dynamic approach, improvising at the piano and vocally, seeking to meet the child where he is, in his frustration, rage, anxiety, apathy or sadness, and to give him the experience of his mood being met and understood in music. Improvised music can respond immediately to any change in the mood of the child, can pick up the slightest clue at the moment it occurs, engage and develop it, so leading the child into a working situation. When intercommunication is established and the child is motivated into meaningful activity, either individually or within a group, then a musical therapeutic process is underway. Throughout the individual sessions the child is encouraged to respond on percussion instruments, on the piano and with his own voice.

In work with groups, this too is concerned with communication; communication between individuals working together in music in a shared activity – not a conditioning process based on automatic responses to an endlessly repeated radio programme or recorded music. Music used in group sessions with integrity and purpose can have far-reaching consequences and penetrates deeply into the child's personality.

It is in this area of group music that the non-specialist, less highly skilled person can do much. It is the enthusiastic joining in and sharing of a musical experience that can encourage and support a diffident or difficult child. They become aware of music and their part in it, they can be supported to meet the challenge in new activities, developing a greater awareness of themselves and others, stimulated through the music to a greater self-confidence. Group music activities help to focus the attention and concentration as the children find themselves drawn into an enjoyable activity.

Sybil Beresford-Peirse

Yoga

The aim of therapeutic Yoga is to maintain healthy minds in healthy bodies, but its practices are being increasingly used to produce cures or alleviations of disease. Yoga works on the premise that most illness is caused by wrong posture, wrong diet and wrong mental attitudes, which imbalances are under the control of the student (patient) himself.

Yoga is a philosophy embracing every aspect of human life, spiritual, emotional, mental and physical. It did not set out to be a therapy, but is being used as such today. It is a system of self-improvement, or 'conscious evolution', which has itself evolved and modified during the 6,000 years of its known existence. People take up Yoga to reduce nervous tension by learning to relax, to slim and to become more agile mentally and physically. Eventually Yoga leads them to meditation, thence to modifications of personal and social behaviour. Students attending regular classes become more relaxed, more supple and clearer headed, and usually begin to question the purpose of life in a way they have not before. This holistic approach leads to better health, and the improvement or eradication of psychosomatic ailments.

When, a century or so ago, Yoga came to the West via soldiers and civil servants returning from India, and via the Theosophical Society, it was in the form of Gnana (spiritual) Yoga, Bhakti (emotional) Yoga, and Raja (mental) Yoga. Only latterly, in the last two decades has Hatha physical) Yoga emerged in popularity. Hatha Yoga was in India also a later development, being only about one thousand years old. Its principal texts are *Hathayoga Pradipika c.* 1500 AD and *Geranda Samita, c.* 1600 AD. Compare these dates to the *Yoga Sutras of Patanjali*, the first text on Raja Yoga, *c.* 300 BC, or the *Upanishads*, the earliest Gnana Yoga texts dating from 1500 BC. The greatest of all Yoga classics is the *Bhagavad Gita, c.* 300 AD, in which all five main systems of Yoga are promulgated: Gnana, Raja, Bhakti, Karma (the yoga of social responsibility) and Hatha in its rudimentory form, before its later development in the *Pradipika* and *Geranda Samita*.

A typical two-hour Hatha class consists of exercises performed standing, kneeling, sitting, lying on the back, lying on the front, and inverted. For every posture (*asana*) there is a counter-posture. So an *asana* performed to the right must be followed by the same to the left. A forward-bending sequence of *asanas* is followed by a backward bending sequence, and so forth. A Hatha class includes a number of relaxation intervals, during which deep relaxation is taught, or some of the breathing exercises (*pranayama*) performed. The students may also be led in meditation, or the teacher gives a short talk. These talks usually deal with the therapeutic aspects of yoga, philosophy and practice (principally the *yamas* and *niyamas*: observances and prohibitions), correct posture, diet or emotional problems. The teacher may also enlarge on other yogas; Gnana, Bhakti, Raja, Karma, or even Siddha, the Yoga of psychic powers. Or again he may speak on the twin doctrines basic to yoga, reincarnation and *karma*, the law of cause and effect.

Introducing the student to some of the inspiring ideas in Yoga philosophy can have beneficial results. He is helped to adopt a correct attitude to life, to his fellow human beings, and to his total environment. After a properly conducted Hatha Yoga session, participants feel relaxed physically and mentally with no subsequent aches and pains from over-exercise. Nor should there be any feeling of having performed badly because yoga is not competitive. The student goes as far with a particular *asana* as he can. If he can do it easily, the teacher will give a variation on it that taxes him further. Generally the furthest point to go is to the threshold of pain, or to the point where the body begins to shake (in the standing postures).

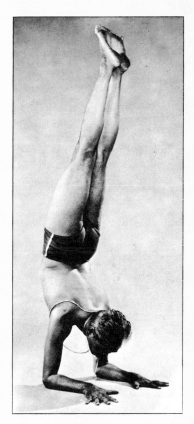

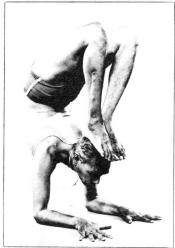

Mr B. K. S. Iyengar, the distinguished Yoga teacher, demonstrating the Scorpion pose *(Vrschikasana).*

Yoga

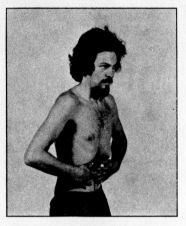

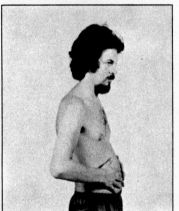

Yogic abdominal breathing.

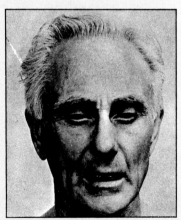

Hissing breath *(Sitkari)*.

Although many qualified Yoga teachers prescribe specific *asanas* and breathing techniques for certain conditions, there are few Yoga therapists operating as such outside India. At present, Hatha Yoga is 'taught' by a 'teacher' and treated as an educational subject. There are very few with medical training taking private patients through a course of remedial Yoga. But plans are emerging for such a development in Britain, principally by the Yoga for Health Foundation.

When we come to specifics, research in India and elsewhere has identified several main areas in which Hatha Yoga practice can ameliorate conditions, and in many cases produce permanent cures. Among them are asthma, bronchitis, dysmenorrhoea, multiple sclerosis, muscular dystrophy, constipation, hypertension, blood pressure, migraine and some kinds of back trouble.

The meditative aspects of Hatha Yoga can be extremely effective in cases of nervous debility, and in mental conditions such as schizophrenia, depression and various phobias. It is in the field of psychosomatic ailments that Yoga therapy can be most effective. The medical profession seem generally agreed that this area accounts for up to 80 percent of medical practice. They are also generally agreed that they can do little about it. This is imbalance in the borderland between mental, emotional and spiritual aspects of human nature, issuing as vague physical symptoms that can prove intractable to drug, and other therapies.

There are three main practices in Hatha Yoga. These are the *kriyas* (cleansings), *asanas* (postures), and *pranayama* – breath control. The kriyas cleanse the whole alimentary tract from mouth to bowel. They also link with pranayama in various cleansing breaths such as *kapalabhati*, *uddiyana* and *nauli*, while *trataka* is a separate exercise which improves eyesight.

Kriyas

In *neti kriya* the nasal passages are cleaned with air, water, cotton or a rubber tube.

In *kapalabhati* the stomach muscles are exercised very forcefully to produce rapid, short exhalations followed by very slow and gentle inhalations. The forceful expulsion of air from the lungs aspirates various secretions, works on the bronchial tubes, and is extremely beneficial for anyone with sinus trouble.

Uddiyana is a breathing exercise which helps constipation. The stomach is drawn inwards and upwards. After a very full exhalation the stomach is drawn in and an attempt is made to inhale. This attempt is largely frustrated because the lungs are restricted by the tightness of the stomach.

Nauli is an extension of this exercise. When in *uddiyana* the abdominal recti are isolated, first one side then the other. With these exercises, very high suction pressures are possible in the intrathoracic and intra-abdominal areas. This can have a beneficial action on the visceral organs.

In *basti* the lower bowel is flushed by drawing water through the anus by creating a vacuum in the stomach by use of the exercises above. This is considered superior to enema as it acts in the same way, but is entirely under the control of the subject.

Trataka is looking at an object with a steady unblinking gaze until the eyes water.

Asanas

When the word *asana* occurs in the earliest Yoga literature, it referred to a suitable pose for meditation, and there still are a wide range of such poses, of which the lotus pose is most familiar. In Hatha Yoga the

Yoga

main body of asanas can be classified as 'corrective', and a smaller group as 'relaxative'. Corrective asanas work mainly on the spine to make it supple. This has led some observers to regard Hatha Yoga as a system of 'spine culture'. However, it is more than that. A large and important group of asanas work on the visceral organs and skeletal muscles, and others work on the joints and ligaments.

Corrective postures can be looked upon as physiotherapeutic measures working locally on a particular part of the body, or as postural patterns of a wide range to modify the whole personality. Personality changes can be brought about in Hatha Yoga by changing the body so that it influences the mind. This is the opposite to normal life where the body is greatly influenced by the mind.

Reviewing asanas in greater detail, we can say that they are postures rather than exercises. When a posture has been taken up correctly (and the stages of taking it up are as important as the posture itself), it should be held for some time, allowing the muscle groups and organs involved to relax into it.

Being postures rather than exercises there is very little energy expenditure. Mostly the asanas work through stretching the muscles. Not just surface but deeper muscles are brought into play, and even ligaments and joints.

In addition to working on the spine, visceral organs and skeletal muscles, the asanas also work on the endocrine system, and the autonomic nervous system. The action on the visceral organs takes place largely through the creation of intra-abdominal pressure. This happens even though the muscles involved are relaxed.

A word must be said about relaxative asanas. These usually work by first tensing, then relaxing the part of the body concerned, or in *sarvasana* the corpse posture, the whole of the body progressively, starting at the toes and moving upwards to the crown of the head. The right type of relaxative asana following a particular set of corrective asanas is very beneficial.

Pranayama

Pranayama is consciously controlled breathing in which the three stages of breathing – inspiration, retention and expiration are varied in a number of ways. In some cases, resistance is offered to inspiration or expiration by closing one of the nostrils, or by partially closing the glottis. The holding phase may be eliminated in some active or cleansing breaths, or be considerably prolonged in others.

Again, during retention of the breath, one of four classical *bandhas*, or 'locks' may be applied. These four locks are:

(a) contraction of the perineal muscles;

(b) contraction of the abdominal muscles;

(c) pressing the chin into the supra-sternal notch;

(d) pressing the tongue against the hard palate so that the teeth are slightly parted.

Expiration is usually twice as long as inspiration. It has been observed that lengthening the expiration compared to inspiration has a tranquillizing effect – most helpful for many subjects.

It is usual to repeat each breathing exercise up to ten times, but beyond that there can be sensations of dizziness due to an excess of carbon dioxide in the bloodstream. The duration of each phase of the breathing cycle can be increased as the student progresses.

It is often the case that one also meditates on the action of air as it is drawn down the nasal passages. The student is invited to imagine that strength is being drawn in with the air, and weakness being expelled on expiration. In this kind of pranayama the gaze is fixed on the tip of the nose, or the eyes look upwards to a point between the eyebrows.

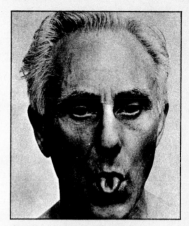

Cooling breath *(Sitali)*.

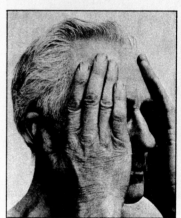

Bee breath *(Bharamari)*; **breathing with closed ears.**

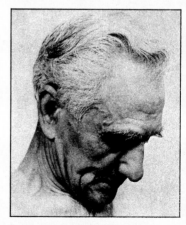

Swooning breath *(Murchha)*. **The chin lock is used during suspension of breath or during exhalation.**

Yoga

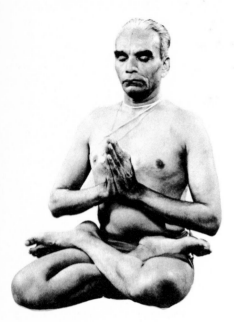

The classic *Padmasana*, or lotus position.

The Eight Limbs

In Patanjali's Yoga Sutras, the Eight Limbs of Yoga are promulgated; their practice is basic to the Yoga way of life and consequent health. They are: *yamas* – restraints, *niyamas* – observances, *asana* – posture, *pranayama* – breath control, *pratyahara* – sense withdrawal, *dharana* – concentration, *dhyana* – meditation, and *samadhi* – heightened awareness. The first two of these, the yamas (restraint from harming other living creatures, from falsehood, from theft, from incontinence and greed), and the niyamas (observances of cleanliness, contentment, simplicity, study and devotion to God) are sure foundations for correct living. They are not moral teachings, though often taken as such, but sound laws for wholesome living. To practise them is to take a first step in self-healing. In many cases it may be the only step needed.

Asana and pranayama have been considered in our treatment of Hatha Yoga. The therapeutic aspects of the final four of the eight limbs are also important. To a person of normal mental health these practices would be looked on as spiritual exercises to be practised in the yogic process of self-conscious evolution.

Interesting experiments have been undertaken in India and USA into the effect of these spiritual/mental exercises on the mentally handicapped and emotionally disturbed. The technique used is that of guided meditation and concentration with the aid of electronic brain-wave scanning equipment, with which the student can readily assess his own progress. Considerable releases of tension have been observed, sufficient to encourage further research along the same lines.

It should be said in conclusion that self-help and self-education are the rule in Yoga therapy. However valuable auxiliary therapies may be, they are outside introductions, not changes generated from within. Auxiliaries include not only drugs and surgery, but hypnotism and psychotherapy, osteopathy and physiotherapy, herbalism and homoeopathy. Yoga students (patients) must not remain passive but participate during the 'treatment'. They must come to a high state of awareness, feeling their way into their bodies and minds, into their emotions and value judgements, and questioning their immediate environment and personal relationships.

They are learning the arts of sensitivity and awareness, and bringing their body and their whole nature into balance.

Vivian Worthington

The Alexander Technique

The Technique to which the late F. Matthias Alexander gave his name has been taught continuously for the past eighty-four years. It has often been wrongly described as a method of relaxation or a form of posture-training, but its scope and purpose lie far beyond the 'release of tension' or even 'the re-education of muscular movement', for it is a way of ensuring that all the potentials of mind and body can be used to their best advantage in the activities of living.

It is a practical Technique, to be applied to all the simple things such as moving and breathing, eating and speaking, lifting and carrying, reading and writing; but is also effective for the safeguarding of health, the avoidance of accidents, the control of habitual reactions, the realization of individual potential and the fulfilment of desires and wishes. It is something that people of all ages have learned to apply in different fields with manifest success, and thus over the years it has been subjected to a continuous process of testing and proving.

Alexander was a man far ahead of his time. Modern scientific research has confirmed his findings and brought to light much supporting data: the validity of his work is due to the rigorous scientific method that he always employed, a full account of which is given in his books, particularly in *The Use of the Self*.

He was born in Wyngard, Tasmania, in 1869. Trained as an actor, he developed a talent for recitation and ballads. At a critical stage in that career he began to have problems with his voice. A long period of medical treatment proved ineffective. It was then that he set out to discover for himself why his voice was not functioning properly, and his success in solving his own problem lead him to apply his method to others. He began taking pupils in 1894.

From the beginning, a few medical men recognized the value of his work and gave him their encouragement and support, and after ten years of teaching in Australia and New Zealand he came to London in 1904 with testimonials and letters of introduction to some of the leading physicians and surgeons of the day. His first book, *Man's Supreme Inheritance*, was published in 1910 and in this he set out the statement of his claim. As he said, there is nothing in it that was not the outcome of his own experience.

His work gained steadily in recognition and acceptance until the outbreak of the First World War, when he paid his first visit to America. For the next ten years he divided his time between London and New York, alternating, in both places, with his brother, A. R. Alexander, who had followed him from Australia to assist him in his teaching.

1924 saw the publication of his second book *Constructive Conscious Control of the Individual* with an introduction by Professor John Dewey, the American philosopher and educationalist, and saw also the opening under his assistant, Irene Tasker, of the little school for children that subsequently became the F. Matthias Alexander Trust Fund School at Bexley, Kent.

Until 1930 there were only four teachers of his Technique, but in that year, with the distinguished support of Professor J. Dewey, the Earl of Lytton (Viceroy of India), Miss E. E. Lawerence (Principal of the Froebel Institute) the numerous doctors and educationalists he decided to open a training course for teachers. From then onwards, his work grew rapidly. His book *The Use of the Self*, containing his account of the evolution of the Technique was published in 1932, and many notable people, including George Bernard Shaw, Aldous Huxley, Professor John Hilton, and Sir Stafford Cripps, became enthusiastic exponents and propagandists.

After the outbreak of the Second World War, he took the children and staff of the Trust Fund School to America and in 1942 published his last book *The Universal Constant in Living*. This was applauded by Sir Charles Sherrington, OM, a Nobel Prizewinner and probably the greatest physiologist in this century. Alexander returned to England in 1943 and from then until his death in 1955 in his eighty-seventh year, he continued actively to teach, to train students, to supervise the work of his assistants, and to develop the Technique further. Since then the Technique has continued to grow rapidly, with more teachers being trained in several countries. There are now four training centres in London alone.

Alexander's Discovery

1. Whatever my life situation, it is *how* I do what I do that decides whether or not I make the best of it. For example, how much strain do I place on my heart, lungs, digestion and how much superfluous and counter-productive muscular effort do I inflict on myself?

Perhaps the greatest disservice that we do to ourselves can be seen in our unconscious bad habits, often so ingrained that they have come to feel right, especially if initially we were encouraged to believe that they were the 'correct' thing to do. In fact these habits come to feel so right that breaking one of them can be a painful and unwelcome experience – ask a long-term smoker to give up and watch the results.

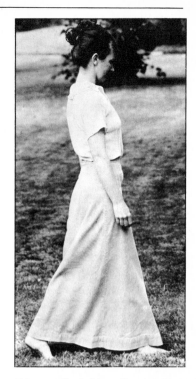

A 'normal' adult's walk. Note that the person is literally 'out of shape'. The feel is awkward and tense.

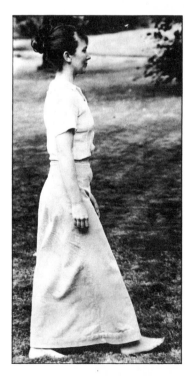

An improved version of an adult's walk after lessons.

The Alexander Technique

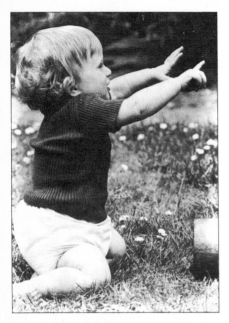

Natural poise is child's play. This child shows it.

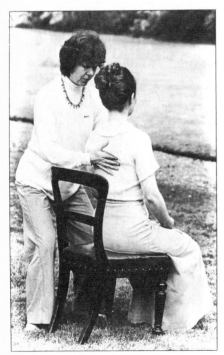

A teacher using her hands to let the student feel the right position.

'Waking up' to this, and to the way in which the results – things like breath holding, indigestion, high blood pressure and so on distort our senses and thinking, is an essential first step.

2. It is all too easy to do something to treat the symptoms, probably wrongly, by externally administered therapy or exercises. Alexander, however, went on to find out *how* we interfere. What are the causes of our ailments, insecurity or bad temper? He was a practical man, working initially on his own voice problems. The first step was to find out *what* caused the trouble. The second step was to find out *how*.

3. Only when he had established just *how* he interfered was he ready to discover how to stop. From experimenting with ways of controlling the interference, he came to the practical skill of maintaining the 'integrity' of self in everything he did. The experience of integrity allows an expansion of consciousness beyond what we want to do to the possibility of finding a new and better way of living. This means that we do not use 'will power' or 'effort', for both of these are an attempt to impose one part of ourself on the rest and are symptoms of a divided self, manifestations of the very interference which caused our problems in the first place. It is a change from blind desire to an ecological state of mind.

Learning the Technique

The Alexander Technique is not a set of exercises. It is concerned with how we go about our activities. A teacher of the Alexander Technique gives a student the opportunity to stop the habit patterns which distort our senses and cloud our thinking. Learning to do this so that we are able to see the wholeness of ourselves in a practical way is not a quick or easy process.

To begin to get useful results, at least thirty individual lessons are usually needed from a qualified teacher. Going to talks on the Technique or reading books does not produce results. By using hand contact, the teacher gives the student a new experience in the co-ordination of himself in carrying out everyday activities. This shows the student that he has a choice in the way he acts. Using speech, the teacher connects 'mental' choices to 'physical' actions, thus demonstrating in practice Alexander's discovery that there is no separation between mind and body. Alexander in fact said that ''you translate everything, whether physical, mental, or spiritual, into muscular tension''.

The Technique is not easy to learn. Because we bring our old habits to everything we do it is very difficult to change – usually, change is just another way of doing things badly. Time is required, and the use of our intelligence and patient persistence in what is so difficult for human beings to do – to stop interfering.

If we begin to make the transition, we find that the human being is not quite what we thought.

Rewards of the Technique

In 1975 Professor Nikolaas Tinbergen, in his Nobel Prize acceptance speech, described the effects of the Technique on himself and his family as ''very striking improvements in such diverse things as blood pressure, breathing, depth of sleep, overall cheerfulness and mental alertness, resilience against outside pressures, and also in such a refined skill as playing a musical instrument''. John Dewey regarded the Technique as the essential practical basis for his 'Child Centered Education'. The support for Alexander by some distinguished scientists was the result of their seeing that the Technique worked. For Coghill and Sherrington, concerned with co-ordination and patterns of movement, it demonstrated, in human beings, what they had discovered in laboratory animal experiments. Since Alexander's early days in London, leading actors, musicians and singers have taken lessons in the Technique. They have found that both the standard and ease of their performances improve. The Guildhall School of Music, the Royal College of Music, and RADA in England and several universities in America use the Technique as part of their curriculum. The sports of golf, horse riding, and athletics have seen some exponents of the Technique demonstrate its utility. A striking example is that of Howard Payne, who, in his forties, dramatically improved the distances for his hammer throwing. Paul Collins, a past Olympic Marathon runner, is using the Technique in teaching running, with some fascinating improvements in running styles. Practising yoga using the Alexander Technique makes for big changes. The postures become a vehicle for greater awareness and naturalness. Sitting up straight, as an example, is achieved without effort and breathing is freer. Breathing exercises and meditation become more open and sensitive. This should not surprise us, for the basis of spiritual work is the removal of the many layers of ignorance which cover our 'true self'. What Alexander found is an essential prerequisite. We have nothing to lose but the chains of our own making.

Christopher Stevens

The Alexander Technique

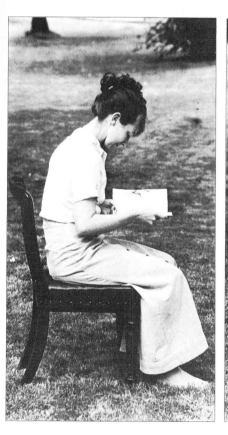 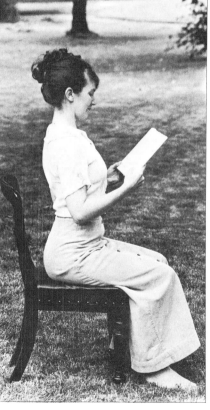 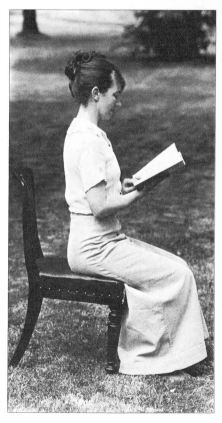

Left and centre are two variations of a sitting position that most people adopt. In the first, the person may say she is relaxed, but you can see the compression of the stomach and the uncomfortable rounding of the shoulders. The second shows an attempt to 'sit up straight'. Notice how curved the back is. The right-hand picture shows an improved sitting position with better head balance and a greater ability to move and act without strain.

Dance Therapy

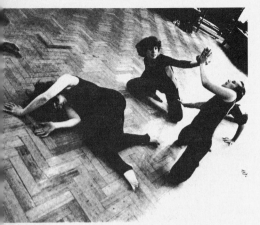

I fear...

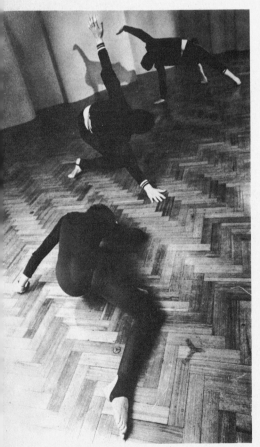

I search...

Evidence of dance as therapy is found widely in human society. The dance has provided both a means of entering abnormal mental states (e.g. the dances of possession and of transcendence of the Asiatic Shaman and of the Whirling Dervish) and a means of cure (e.g. West African cults). From the very origins of dance, the activity has been linked with the release of energy, the unifying of spirit and body, the ecstatic principle evolving through movement.

Dance in its modern Western therapeutic aspect may be traced back to Rudolph Laban (1879–1959). Laban, who initially worked in theatre dance in Germany developing his concept of the complete individuality of man's movements, fled to England at the outbreak of war where he involved himself in the educational and therapeutic aspects of dance. Dance, he believed, could create a beneficial effect on the mental condition of the individual: "Man must be made conscientious enough to occupy himself with that means of recovery which is so cherished by living beings, namely with dancing." He created new and freer dance forms that were able totally to involve the individual, body and mind becoming a harmonious whole. The dance thus became a vital art that concerned itself with authenticity, awareness of body sensation and individuality.

In the context of this article, dance is used in a curative way with the psychiatric patient. The key is to see each patient as a unique individual with his own range of movement energy and form of expression. Each person organizes this energy differently, and the movement quality (Laban's "effort") can be recognized and modified by the therapist.

There are other approaches to dance therapy besides that which has developed from Laban. Some emphasize the rhythmic accompaniment of music and its socializing effect, while others work from a more general dance background.

Dance therapy possesses links with other creative therapies used in the psychiatric field, such as music and art. What do they have in common? The diagnostic aspect of the art form is one area. Just as the subject-matter of a painting made by a patient may be analysed, so effort theory analyses the content of movement. Another common aspect is the cathartic, emotion released yet held in the form of the art symbol; and it is the symbol which may touch the unconscious. The exploration of the unconscious is a vital part of psychotherapy; as Jung says, the unconscious is at least half of man's existence, thus the more diverse ways one can approach the unconscious, the clearer will be the analysis. The arts also involve the act of creation, an actualization which may help to reinforce the self.

There are two important psychological foundations to the theory of dance therapy which have recently developed:

1. Body image – the building up of an accurate mental picture of the body, which in turn forms the bodily ego, the basis of self-concept. For example: the depressive with an enfeebled body image and self-concept; the severe schizoid often grossly lacking self-image and identity. It is in the intense relationship of self and body life that the power of dance therapy lies.

2. Non-verbal communication (NVC). NVC may be the most authentic expression of man: "If his lips are silent he chatters with his finger-tips; betrayal oozes out of him at every pore" (Freud). In mental disorder, NVC becomes disturbed and leads to a negative feedback from others. Movement may be the best way to restore relationship in life. If the patient is able to relate more effectively, he becomes accessible to psychotherapy and his self-concept may be reinforced.

Other aspects which form part of the content of the dance therapy session may include: emotional release, direct attempts to embody

Dance Therapy

fantasy in dance, regressive movement patterns and re-experience of actions, the balance of personality opposites such as open-closed and excited-apathetic, relationship creation in dance sublimation.

A brief account of a dance therapy session may illustrate some of these ideas. Imagine a group of eight to ten depressed patients; the aim is to give them a sense of life, of purpose and of positive identity. The dance session may begin by working from the kinaesthetic sensations within the body (e.g. rising and sinking using the floor for support, and stretching to the sky as if to lift the face to the sun). Working from interaction (e.g. a musical rhythm captured in a single body part, even just a finger initially) relationship can grow through the whole body and into the group creating a belonging in unison.

A group with some experience of dance might go on to a simple sequence with appropriate music that may appeal through kinaesthesia or mental imagery: touching fingertips with a partner, increasing the pressure of the hands; one leading, one following, gradually growing into a simple dance of meeting and parting, involving trust and responsiveness.

Effective therapy depends on the characteristics of the therapist to a great degree because of the personal nature of the situation. He or she must be sensitive, flexible, positive and cheerful. It is necessary to be able to identify with the patient without losing objectivity and to have a good repertoire of social skills in order to control the interaction.

Dance therapy is at an exciting stage of development, yet further work needs to be done to substantiate the way in which it can provide help. There is a need for better training courses, with the emphasis placed upon the selection of the appropriate personality to work in this field; a need for both a proven and theoretical base and demonstrable success in practice. (A therapeutic dose of scepticism here!)

In Britain, dance therapy is often regarded with suspicion. It is only through persistence and sometimes a willingness to work in a voluntary capacity or to accept the label of 'keep-fit teacher' or 'recreational therapist' that the opportunity arises to practise in an appropriate environment and thus to convert the unbelieving. In the United States, dance therapy is accepted as a valid part of treatment; in many psychiatric institutions, a dance therapist is employed in the professional clinical team.

Within such a context, dance therapy may aim not only at the relief of clinical symptoms but also the recovery of joy in being human.

Felicity Ling

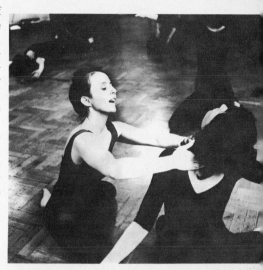

Out from me . . .

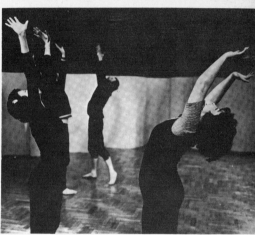

. . . I make me.

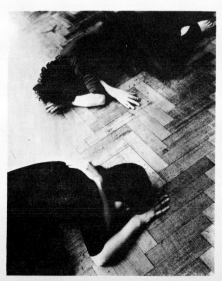

I am alone . . .

. . . We are together.

Curative Eurythmy

"If we wish to enter into the true nature of Eurythmy, we must perforce enter into the true nature of the human being. For Eurythmy, to a far greater extent than any other art, makes use of what lies in the nature of the Human Being"
– Rudolf Steiner,
Eurythmy as Visible Speech.

'All therapies related to Anthroposophical medicine arise out of artistic trainings which develop intuition in the therapist to know which movement, colour or sound should be used for healing not a specific illness, but each individual within that illness.

Eurythmy movements arise out of the sounds of speech: on the one hand the consonants and on the other the vowels. The forming quality of the consonants can be recognized in organic nature – the vibrating 'R', the enveloping 'B', the ebbing and flowing of 'L' and so on. The vowels are the expression of our inner mood. We say 'Ah' in wonder, or 'Oo' when we feel chilled. A little child will open its arms to the world in 'Ah', we cross our arms in 'Eh' as we grow older, shutting out the world and achieving consciousness. With 'I' we become upright.

Man learns to stand upright within the forces that work from the earth. These forces are called out-raying forces. The forces coming from the periphery are described as in-raying forces; they are active not in heaviness, but in buoyancy, and we become aware of them by their effect on the fluids of the body, in the circulation and the functions of the organs. In curative eurythmy we use the inflowing forces, that is the consonants, where there is a disturbance of *form*, e.g. in arthritis or paralysis. We would work with the vowel movements where the *function* of the organ is disturbed. The curative eurythmist should mediate between the irregular movements of a sick organism and the ideal healthy movement and should move as perfectly as possible, so that the movement can work on the maladjusted movement of the patient. The growing number of patients suffering from movement handicaps shows in what danger the movement is.

In her book *Foundations of Curative Eurythmy*, Margarete Kirchner-Bockholt writes:

"As a result of our civilization, a greater danger arises that the connection with natural movements will be lost. A repetitive movement on a machine can jostle out of existance those movements inspired by our life of soul and spirit. As the movements and gestures become altered through minding a machine, we see how thinking, feeling and willing come into them less and less, we become more and more dulled in our movements. We can also observe in children with damage of the middle brain, meaningless, chaotic unrhythmical movements which have no real purpose – in such cases curative eurythmy can be of special significance."

Dr Kirchner-Bockholt worked with Rudolf Steiner and was present when he gave the first curative eurythmy lectures to the doctors, at their request, in April 1921. The following year he gave therapeutic eurythmy into her care. In many different cases doctors asked Steiner's advice concerning curative eurythmy, and consequently we have exercises for: the digestive tract, the kidney and urinary tract, rheumatic illnesses, the heart and circulatory system, the respiratory system, the skin and cancer.

There are also special exercises which are used in connection with psychiatric treatment.

Since its inception in the 1920s the practice of curative eurythmy has grown considerably. Several hundreds of curative eurythmists have been trained and are active in schools for normal children and with those in need of special care. They also work in adult clinics and in private practice, always in association with a doctor. Remarkable results have been achieved and new ways of healing discovered.

Valerie Soukup

Sport as Therapy

A characteristic of many cultures has been their celebration of a relationship between sport, philosophy and religion. The Greeks, Mayans and Celts all held sacred games to evoke and re-enact the deeper truths of life; the Sioux had a game, *Tapa Wanka Yap* – the throwing of the ball, in which God's presence was revealed to the players; in Tibet there were the *lung gom* walks – steady-paced walks that lasted for thousands of miles, day and night, and which expressed the individual's mastery of the inner life. In addition to these, there was the Mayan ball-game and the martial arts of China, Japan and Korea.

Such ritual games now no longer exist in the West and sport has developed into little more than competitive games. Just as, however, the monk on a long gom walk, or the young Sioux in his ball-game would experience altered states of consciousness (ASCs) which allowed them new insights into themselves and their culture, there is considerable anecdotal evidence to suggest that spontaneous altered states of consciousness are sometimes experienced by contemporary sportsmen. Almost invariably these states allow them to perform with a degree of skill and insight that would not usually be possible. Examples of these experiences occur throughout a range of sports: racing driver, Jackie Stewart has described a sense of things slowing down during a race permitting manoeuvres which would not otherwise be possible. Golfer, Tony Jacklin has described "a pure, vividly clear state . . . living fully in the present and not moving out". In this state he was aware of every single movement of his body and club during the stroke, and which lead to him hitting the ball further and more accurately than before. David Meggyesey, the American line-backer has spoken of seeing auras around his opponents which allowed him to anticipate the moves they were about to make. There is increasing evidence that this type of experience is far more widespread than was originally thought, and it is only the understandable reluctance of sportsmen to talk about their experiences that has lead to the assumption that such states and transformations are rare.

Three researchers at the Washington Street Research Center in San Francisco, James Hickman, Michael Murphy and Mike Spino, believe that one key to optimal performance in sport lies in these altered states of consciousness. Considered in this light, sport becomes more than a competitive situation focused on winning; it offers ultimately a means for integrating and balancing mental and physical discipline. These three researchers also believe that man's consciousness is still evolving, and that the altered states experienced by sportspeople suggest that the next step in evolution is one in which altered states of consciousness produce bodily transformations. Earlier stages in evolution saw gradual transformations in consciousness occurring as a result of physical evolution. In pursuit of this theory, they have developed a workshop program in which they are attempting to "uncover the modalities through which the evolution of consciousness effects evolutionary transformations of the body . . . and to develop physical disciplines to support them". They chose jogging, an increasingly popular and easily accessible sport for most people, as the focal point for their experiments. Sponsored by the Esalen Institute Sports Center, a five-day group training program was recently conducted to explore their ideas. A combination of mind/body conditioning techniques were used to enable participants to expand their awareness and experience new limits of mental and physical fitness.

The first day's training began with a period of meditation designed to cultivate in each participant an awareness of the 'witness self', an idea used in yoga to teach a person to observe himself as if he were another person, to notice exactly what he is doing and so invest ordinary activity with attention. Developing the 'witness self' the group was

Sport as Therapy

told, allows a clearer expression of each individual's sense of form and beauty. At the end of the meditation period each person was asked to remain in this ASC but to open their eyes, stand up and gradually begin to move. This was later extended into the actual jogging. Most participants found even on the first morning that they were able to run further after this meditation. Later on the first day, a variety of running gaits and tempos were taught with the object of strengthening the body's aerobic and anaerobic functioning.

The second day's training concentrated on using particular visualizations to support the running experience. For example, the group was asked to visualize their bodies being filled with a heavy oil, to experience the heaviness and then to replace the oil with a substance lighter than air. The feeling of lightness and clarity was carried over into the running with the instruction only to run when the lightness was present. Also during the second day, the group was encouraged to discuss interpersonal issues which affected their running abilities, such as feelings of inadequacy when passed by another runner. After discussion, most members were able to visualize better.

The third day's training was designed to teach an ability to sustain focused awareness while running. After a period of meditation to create a sense of inner stillness, members were asked to visualize a quiet grassy meadow and then to see a human form emerging in the distance. The group was told that this form was the 'perfect runner' which carries perfect knowledge of each member. They were to observe the way it ran and surrender to its lead. Holding this image in their minds, participants were asked to stand up and begin running, and to run only while this image was in their mind. While some members had difficulty in focusing on the image, others found themselves able to run without fatiguing. One member described merging with his 'perfect runner'.

By the fourth day, the running abilities of the group had improved dramatically with some members, who had only jogged occasionally, running several miles without becoming fatigued. The fourth day was designed to explore the limits of their new physical abilities. Some felt they could run all day, while others had to hold back from exceeding their margins too widely; others reported a sense of ''blissful fatigue'' at the end of their run.

The fifth day was devoted to an easy workout, primarily to aid the group's re-entry into their personal worlds. The afternoon was devoted to a gestalt session in which everyone was asked to reexperience the most unhappy and the most rewarding sporting experience of their lives.

There is a growing movement, particularly in California, to reestablish the connections between inner mental states and sport. Transcendental meditation has been investigated in relation to running speed, jumping ability and agility with promising results. While many of these investigations are aimed primarily at producing optimal performance for sportsmen, the results already suggest that here is yet another useful key to psychological as well as physical well-being and more perfect self-expression.

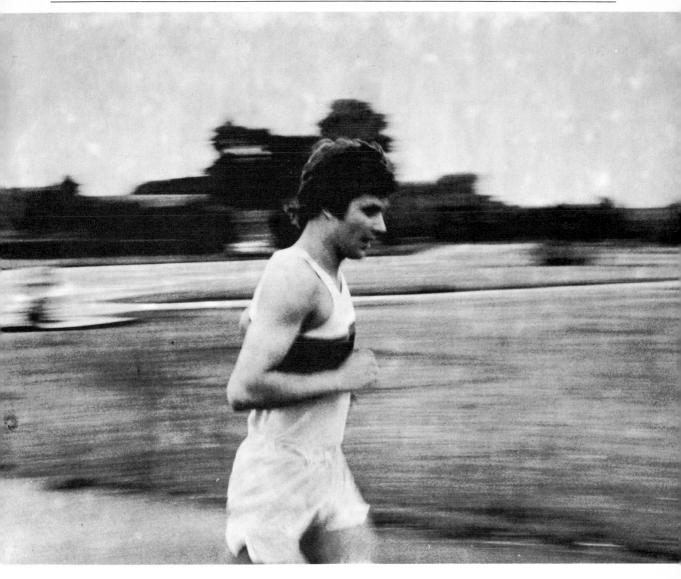

Postscript

Michael Murphy published his first novel, a metaphysical golf fantasy called *Golf In The Kingdom*, in 1972. In response to the book many sportspeople wrote to Murphy about their extraordinary experiences in sport. The enormous amount of material he collected over the ensuing five years led Murphy to discern similarities between sport and traditional contemplative disciplines (Murphy, 1977). With Rhea White, a noted paraphychologist and sport enthusiast, he is currently writing a book, *The Psychic Side of Sports*, that explores these similarities. In it, Murphy and White maintain that sport can be a liberating discipline or a kind of yoga which sometimes unlocks extraordinary capacities in the participants. But when these unusual experiences emerge in sport, there is usually no context or insight to support them and they are repressed, ignored, or forgotten. The book dramatizes how widespread these types of experience are.

Prepared from information supplied by the Washington Street Center, San Francisco, CA and by the Esalen Institute, Big Sur, CA.

Sport as Therapy

T'ai Chi Ch'uan

The first documents about T'ai Chi in China date from around our first century, but even at that time these and related exercises were called 'ancient'. There was once a Taoist hermit who, after long hours of sitting meditation each day, would leave his cave in the mountains and perform a series of movements that would increase his circulation and restore his vigour without disturbing his deep meditative concentration. The movements he made imitated what he saw in Nature: the movements of birds, animals, streams, clouds and wind. For centuries, the practice was transmitted and modified from generation to generation remaining the 'secret' possession of various religious sects and wealthy families. In the last century, through the enlightened teaching of a Mr Yang (from whom almost all modern systems of T'ai Chi received inspiration) T'ai Chi has become a popular practice. Even today in Mainland China and in the many overseas Chinese communities, T'ai Chi is a part of millions of people's daily fitness programme. In the West over the last ten years an ever-growing interest has brought many teachers to America and Europe. There exist many schools of T'ai Chi, each with its own lineage and style, but all share a legendary origin.

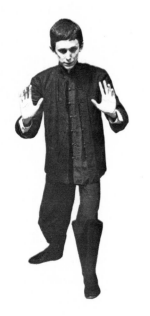

Fundamental to all traditional Chinese medicine is the idea that sickness is simply the inhibition of Chi flow (the flow of Life Force). Since through the routine practice of T'ai Chi such inhibition is prevented, T'ai Chi has often been considered a part of Chinese medicine (traditionally including: diet, yogic breath control, acupuncture and herbalism). Like all sound medical practices, T'ai Chi does not treat symptomatically; that is, no special or manipulative exercises are employed, but a routine of continuous movements involving one's whole Being.

In addition to its restorative and therapeutic qualities, T'ai Chi has long been part of the integrated path of the Shen Jen – Spiritual Man or Sage. Some modern school of Kung Fu and Karate look upon T'ai Chi as an ancestor, because of its enormous contribution to the 'internal' aspects of self-defence in the Martial Arts.

In the Chinese languate *T'ai* means great or original, *Chi* means life force or energy, and *Ch'uan* means fist or boxing, also implying way. T'ai Chi Ch'uan (or T'ai Chi for short) appears to the observer as a 'dance' or continuous yoga postures set to the rhythm of slow, deep breathing. The relaxed and flowing movements stimulate the even flow of blood, breath and Chi, completely 'nourishing' the body, mind and spirit and bringing them into a harmonious state of balance.

Charles Belyea

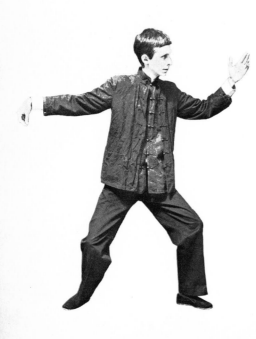

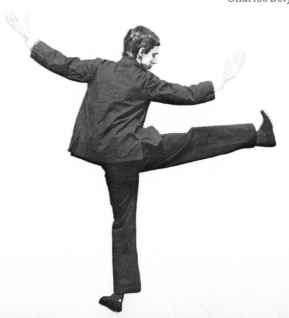

Resources

Information on individual therapies can be obtained from the following sources. If written replies are required, it is advisable to enclose a stamped addressed envelope.

Oriental Medicine

US
East West Foundation
359 Boylston Street
Boston
Massachusetts 02116

UK
Community Health Foundation
188–194 Old Street
London EC1V 9BP

Homoeopathy

US
National Center for
Homoeopathy
Suite 506
6231 Leesburg Pike
Falls Church, Virginia 22044

UK
British Homoeopathic
Association
Basildon Court
27a Devonshire Street
London W1N 1RJ

Society of Homoeopaths
59 Norfolk House Road
Streatham, London SW16

Anthroposophy

US
c/o The Fellowship Community
241 Hungry Hollow Road
Spring Valley, New York 10977

UK
Anthroposophical Medical
Association
Rudolf Steiner House
35 Park Road, London NW1

Aura Diagnosis

UK
Karl A. Francis MFPhys
Acacia House Centre
Centre Avenue
The Vale
Acton Park, London W3 7JX

Ronald Beesley
College of Psychotherapeutics
White Lodge
Stockland Green Road
Speldhurst
Tunbridge Wells TN3 0TT
Kent

Harold Sharpe
Craigside
207 Scar Lane
Milnsbridge
Near Huddersfield, Yorkshire

Kirlian Diagnosis

US
c/o 10 South Road
Bronxville, New York 10708

UK
Brian Snellgrove
56 Carshalton Park Road
Carshalton, Surrey

Acupuncture

British Acupuncture
Association
34 Alderney Street
London SW1V 4EU
(The International Organization of Acupuncture Associations can be contacted at the above address and can furnish individual addresses in the United States)

UK
College of Acupuncture
c/o 118 Foley Road
Claygate, Surrey

Reflexology

UK
Doreen E. Bayly
107 West Kensington Court
London W14 9AB

Osteopathy

There are ten Osteopathic schools in the US. Each teaches the full orthodox medical course, including surgery and graduates of each take their own State Board examination. Each course is for seven years and all graduates enjoy State recognition.
Chicago College of
Osteopathic Medicine
College of Osteopathic
Medicine and Surgery, Des
Moines, Iowa
Kansas City College of
Osteopathic Medicine
Kirksville College of
Osteopathic Medicine
Michigan State University
College of Osteopathic
Medicine
Ohio University College of
Osteopathic Medicine
Oklahoma College of
Osteopathic Medicine and
Surgery
Philadelphia College of
Osteopathic Medicine
Texas College of Osteopathic
Medicine
West Virginia School of
Osteopathic Medicine

UK
In England there are three full-time schools:
The British School of
Osteopathy
16 Buckingham Gate
London SW1

The British School of
Naturopathy and Osteopathy
6 Netherhall Gardens
London NW3

L'Ecole Européene
d'Ostéopathie
28–30 Tonbridge Road
Maidstone, Kent

Shorter courses are given at:
The Andrew Still House
Dorset Square, London W1

College of Osteopathy
c/o Manor Road North
Wallington, Surrey

Cranial Osteopathic
Association
c/o Hatton House
Church Lane
Cheshunt, Herts
EN8 0DW

Chiropractic

US
International Chiropractors
Association
741 Brady Street
Davenport, Iowa 52808

National College of
Chiropractic
200E Roosevelt Road
Lombard, Illinois 60148

UK
Anglo-European College of
Chiropractic
1 Cavendish Road,
Bournemouth

Impact Therapy

UK
John B. Tracey MB BChir
Gipsy Lane Gardens
Pinhoe, Exeter

Rolfing

US
Rolf Institute
PO Box 1868
Boulder, Colorado 80302

Touch for Health

US
1194 North Lake Avenue
Pasadena
California 91104

UK
Brian Butler
42 Worthington Avenue
Surbiton, Surrey KT6 7RX

Manipulative Therapy

UK
The Northern College of
Physical Therapies
(Northern Institute
of Massage)
100 Waterloo Road
Blackpool FY4 1AW

Bates Method of Eyesight Training

UK
Michael Ronan
Secretary: Bates Association
of Eyesight Training
39 Smith Street, London SW3

Naturopathy

US
National College of
Naturopathic Medicine
Room 413
510 SW Third Avenue
Portland, Oregon 97204

UK
British Naturopathic and
Osteopathic Associations
6 Netherhall Gardens
London NW3

Research Society for Natural
Therapeutics
c/o 8 Stokewood Road
Bournemouth

Medical Herbalism

UK
National Institute of Medical
Herbalists
68 London Road, Leicester

Society of Herbalists
21 Bruton Street, London W1

Bach Flower Remedies

UK
Dr Edward Bach Centre
Mount Vernon
Sotwell
Wallingford, Oxon OX10 0PZ

Exultation of Flowers

UK
Seaweed Croft
Geddes
Nairn IV12 5QZ, Scotland

Aromatherapy

UK
Aromatic Oil Company
12 Littlegate Street
Oxford OX1 1QT

Vita Florum

UK
Cats Castle
Lydeard St Lawrence
Taunton, Somerset

Nutrition

UK
The McCarrison Society
(founded to study the relationship between nutrition and health and named after Sir Robert McCarrison 1878–1960)
Carrow
Shinfield Road, Shinfield
Reading, Berkshire RG2 9BE

Soil Association of Great
Britain
Walnut Tree Manor
Haughley
Stowmarket, Suffolk IP14 3RS

Veganism

US
The Vegan Society, Box H
Malaga, New Jersey 18328

The Farm
Summertown, Tennessee
38483

UK
The Vegan Society
47 Highlands Road
Leatherhead, Surrey

Vegetarianism

US
North American Vegetarian
Society
501 Old Harding Highway
Malaga 08328, New Jersey

UK
The Vegetarian Society
53 Marloes Road, London
W8 6LA

Resources

Food Allergy and Clinical Ecology
US
Human Ecology Action League
4051 McKinney Avenue
Suite 310
Dallas, Texas 75204

UK
Food Allergy Association
9 Mill Lane
Shoreham, Sussex

Action Against Allergy
31 Abbey Parade
Merton High Street
London SW19 1DG

Macrobiotics
see Oriental Medicine

Psionic Medicine
UK
Psionic Medical Society
Beacon Hill Park
Hindhead, Surrey

Radiesthesia
US
The American Society of
Dowsers
Danville, Vermont

UK
British Society of Dowsers
19 High Street
Eydon
Daventry, Northants

Radionics
UK
Radionic Association
16a North Barr
Banbury, Oxon OX1 0GF

Pyramid Energy
US
Pyramid Power V; Inc
PO Box 66092
Los Angeles, California 90066

UK
Pyramid Energy Products
20 Bride Lane
Ludgate Circus
London EC4Y 80X

Healing
US
American Healers Association
PO Box 213
Princeton, New Jersey 08540

UK
National Federation of
Spiritual Healers
Shortacres
Church Hill, Loughton, Essex

Psychosynthesis
US
Psychosynthesis Research
Foundation
Room 1902
40 East 49th Street
New York, NY 10017

UK
Institute of Psychosynthesis
Highwood Park
Nan Clark's Lane
Mill Hill, London NW7

Human Cybernetics
UK
Dr George Hall
9 Thruxton Way
London SE15 6ED

Autogenic Training
UK
Centre for Autogenic Training
12 Milford House
7 Queen Anne Street
London W1M 9FD

Biofeedback
US
Coherent Communications
13733 Glen Oaks Boulevard
Sylmar, California 91342

UK
Audio Ltd
26–28 Wendell Road
London W12

Transcendental Meditation
US
Capital of the Age of
Enlightenment
South Fallsburg
New York, NY 12779

UK
Maharishi International
College
Roydon Hall
Seven Mile Lane
East Peckham, Kent TN12 5NH

Arica
US
Arica Institute
24 West 57th Street
New York, NY 10019

UK
57 Marlborough Mansions
Cannon Hill, London NW6 1JS

Somatography
UK
H. Bryn Jones
1 Challoner Street, London W14

Biodynamic Psychology
UK
Centre for Bioenergy
Centre Avenue
Acton Park, London W3 7JX

Bioenergetics
US
Institute of Bioenergetic
Analysis
144 East 36th Street
New York, NY 10011

UK
British Association for
Bioenergetic Analysis
The Meeting House
University of Sussex
Brighton BN1 9RH

Psychodrama
US
Moreno Institute
Beacon Hill
Beacon, New York

UK
c/o 83a Oxford Gardens
London W10

Primal Integration
US
International Primal
Association
15 East 40th Street, Room 306
New York, NY 10016

UK
The Churchill Centre
22 Montagu Street, London W1

Gestalt
US
Gestalt Centre of
Psychotherapy and Training
150 East 52nd Street
New York, NY

UK
Ursula Fausset
7 Parliament Hill
Hampstead, London NW3

Co-counselling
US
Dodie Pratt
492 Grant Hill Road, Coventry
Connecticut, 06238

UK
London Co-counsellors
c/o Anne Dickson
83 Fordwych Road, London
NW2

Encounter
US
Esalen Institute
Big Sur, California 93920

UK
Quaesitor
137 Biddulph Mansions
Elgin Avenue, London W9

Sensitivity Training
US
National Training Laboratories
NTL Institute for Applied
Behavioural Science
PO Box 9155 Rosslyn Station
Arlington, Virginia 22209

UK
Group Relations Training
Association
3 St Hilda's Road
London SW13

Transactional Analysis
US
International Transactional
Analysis Association Inc
1772 Vallejo Street
San Francisco, California 94123

UK
European Association for
Transactional Analysis
40 Stavely Road
Dunstable, Beds L9 3QQ

Colour Therapy
US
Spectro-Chromo Institute
Malaga, New Jersey

UK
Hygeia Studios
Colour-Light-Art Research
Ltd
Brook House
Avening
Tetbury
Gloucestershire GL8 8NS

Music Therapy
UK
British Society for Music
Therapy
48 Lanchester Road
London N6 4TA

The Nordoff Music Therapy
Centre
Goldie Leigh Hospital
Lodge Hill
Abbey Wood, London SE2 0AY

Yoga
US
Oki Yoga Dojo
Apt 103
373 Commonwealth Avenue
Boston, Massachusetts 02115

UK
Yoga for Health Foundation
Ickwell Bury
Northill, Bedfordshire

The Alexander Technique
US
The American Centre for the
Alexander Technique
142 West End Avenue
New York, NY 10023

UK
Society of Teachers of the
Alexander Technique
3 Albert Court
Kensington Gore, London SW7

Dance
US
Dance in Psychotherapy
Dance Horizons
1801 East 26th Street
Brooklyn, New York 11229

UK
Felicity Ling
20 Dartmouth Hill, London SE10

Curative Eurythmy
see Anthroposophical
Medicine

T'ai Chi Ch'uan
UK
International T'ai Chi Ch'uan
Association
40 Hillcroft Crescent
Wembley Park, Middlesex

Index

Page numbers in **bold type** refer to places in the text where the subject is treated in detail. Page numbers in *italics* refer to illustrations. (The majority of illustrations, however, will be found under the **bold type** entries.)